Contraception
Your questions answered

Contraception

Your questions answered

Second Edition

John Guillebaud MA FRCSE FRCOG
Professor of Family Planning and Reproductive Health,
University of London
Medical Director of the Margaret Pyke Centre,
London

CHURCHILL LIVINGSTONE
EDINBURGH LONDON MADRID MELBOURNE NEW YORK AND TOKYO 1993

CHURCHILL LIVINGSTONE
Medical Division of Longman Group UK Limited

Distributed in the United States of America by
Churchill Livingstone Inc., 650 Avenue of the Americas,
New York N.Y. 10011, and by associated companies,
branches and representatives throughout the world.

First edition 1985 (Pitman Publishing Ltd)
   Reprinted 1986
   Reprinted 1987 (twice)
   Reprinted 1988
   Revised and reprinted 1989
   Reprinted 1991
   Reprinted 1992
Second edition 1993
   Revised and reprinted 1994

ISBN 0-443-04070-2

British Library Cataloguing in Publication Data

A catalogue record for this book is available from
the British Library

Produced by Longman Singapore Publishers Pte Ltd
Printed in Singapore

Preface to the Second Edition

We have not inherited the earth from our grandparents – we have borrowed it from our grandchildren. (Attributed to the ancient Chinese)

Although the first edition of this book was adequately revised in 1989, a glance at the very first question (see Q 0.1) herein shows the urgency of a more comprehensive update. Frighteningly, we have three quarters of a billion more humans on the planet since the first edition, an increment close to the total world population when Rev. Thomas Malthus first drew attention to the problem of exponential growth on a finite planet. It has never been more true that 'Whatever your cause, it is a lost cause.... unless we stabilise human numbers'.

Population is *the great multiplier* of those vast problems – the environment, the extinction of other species, poverty, global security – facing our children as the human race approaches the next millenium. All likely future scenarios, varied as they are, share this: so much misery to be suffered by so many, and so much of it so *avoidable*. I only wish that more might share with me the ability to say, whilst still fighting on every relevant front for both social justice and sustainability: 'God is still on the throne'. If we truly loved the Creator, we would love and care for what he has created. If we truly loved our neighbour, we would love and serve our future neighbour (not to mention, right now, our neighbour overseas). But more on that is for another book!

Since the first edition the methods actually available to most couples even in the privileged West have, disappointingly, changed very little. Q 5.137, on the subject of the LNG-ring, reads strangely in 1993: 'due to reach Britain by early 1986'. We are still waiting for that, the implant and the LNG-IUD – and for any form of 'male pill'. At least the female condom has finally made it, and the existing methods have undergone some further refinement, for example a greater choice of low-dose pill formulations.

But perhaps more significant is some highly reassuring epidemiology (reviewed in Ch. 4–6) which effectively demolishes some persistent myths about available medical methods. In summary: the combined oral contraceptive (COC) has been blamed for too long for arterial disease events which were primarily due to smoking by COC-takers; and the intrauterine device (IUD) has been blamed for pelvic infections and ectopics nearly always caused by sexually transmitted diseases acquired from their partner by IUD-users.... Nearly all the anxieties about injectables and cancer have evaporated (see Q 5.105). The new facts, that these methods are much closer to hazard free than used to be thought, deserve maximum publicity – spearheaded by doctors and nurses.

I would stress again that, among the other important topics listed above, the omission of detailed consideration of emotional and psychosexual aspects is only for reasons of space. They are implicit in every chapter, since contraception has everything to do with sex! Sexuality and communication influence crucially both strong and weak motivation for effective contraception (see Q 8.4), and we forget that whole area at our peril – and too often.... We must be perpetually on the look-out for relevant verbal and non-verbal clues, particularly at the 'moment of truth' during any vaginal examination. We must assiduously avoid the busy doctor's knee-jerk reaction of reaching for the prescription pad (even if there is logic in the offer of a less progestagenic pill – Q 4.229), when the complaint is loss of libido! You have no time, I hear you say....OK, bring them back later, or make a brief assessment and then refer, to someone else with the time and the counselling skills.

To promote accessibility to the facts in this new edition, the figures and tables are listed on pages xiii–xviii and the main headings appear at the start of each chapter.

In addition to those already acknowledged, who helped particularly with the first edition, I wish to thank Drs Elphis Christopher, Ron Kleinman, Sam Rowlands and Anne Szarewski; also my secretary Mrs Helen Prime and my son Jonathan whose keyboard skills have been invaluable. Toni Belfield, Head of Information of the UK FPA, helped in the writing of Chapter 8. Dr Hilary Luscombe of the National Association of Family Planning Doctors assisted with literature searches and lists of the topics about which questions are most commonly asked. Among many others at Churchill Livingstone, Lucy Gardner and Pat Croucher succeeded, as you can see, in turning my typescript, computer disks, rough notes and faxes into the completed book. All of these are most warmly thanked.   **John Guillebaud**

1993

Preface to the First Edition

As its title suggests, this book is designed as a ready source of answers to the many questions which are being asked, always with interest and often with a hint of anxiety, both by the consumers and the providers of modern reversible birth control methods. I have acquired experience in answering most of them as a result of lecturing in family planning very widely, in this country and abroad, and also on the postgraduate lecture courses held regularly at the Margaret Pyke Centre. In these, upwards of 600 doctors and 200 nurses are trained each year. The book is intended primarily for general practitioners and family planning doctors, working in a developed country such as Britain, but it will also be of value to other health care professionals, and medical students.

The questions about each method are arranged so far as possible in a logical order. They are mostly based on the questions which doctors ask of a specialist colleague like myself, arising from their clinical experience and the questions they have been asked by patients. In a concluding section of most chapters there is an assortment of the very practical questions which are asked by patients, some of which can be demanding to the unprepared (see, for example, Qs 4.250 and 6.165).

Reasons of space have required me to concentrate almost entirely on answers to questions about the technology of reversible birth control, with little discussion of and male and female sterilization and induced abortion, as well as essential subjects such as counselling, social factors affecting contraceptive use, medico-legal aspects, sexual problems and health screening. Most of these are dealt with in other texts in the Further Reading section, notably the *Handbook of Family Planning* edited by Nancy Loudon and published by Churchill Livingstone.

For reading and commenting on sections of the text, I am most grateful to the following: Walli Bounds, Ken Fotherby, Susan Hatwell, Sam Hutt, Howard Jacobs and Pram Senanayake. Special thanks are due to my deputy at the Centre, Mr Ali Kubba, who has read and constructively criticized the whole book: but I must be held responsible for any errors that remain.

Ray Phillips and his staff of the Middlesex Hospital Department of Medical Photography and Illustration, especially Stuart Nightingale and Angela Scott, have been most helpful in the preparation of figures – apart from some separately acknowledged in the figure captions and tables. Toni Belfield contributed a list of questions which have been asked of the Family Planning Association's Information Service by the general public. My publishers have been most understanding, notably Katherine Watts and Howard Bailey. I also acknowledge the help of Mr John Adkins, Headmaster of Egerton-Rothesay School, in providing me with a haven of quiet for much of the writing. Last, but not least, I record my thanks to my select team of typists: Margaret Bailón, Diane Berry, Sue Nickells and Georgina Tregoning.

My wife Gwyneth as usual has been enormously supportive. She and our young children have been most tolerant of their recent one-parent family status.

John Guillebaud
September 1985

Contents

Glossary

AIDS	acquired immune deficiency syndrome
ALO	*Actinomyces*-like organisms
BBD	benign breast disease
BBT	basal body temperature
BMI	body mass index
BP	blood pressure
BTB	breakthrough bleeding
CASH Study	Cancer and Sex Hormones Study
CDSM	Committee on Dental and Surgical Materials
CIN	cervical intraepithelial neoplasia
COC	combined oral contraceptive
CVS	cardiovascular system
D&C	dilatation and curettage
DES	diethylstilboestrol
DM	diabetes mellitus
DMPA	depot medroxyprogesterone acetate
DVT	deep venous thrombosis
EE	ethinyloestradiol
FOC	functional ovarian cysts
FPA	Family Planning Association
FSH	follicle stimulating hormone
HDL-C	high-density lipoprotein-cholesterol
hCG	human chorionic gonadotrophin
HIV	human immunodeficiency virus
HRT	hormone replacement therapy
IMB	intermenstrual bleeding
IPPF	International Planned Parenthood Federation
IUD	intrauterine device
IUD	intrauterine death
LA	local anaesthesia
LH	luteinizing hormone
LNG	levonorgestrel
JCC	Joint Committee on Contraception
MPA	medroxyprogesterone acetate

MPC	Margaret Pyke Centre
NAFPD	National Association of Family Planning Doctors
NET EN	norethisterone oenanthate
NFP	natural family planning
NMR	nuclear magnetic resonance
OC	oral contraceptive
PC	postcoital
PCO	polycystic ovary/ovaries
PD	peak day
PFI	pill-free interval
PG	prostaglandins
PGSI	prostaglandin synthetase inhibitor
PID	pelvic inflammatory disease
POP	progestagen-only pill
PPA	post-pill amenorrhoea
RCGP	Royal College of General Practitioners
RCOG	Royal College of Obstetricians and Gynaecologists
SAH	subarachnoid haemorrhage
SEM	scanning electron microscope
SHBG	sex hormone binding globulin
SLE	systemic lupus erythematosis
STD	sexually transmitted disease(s)
TSS	toxic shock syndrome
UC	ulcerative colitis
UK NCCS	UK National Case Control Study
US	ultrasound
USA FDA	USA Food and Drug Administration
WHO	World Health Organization
WTB	withdrawal bleeding

Figures

Tables

Introduction: The population explosion and the importance of fertility control

0.1 What is the population explosion?

See Figure 0.1. According to the figures of the Population Reference Bureau, and in round numbers, during the early 1990s every 2 seconds somewhere on the globe there are nine births and three deaths. Those six extra births mean 1 million arriving every 4 days, or the equivalent of 1000 jumbo jets arriving every day at London Airport. The doubling time is projected as about 40 years; in so little time we must expect the arrival of a complete new world, when even now many of the existing 5500 million are grossly deficient in the bare necessities of life: food, clean water, clothing, housing, health care, education and recreation....

0.2 But isn't this primarily a Third World problem?

Certainly, more than 90% of the growth in human numbers is occurring in the poor countries of the world. But it has been calculated that every new birth in the developed world is likely to lead, in the lifetime of that individual, to up to 40 times more damage to the fragile environment, with inevitable destruction of the habitats of other animals and plants. According to the Worldwide Fund for Nature, total extinction now proceeds at the rate of several species per day, and rising. All this, and more, results from the wastefulness of our 'high-tech.' affluent lifestyle which causes pollution and resource depletion – exacerbated by the increasing number of polluters and resource-depleters.

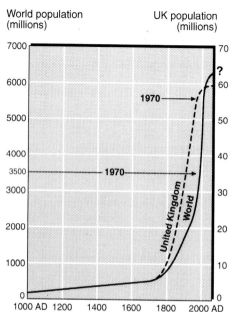

Figure 0.1 Estimated rate of population growth, AD 1750–2000. Q 0.1
Note: the UK differs from the rest of the world mainly by having had
its population explosion slightly earlier. England too was once covered
by forest

Moreover, as was shown by the two reports of the Brandt Commission, the developed countries of the world cannot consider themselves forever immune to events elsewhere on this small finite planet. No wall will be high enough to stop the flood of 'economic migrants', for one thing. The rich 'north' ought to give far more and far more appropriate aid to the 'south', out of simple humanity. But even without that motivation, their own calculated self-interest should force voters and therefore politicians, world-wide, massively to increase the help they give to the poor countries.

If we are not part of the solution, we are part of the problem.

0.3   What changes birth rates?

As shown in Figure 0.2, a great deal more is necessary than simply the provision of family planning. Three of the most important items in the figure are:

1   Better health and fewer child deaths, since it has been calculated that in rural areas of India a couple need to have five children

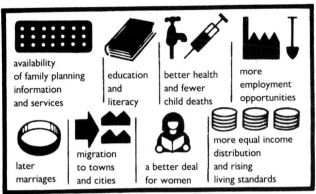

Figure 0.2 What changes birth rates? Q 0.3.
(From The shape of things to come. 1982 Population Concern, 231 Tottenham Court Road, London WC1)

in order to have a 95% chance of one son reaching maturity. There is a vicious circle here though, as child mortality is itself greater in the absence of effective family spacing, now being exacerbated by the worldwide decline in breastfeeding without enough alternative contraception.

2 Secondly, there needs to be a better deal for women. In too many societies worldwide women remain second-class citizens, and have little choice in their destiny or that of their family. They are forced by their male-dominated society in general, and their husbands in particular, as well as by their biology (see Qs 1.1– 1.10), to have far more children than they desire. This was clearly shown by the World Fertility Survey, which during the 1980s found that almost 50% of married women in the developing world wanted no more children. So for them at least family planning has now become a *perceived* unmet need.

3 Thirdly, implicit in the whole of Figure 0.2, are two slogans or sayings. The first is an ancient proverb referring to the inhabitants of rural areas: 'Every mouth has got two hands.' In rural poverty the hands are far more noticeable than the mouth, in that the labour and support which a child can give to its parents, especially in their old age or during disease, are far more important to them than the extra cost that may be incurred. Given the same inputs into decision-making, let us admit that we would make the same decisions with regard to family size, which are entirely logical on the microlevel.

It is hard for individuals to see how the macroproblem – that burgeoning numbers in large tracts of the Third World leading to excessive tree-cutting, desertification, salinization, malnutrition and ultimately disaster – is in any way their business.

Apart from the 'Big Brother' Chinese solution – enforcing one-child families – what can be done? Even the Chinese agree that was a draconian and not very successful measure forced on them mainly because they did not bring in a much less restrictive two-child policy when they had half as many people only 50 years ago. The best answer is summarized in the second slogan: 'Take care of the people and the population will take care of itself.'

0.4 Does this mean that development is the best contraceptive, so family planning does not matter?

Far from it; many people have misinterpreted the slogan in this way, overemphasizing for example improved child survival as a prerequisite for family planning acceptance (which experience in Bangladesh and elsewhere has disproved). The result is that in large areas of the world the basic tools for the family planning job are just not available, in the slums and rural areas where people actually live, at a price that they can afford. 'Population will take care of itself' only when 'taking care of the people' includes every item in Figure 0.2 as part of an integrated solution. Family planning services must be locally, comprehensively and appropriately pro-vided, as a human right, on an equal basis at least with all the other items illustrated.

Such services must also try, vigorously but with understanding of the employment and other pressures which cause it, to coun-teract the flight from breastfeeding which is a sad fact of urban life almost everywhere. Lactation, as well as being so good for babies, has until now prevented more births than family planning – and the take-up of the latter in some places will barely compensate for the decline of the former, leave alone lead to any reduction in birth rates. (For more about breastfeeding as a contraceptive, see Qs 1.31 and 1.32.)

At present the proportion of aid for the Third World spent on the provision of voluntary birth control is around 1%. Now I have never stated that family planning is a panacea, the whole answer: but it is surely much more than 1% of the answer!

0.5 If everything were done that could and should be done, what is the most likely future total world population at stabilization?

Realistically, twice its present size. Short of a cataclysm, this is a demographic certainty. Why? – Because world population, like a super-tanker, has so much inbuilt momentum. 1700 million of the world's inhabitants are under 15, and *that means very nearly all of tomorrow's parents are already born.* They will be responsible for a doubling even if they have only an average of two children each. To me, this is the most frightening among all alarming eco-statistics.

So everything we must do as in Qs 0.3 and 0.4 can only stop world no. 3 arriving; the arrival of world no. 2 is inevitable. Scientists can see some chance of a passable if perilous future for 11 billion humans. However, 16 plus billion really does risk collapse of life-support mechanisms in the ecosystem – and misery on an unheard-of scale.

0.6 Is the population crisis as dangerous as you imply?

The trouble about the population/development/resources/pollution story is that it is based on trends rather than catastrophic events. Our social evolution depended on our reacting to obvious inputs to our special senses, like the roar of a sabre-tooth tiger. We are much less inclined to worry about dangers which are at least as great if they are insidious and silent – take cigarette smoke for instance!

Secondly, the crisis is not caused by 'evil', only ignorance. It happens through millions of people 'doing their own thing'. They are, directly or indirectly, and most understandably, using technology to improve their families' material environment: oblivious to the fact that, with more and more people doing the same and continuing for long enough, the consequences are capable of rendering the world as uninhabitable as that following nuclear war. Somehow we must all learn that we must stop treating the fragile planet as an inexhaustible 'milch-cow' for our wants and as a bottomless cesspit for our wastes.

There is a Chinese proverb: 'we have not inherited the world from our grandparents – we have borrowed it from our grandchildren'. I believe that our own children's children will brand this generation, living in the last quarter of the twentieth century, as the worst ever: in that it was the last to have some chance of preventing the environmental wasteland which they will have inherited, but too little was done far too late. We will be seen as having selfishly mortgaged their future for our present gain.

The disease smallpox was eradicated from the face of this planet by an equivalent amount of money to that which was then spent by the world's armed forces every 8 minutes. It has been estimated that the money required to provide adequate food, water, education, health and housing for everyone in the world could be provided by as little as one month's-worth of worldwide defence spending!

0.7 In view of the urgency of these matters, and the inbuilt momentum of population growth, why is so little being done?

The main problem is, as the politicians say, 'politics is the art of the possible'. Voters worldwide faced with the challenge of less 'jam' today in order that their children may inherit a tolerable world in the future, invariably vote instead to have at least as much 'jam' as they currently have, and preferably more. Human perspectives are remarkably insular in terms of space and brief in terms of time. The following sayings summarize things well: 'my car is my car, everyone else's car is traffic'; 'my visit to the seaside is my holiday, everybody else is a tripper'; and 'my baby is my baby – everybody else's baby is overpopulation'. These attitudes are reinforced by ignorance, by apathy and often by a hint of racialism: 'the death of one baby, in London, is a tragedy – the death of millions of babies, somewhere overseas, that is a statistic'.

0.8 What can we do, as doctors or other health workers?

We are bound to feel impotent in the face of the major trends discussed above. However, 'the ocean is made up out of drops' .... we should not underestimate our influence on those around us, our patients and our peer groups, and through them our politicians. More immediately – and here we come to the reason why this book has been written – we can ensure that we are so well informed about the whole subject of contraception, that we can answer the questions of the women and the men who come to us for contraceptive advice and help. In so far as we are able to influence events, the aim is to authenticate the maxim 'every child a wanted child'.

0.9 Is it enough to be able to answer the questions?

No – 1 g of *empathy* is worth 1 kg of *knowledge*.

1 There are practical *skills* to be learnt and maintained: notably in the fitting of intrauterine devices, and the fitting and the training for women who wish to use female barrier methods.

2 Almost more important, it is essential for health care professionals to have the correct non-directive counselling *attitude* and approach. Couples must decide for themselves what aspects of the list in Q 0.10 below are most important in their situation. It has been well said that in the field of birth control: 'we are advisers, we are the suppliers but we are not the deciders'.

It is no good just blaming the user when conception occurs 'because she fails the method'. As many studies have shown, compliance can depend as much on aspects of counselling, instruction and provision of a chosen method as on its inherent effectiveness. The mare may not have drunk the water: but did we really take her right to it?! And how can we help to prevent a recurrence? (after pill failure, for example, perhaps by suggesting tricycling of a monophasic pill – see Q 4.24 and Qs 8.1–8.16.)

0.10 What are the features of the absolutely ideal contraceptive?

The list below is modified from Table 13 in my book *The Pill* (see Further Reading). The first three are the most important. The ideal method would be:

1 100% *safe*, with neither dangerous nor annoying unwanted effects;

2 100% *effective*;

3 *independent of intercourse*;

4 reversible;

5 effective after acceptable, simple and painless procedure(s) not relying on the user's memory: so the 'default state' is one of contraceiving not conceiving!

6 reversed equally simply, without having to 'ask permission to stop';

7 cheap and easy to distribute;

8 independent of the medical professions;

9 acceptable to every culture, religion and political view;

10 used by or obviously visible to the woman (whose stakes in effective contraception are obviously greatest).

Since we are talking of the ideal, it would be useful to have also one or more beneficial non-contraceptive side-effects. Among the latter the most relevant in today's world has to be the great bonus of the condom (male or female), namely protection against sexually transmitted diseases including viruses.

0.11 How do the available reversible methods perform when tested against the list in Q 0.10?

Badly, all fail on at least one of the critical first three criteria. Maximum effectiveness and independence from intercourse tend to go together and, unfortunately, to be inversely linked with freedom from health risk. So in practice, when counselling most couples one can explain that there is always a dilemma, a 'Hobson's choice', as depicted in Table 0.1. We shall return to this table in discussing the female barriers (see Ch. 3), and the best direction for future birth control research (see Ch. 8).

0.12 How is the effectiveness of any method commonly reported?

The data about efficacy, particularly of the non-medical methods, have shown extremely variable results. In clinical investigations an effort is usually made to make the (in practice very difficult) distinction: between pregnancies that occurred despite the fact that the method was used correctly during every act of intercourse (method-failures), and those that resulted from incorrect use or

Table 0.1. The contraceptive dilemma

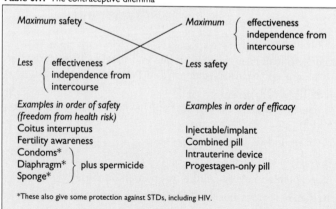

Examples in order of safety (freedom from health risk)	Examples in order of efficacy
Coitus interruptus	Injectable/implant
Fertility awareness	Combined pill
Condoms* ⎫	Intrauterine device
Diaphragm* ⎬ plus spermicide	Progestagen-only pill
Sponge* ⎭	

*These also give some protection against STDs, including HIV.

non-use on one or more occasions (user-failures). Hence are derived estimates of the theoretical or method-effectiveness and of the actual use-effectiveness.

1 Method-effectiveness rates vary because of physiological differences between individuals, notably increasing age which diminishes fertility.

2 Use-effectiveness is a function of the motivation of the study population, the acceptability of another baby, the adequacy of counselling, the difficulty of using the method, the effect of experience from increasing duration of use, and other factors. Hence the findings are even more variable and it is very difficult to compare data from different studies among deferent populations.

3 Extended use-effectiveness is a measure of all the pregnancies occurring in a large population based on their initial intention to use a particular method. It includes individuals who abandon the method which they initially set out to use. Failure rates calculated on this basis tend to be very high indeed, even for a highly effective method such as the combined pill, since side-effects or anxiety about side-effects can lead to it being abandoned without any effective replacement, in a large proportion of the initial users.

0.13 How are the effectiveness rates measured and expressed?

Both method- and use-effectiveness rates are usually expressed as failure rates/100 woman-years of exposure. The basis for calculations is know as the Pearl pregnancy rate, calculated from the formula:

$$\text{Failure rate} = \frac{\text{Total accidental pregnancies} \times 1200}{\text{Total months of exposure}}$$

When applying this formula every known conception must be included, whatever its outcome. The figure 1200 is of course the number of months in 100 years. By convention 10 months are deducted from the denominator for each full-term pregnancy and 4 months for any kind of abortion.

Trussell (of Princeton, USA) points out that the usual convention of using the same denominator (total number of months) whether the numerator is the number of method-failures or user-failures is wrong. It fails to account for the fact that many contraceptive-users make errors and 'get away with it'. Any such method-failure rate is artificially lowered by the larger denominator. The true rate would use for the denominator only the months of total compliance. Very few studies, in which all users kept coital diaries, have had any chance of computing this true rate. Because errors in compliance are so common and vary so widely, this means that ordinary method-failure rates ought not to be compared between populations.

The risk of contraceptive failure tends to fall with the duration of use because of changes in the population under study, as women drop out for whatever reason. Long-term users obviously tend to be those who use the method efficiently and also include those of lower fertility. The life-table method of analysis has been adopted to overcome these problems. The method takes into account all the reasons for contraceptive discontinuation, and permits the calculation of failure rates (or the rates for other events such as expulsion of an IUD) for specified intervals of use. The Pearl rate pools the data and can only give one common measurement.

0.14 What effectiveness rates can be quoted, for potential users?

As just implied the epidemiology of contraception is not an exact science. Vested interests (especially by advertisers) readily lead to misuse of the data on effectiveness of particular techniques. Failure rates should not be quoted as exact measurements, but rather as ranges as in Table 0.2. They need to be interpreted by the provider to each potential user, in the context of the woman's age and factors such as the steadiness of the relationship and the frequency of intercourse. Despite all the pitfalls the table clearly shows that there is a ranking order, with pills being more effective than IUDs, and these in turn are less likely to fail than the barrier methods. But note the considerable overlap: careful condom-users have been known to do better than poor pill-users.

In interpreting Table 0.2 to couples at counselling, it is often helpful to divide 100 by the figures given for the rates. This calculation gives the number of years of regular intercourse, carefully using the method, which would be expected to lead to one conception. For example, if per 100 woman-year rates of 20,10 and 1 were being compared, the couple could be told that regular use of the method would give an 'evens' chance of one pregnancy by the end of 5 years, 10 years or 100 years of fertility, respectively. This clearly shows the difference, though for any method it is

Table 0.2. User-failure rates for different methods of contraception/100 woman-years

	Range in the World literature*	Oxford/FPA Study (Lancet report in 1982; all women married and aged above 25)		
		Overall (any duration) use)	Age 25–34 (≤2 years use)	Age 35+ (≤2 years use)
Sterilization				
Male	0–0.2	0.02	0.08	0.08
Female	0–0.5	0.13	0.45	0.08
Levonorgestrel implant				
(Norplant)	0–1			
Injectable (DMPA)	0–1	–	–	–
Combined pills				
(50 µg oestrogen	0.1–3	0.16	0.25	0.17)
<50 µg oestrogen	0.2–3	0.27	0.38	0.23
Progestagen-only pill	0.3–4	1.2	2.5	0.5
IUD				
Copper T 200	>2			
Nova-T/Multiload Cu250	1–2			
Multiload Cu 375	0.5–1			
Cu-T 380 (Slimline)	0.3–1			
Levonorgestrel IUD-20	<0.5			
Diaphragm	2–15	1.9	5.5	2.8
(Male) condom	2–15	3.6	6.0	2.9
Female condom	Believed comparable to male condom			
Coitus interruptus	8–17	6.7	–	–
Spermicides alone	4–25	11.9	–	–
Fertility awareness	6–25	15.5	–	–
Contraceptive sponge	9–25	–	–	–
No method, young women	80–90	–	–	–
No method at age 40	40–50	–	–	–
No method at age 45	10–20	–	–	–
No method at age 50 (if still having menses)	0–5	–	–	–

*Excludes atypical studies giving particularly poor results and all extended-use studies.

Note: 1 Ranking of efficacy, but overlap of ranges in the first column.

    2 Influence of age: all the rates in the fourth column being lower than those in the third column. Lower rates still may be expected above age 45.

    3 Much better results also obtainable in other states of relative infertility, such as lactation.

important to add something like: 'Of course that one pregnancy could occur at any time, even in the very first year.'

It is also helpful to put things in the context of 'the failure rate of no contraception at all'. Among 100 young couples setting out to achieve a pregnancy, that 'failure rate' will be 80–90/100 woman-years, but that rate would be halved for 40 year olds (meaning that the less effective methods will be 'stronger', for them).

In the complete absence of birth control practices, but allowing for times of natural infertility during pregnancy and lactation, the average annual rate again drops to about 40/100 woman-years. This corresponds to about 10–12 liveborn children in 25 years of marriage.

0.15 Knowing that failure rates depend so much on motivation and compliance, what can I as a prescriber do to identify and to minimize problems?

It is no good just blaming the method-users. Prescribers can fail them in a number of ways, both by errors but more commonly by omissions: for example, simply not allowing enough time for basic instructions and for them to ask questions. 'You cannot make the horse drink'.... but in the first place have we *properly* 'taken the horse to the water?' More on this follows in Chapter 8 (see Qs 8.3–8.16): we need first to be fully informed about the methods available.

Table 0.3 shows current usage of the methods in Great Britain (1991).

Table 0.3. Percentage of women aged 16–49 using the pill, sterilization and the condom as main method, by age (Great Britain, 1991)

Method of contraception		Age					
		16–17	18–19	20–24	30–34	40–44
Sterilisation	25	0	0	1	21	50
Pill	23	16	46	48	25	4
Condom	16	10	15	14	17	13
IUD	5					
Other birth control or sterile after hysterectomy	6					
Pregnant or wanting pregnancy	9					
Abstinence/no partner	16					

General Household Survey. Preliminary results for 1991, OPCS 1992.

1

Aspects of human fertility and fertility awareness: Natural birth control

BACKGROUND CONSIDERATIONS

1.1 How fertile are human beings?

Although we break no records in the animal kingdom, we are fertile enough to become numerically by far and away the most successful vertebrate that this planet has ever known. The first half of this chapter deals with physiological factors which either promote conception or make the devising or the practising of contraception difficult. We have first to consider aspects relating to intercourse, then the sperm, the ova, fertilization and implantation.

Returning to the question, we can at least be grateful that the fertility of average couples is not as great as the human maximum, which must have been approached by the couple described in the *Guinness Book of Records*:

> The greatest officially recorded number of children produced by a mother is 69 by the first of the two wives of Feodor Vasilyev (b. 1707), a peasant from Shuya, 241 km east of Moscow. In 27 confinements, she gave birth to 16 pairs of twins, 7 sets of triplets and 14 sets of quadruplets ... Almost all survived to their majority.

1.2 What features of human intercourse are particularly favourable to fertility?

1 Obviously it is very pleasurable, and the human female is exceptional in having no breeding season and in being potentially receptive on most days of the cycle.

2 Some indication of the power of the human sex instinct is provided by the calculation (never mind the assumptions) by WHO, that intercourse takes place about 42 000 million times per year. This works out, somewhere in the world, to over 1300 ejaculations per second ....

3 The drive towards copulation in both sexes is such as to militate against forward planning, and to the successful use of intercourse-related methods.

4 In many women maximum desire coincides with the most fertile phase, when there is an abundance of oestrogenic mucus, very favourable to sperm survival.

5 The outpouring of vaginal transudate described by Masters and Johnson raises the pH of the vagina so that it becomes favourable to sperm.

6 There is evidence that, at least in some women, there is a negative pressure in the uterus at orgasm which may promote physical aspiration of sperm into the cervix and uterus. Sperm are found in the cervix within 90 seconds of ejaculation.

1.3 How do the mechanics of intercourse interfere with the efficacy of vaginal methods?

1 The ballooning of the whole upper two-thirds of the vagina, also described by Masters and Johnson, leads to:
   (a) an increased risk of sperm passing over the rim of a diaphragm or other cervical cap, and
   (b) the risk of displacement of any cervical device into a fornix, e.g. the contraceptive sponge.
2 The penile thrusts themselves lead to:
   (a) the potential to dislodge all forms of female barrier, particularly in certain positions of intercourse, and
   (b) if a vaginal spermicide is used, it is probable that the spreading effect of intercourse means that there is ultimately too little spermicide around the external os of the cervix at ejaculation. This may in part explain how spermicides have usually appeared far more effective in vitro than in vivo (see Q 3.74).

1.4 What are the relevant facts about cervical mucus?

Cervical mucus is only the most obvious component of the genital tract mucus and fluid, which extend right through the cavity of the uterus and both tubes. Under the influence of unopposed oestrogen in the follicular phase it becomes increasingly fluid and receptive to sperm, with a marked Spinnbarkeit. It helps to capacitate sperm and provides an optimum environment for them to proceed to the upper tract. The ability to promote sperm survival for prolonged durations varies from woman to woman and from cycle to cycle, as does the length of time within the cycle that ovulatory mucus is present.

The characteristics of mucus change abruptly under the influence of progesterone, even though the corpus luteum continues to secrete oestrogens. It rapidly becomes impenetrable and hostile to sperm. Women can be taught to feel the change from the earlier slippery 'ovulatory' mucus to the sticky mucus of the luteal phase.

But before ovulation WHO found (1983) 'a substantial probability of pregnancy if intercourse occurs (even) in the presence of sticky mucus ...'. See Q 1.25.

1.5 What other changes occur at the cervix during the cycle?

Continuing research into birth planning by methods of fertility awareness has shown that women can be taught to detect the changes occurring in the size of the external cervical os, and also in its position relative to the introitus. The cervix starts low and rises appreciably during the follicular phase, until around ovulation it reaches peak height from the introitus with maximum softness and sufficient dilation to admit a finger tip. The cervix then descends and narrows rapidly early in the luteal phase, becoming once more closed, firm and close to the vulva. It is reported that daily autopalpation of these cervical changes can be of particular value in the detection of the return of fertility towards the end of lactation (see Q 1.31).

1.6 Which are the most important physiological facts about sperm which promote conception?

All of us whose work involves family planning rapidly develop an enormous respect for these little swimmers! There is great individual variation between men, and between individual sperm within the same man's ejaculate. From the point of view of preventing pregnancy we have to consider the very best sperm with regard to motility, survival and fertilizing ability, rather than those exhibiting average qualities; and there are an incredible number of them, produced by spermatogenesis at rates of the order of 1000 per second from each testicle!

1.7 How many sperm are present, and what are the implications?

It is worth recalling that, with a count of say 80 million/ml being not unrepresentative, it would not be unusual for there to be 350 million sperm in the 3–5 ml of a man's ejaculate. If each sperm could find an egg this would be enough to populate most of North America! One per cent of this number might very well cause a pregnancy (see Q 1.9) and yet would be contained in the hardly visible volume of less than 0.05 ml.

This has obvious implications for coitus interruptus (see Q 2.7) and also for any lack of care when using the sheath (see Q 2.19). It should be more widely known that in contraceptive terms semen is a dangerous fluid!

1.8 What is the extreme limit of sperm survival in genital tract mucus, and what are the implications?

This has proved very difficult to study directly, since the studies themselves are liable to alter what is being observed. It seems clear that sperm normally survive no more than 6 hours in the vagina, as its pH reverts to its normal low value subsequent to intercourse. Motile sperm have been found even in the vagina up to 16 hours after intercourse, however, and survival in the cervical, uterine and tubal fluid appears very variable. Survival depends on features of the sperm themselves, the seminal fluid, and to what degree the oestrogenic mucus approaches the ideal – in that woman or in that particular cycle.

In the past most authorities have talked in terms of average survival times of about 3–4 days. However, with so many millions ejaculated (see above) one must be concerned not with average sperm survival but lunatic fringe sperm survival! It is the duration of the ability to fertilize of the first centile of the sperm (i.e. the most vigorous 3 million or so) which is the relevant figure. This is not known; but both direct studies and indirect studies such as that of Barrett and Marshall (see Qs 1.14 and 1.15) suggest that this can certainly exceed 5 days. On some rare occasions in some rare couples, particularly where the woman produces good mucus for an unusually long time, it might even reach 7 days. Mucus assessment (see Qs 1.4 and 1.24) should theoretically give more advance warning of ovulation than usual in those very cases, but it may fail to do so.

The main implication is the likely ineffectiveness, in long-term use by most couples, of the first phase of the so-called 'safe period' (see Q 1.16).

1.9 How can it be that 1% of a man's ejaculate (i.e. about 3 million sperm) could cause a pregnancy, when men with that number of sperm/ml are commonly held to be infertile?

This question implies a common misunderstanding of the nature of semen analysis in an infertility clinic. For a start, an excessively high count can actually be associated with male subfertility. And when a low count is present, it is mainly acting as a marker for other much more important features of the sperm which are causing the subfertility, such as poor motility, frequent abnormal forms, or the presence of antibodies. The paucity of sperm signifies that they are also pretty poor individuals. This does not apply when 3 million good sperm from a fertile man are deposited at the cervix because of too late use of a condom.

Evidence for the above comes from routine sperm counts in men having vasectomies who have fathered children. Counts less than 2 million/ml are not uncommon; and in a study of late recanalization reported from Oxford, it appeared that one man with counts of only 500 000 and 750 000/ml (with motility demonstrated) was responsible for his wife's pregnancy.

1.10   What are the relevant physiological facts about ova?

1   More often than expected by many couples, ovulation occurs early. Remarkably few women claiming 28-day menstrual cycles do not sometimes have 26-day cycles, and some can feature fertile cycles as short as 21 or 22 days in length (see Q 1.15 for the implications).

2   Ovum fertilizability is short – practically the only physiological fact so far discussed which helps contraception. From in vitro fertilization research, maximum ovum survival is believed to be 24 hours but successful fertilization appears to be unlikely beyond 12 hours. This means that if a pregnancy is desired, the best chance of successful fertilization is when that fragile ovum arrives at a tube which is already populated with adequate numbers of vigorous, motile sperm.

1.11   Can human females be like rabbits, ovulating on intercourse?

I think the answer to this question which is often asked can (fortunately) be a fairly definite 'no'. First there is no need whatever to postulate any such mechanism, when one adds together the data mentioned above concerning sperm survival and the frequent occurrence of ovulation earlier than usual. Intercourse can be fertile almost any time, not excluding during the menses, if sperm may survive for up to 7 days and ovulation can be unexpectedly early or late.

A more important reason for rejecting this hypothesis is the fact that, were it to be true, newly married women would have shorter menstrual cycles than women who were abstaining from intercourse (such as nuns). Such a shortening of the mean duration of menstrual cycles has not been observed.

1.12 After fertilization how much preimplantation wastage occurs?

Here we have one more fact which reduces the size of the contraceptive task. Assessments of postfertilization wastage vary considerably, but a good modern estimate would be around 30–40%. Frequently there are chromosomal abnormalities, but local factors affecting the receptivity of the endometrium to the blastocyst are also important. These can be enhanced by contraceptive methods (see Qs 5.4 and 7.6).

Fertility awareness and natural family planning

BACKGROUND AND MECHANISMS

1.13 Putting the above physiological facts together, how long is the potentially fertile phase in the human female?

This had traditionally been termed 'midcycle', or say days 10–17 of a 28-day cycle; but recent in vivo and in vitro studies, which form the basis of the physiology described in the last ten questions, clearly indicate that the fertile phase both starts and finishes earlier. The latest work would imply that under optimal conditions for sperm survival the potentially fertile phase comprises days 7–14 (i.e. *the whole of the second week of a 4-week cycle*) with ovulation taking place on day 14–15 plus a further 1 plus days to allow for maximum ovum survival – i.e. in all from *day 7 to day 16* – adjusted of course, as appropriate, if the cycle is longer or shorter than 28 days. It is fascinating that recent in vivo work on sperm and ovum survival reflects so accurately the findings of Barrett and Marshall which were reported as far back as 1969 (Fig. 1.1).

1.14 How was the Barrett and Marshall study designed? What is the risk of conception on each day of the cycle (Fig. 1.1)

In brief, 241 previously fertile women who had been fully trained to keep basal body temperature (BBT) charts also kept a careful record of every act of intercourse. Whether conception took place in a given cycle was also known. Some were attempting to conceive; others to avoid pregnancy. All the data on 1898 cycles and 6015 acts of coitus were fed into a computer, and for each woman the day of BBT shift, and hence presumed ovulation, was identified in a standard way for that cycle.

The analysis gave figures for the percentage risk of conception for intercourse on each day of the cycle relative to the BBT shift, and these have been charted to produce Figure 1.1 (0 represents the BBT shift). The continuous line joins the points for which the data were sufficient for an estimate of percentage risk of conception to be made; the dotted lines are no more than approximate projections down to the horizontal axis.

1.15 What are the main observations from Figure 1.1?

1 The percentage risk of conception exceeds zero between days 7 and 16 of a 28-day cycle, as predicted from sperm and ovum survival studies (see Q 1.13).

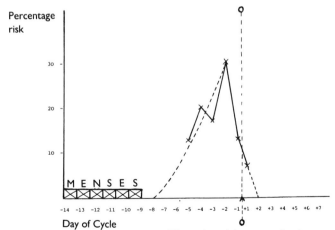

Figure. 1.1 The risk of conception on different days of the menstrual cycle (Barrett JC & Marshall J 1969) (See text Q 1.14–1.16).
(Redrawn from Table 2 in Population Studies 1969; 23: 455–461)

2 Peak fecundability occurs well before ovum release, again congruent with the notion that it is best for the sperm to be waiting in the tubes in advance of ovulation.

3 The first phase of the so-called 'safe period' is shown to be exceedingly short, even in a woman who never ovulates earlier than day 14. Since it is well known that very many women do occasionally ovulate earlier in the cycle, in a 24-day cycle intercourse any later than day 3 might, on the basis of these data, sometimes result in conception!

4 The good news from Figure 1.1, however is that the second phase of the 'safe period' is dependent only on the reliability of ovulation *detection*. There is only one ovum, and it is fertilizable for a predictable, short time. This is quite unlike the first phase which is beset by problems: the millions of sperm, the capriciousness with which enough of them may just survive on occasion for as much as a week, coupled with the possibility of a random, early ovulation. So far no effective means have been devised of *predicting* ovulation accurately as far as 5, leave alone 7 days ahead.

1.16 What are the implications of the fecundability curve (Fig. 1.1) for family planning?

In my view, with any combination of present technologies, only the second phase of the 'safe period' should ever be relied on by a woman who feels that she must avoid pregnancy. The first phase is only suitable for those who are delaying a wanted pregnancy ('spacing'). The one exception to this recommendation might be a woman with very regular longish menstrual cycles (never less than 28 days) who is good at detecting mucus and cervical changes. But the capriciousness of sperm survival under occasional optimal conditions in the female reproductive tract still means that, whatever methods based on fertility awareness are used, the preovulatory phase will be 'in a different ball-park' of potential efficacy, as compared with the postovulatory phase.

1.17 Why have family planning specialists traditionally decried natural family planning methods? What should be their modern attitude?

The bad reputation of these methods followed from the high failure rate of the old calendar/rhythm approach (see Q 1.18), coupled with a lack of awareness of the fundamental difference in effectiveness potential between the first and the second infertile phases, however they might be determined. That lack of awareness is still common today among both the opponents and the proponents of the methods.

The correct attitude today should be a very positive one to the second infertile phase, based on the most accurate currently practical detection of ovulation. As far back as 1968 Marshall showed that correct use of BBT temperature charts with unprotected intercourse only in the postovulatory phase had a method-related failure rate of only 1.2/100 woman-years and the overall failure rate was a creditable 6.6/100 woman-years.

1.18 For the record (since it is not recommended), what calculations are required for the calendar/ rhythm method?

1 First the woman should define the shortest and longest menstrual cycle over the previous 12 cycles.

2 Secondly she should subtract 20 days from the length of the shortest cycle to derive the first day of the fertile phase. This allows 14, 15 or 16 days for the maximum length of the luteal phase plus 6, 5 or 4 days for maximum sperm survival. Sadly both these durations may sometimes be longer!

3 Thirdly, subtract 11 from the longest cycle observed to derive the last day of the fertile phase, so allowing 12–14 days for minimum length of a fertile luteal phase and 1 day for the duration of ovum fertilizability. Even with good compliance this method has a high failure rate. Compliance is also difficult, because few women have regular menstrual cycles so the amount of abstinence required becomes intolerable to many couples.

1.19 How are the phases of the fertility cycle defined? See Figure 1.2.

1 The first infertile phase starts on day 1 of the menses and ends with the earliest time that any sperm could survive to cause a pregnancy. It varies very much in length depending on the rapidity of the follicular response to the pituitary hormones.

2 The (true, as opposed to detectable) fertile phase extends from the end of phase 1 until that time following ovulation when the ovum is incapable of being fertilized. Its duration is therefore the sum of the maximum number of days of sperm survival (say

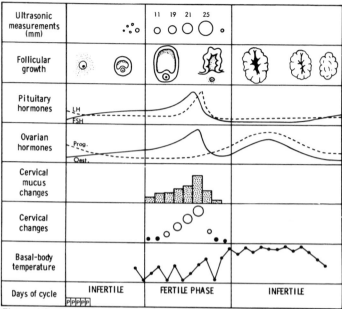

Ultrasonic measurements (mm)			11 19 21 25		
Follicular growth					
Pituitary hormones	LH FSH				
Ovarian hormones	Prog. Oest.				
Cervical mucus changes					
Cervical changes					
Basal-body temperature					
Days of cycle	INFERTILE PPPPP		FERTILE PHASE		INFERTILE

Figure. 1.2 The relationship during the cycle of serial ultrasound measurements, hormonal control and clinical indicators of fertility. Q 1.19.
(Reproduced courtesy of Dr A. Flynn, Birmingham Maternity Hospital, Queen Elizabeth Medical Centre, Birmingham)

7 days) and the maximum duration of fertilizability of the ovum (say 24 hours).

3   The second infertile phase extends from the end of the fertile phase until the onset of the next menstruation. This phase has a mean duration of 13 days with a range, in likely fertile cycles, of about 11–15 days. It is often called the 'absolute' infertile phase as significantly delayed superovulation never occurs in the human. (If two or more eggs are released this is believed to be always on the same day.) Provided ovulation is accurately determined and sufficient time is allowed for the ovum to succumb, conception really is impossible in this phase.

1.20   How may the phases be determined, in practice?

We must distinguish carefully between:

1   The biological events which delineate the phases – these are clear-cut and defined in Q 1.19. But they are not the same as:

2 The biological indicators of the events. These can be further classified into:
   (a) biophysical methods (e.g. serial ultrasonic monitoring of follicular growth, changes in vaginal, ovarian or hand blood flow, etc.);
   (b) biochemical methods which detect the change in concentration of the sex steroids or their metabolites in body fluids such as urine or saliva;
   (c) clinical indicators such as BBT, mucus and cervical changes.
   The accuracy of these indicators of the events at 1 varies, and must also be distinguished from:

3 The ability of the woman accurately to detect the indicator. And finally after detection and recording of the indicator we have to consider:

4 The compliance of the woman and of her partner, which is a different matter again.

The importance of numbers 3 and 4 was well shown in a celebrated study, which apparently showed that the pregnancy rate was higher when charts of clinical indicators were interpreted by the woman's husband than when the woman decided when it was safe to have intercourse!

1.21 What are the major clinical indicators of fertility?

1 Changes in the cervical mucus (see Qs 1.4 and 1.24).

2 Changes involving the cervix itself (see Q 1.5).

3 Changes in the BBT (see Q 1.22).

1.22 How are the changes in the BBT used?

The biphasic nature of the temperature cycle is caused by metabolites of progesterone, hence this can only be used to detect the onset of the second infertile phase. A woman must measure her temperature under basal conditions after a period of sleep, without getting out of bed, having a drink or smoking a cigarette. The shift of temperature is small (0.2–0.6°C), hence a special expanded-scale mercury thermometer should be used, or better still a modern, direct-reading, electronic version. The temperature should be taken orally or vaginally for an absolute minimum of 3 minutes, sticking to the same orifice for any given cycle.

The results are plotted daily on a special chart. To detect the shift a cover line is drawn 0.05°C over the lower phase temperatures of which there should be a minimum of six. The second infertile phase is held to begin on the morning of the third consecutive high temperature after the temperature shift; each being a minimum of 0.2°C higher than those six earlier temperatures covered by the line drawn as just described.

1.23 What are the difficulties of BBT assessment?

Some women have problems with using and reading thermometers, and with keeping interpretable charts. But the main danger is of a mild infection occurring prematurely say around day 10, so raising the temperature before ovulation in what is actually going to be a relatively long cycle.

1.24 How are the mucus changes used to detect the fertile and infertile phases?

At every micturition the woman is instructed to observe the quantity, colour, fluidity, glossiness, transparency and stretchiness of the mucus. The most fertile characteristics of the mucus over the entire day are charted each night. The client fills in either a colour (green for dry, yellow for mucus, and red for bleeding) or writes in a description of the mucus seen.

The peak mucus day can only be identified retrospectively, and corresponds closely with the peak secretion of oestrogen in the blood. This is the last day during which the mucus is slippery with an elastic quality allowing it to be stretched for several centimetres before it breaks, like raw egg-white. After ovulation, the rise in progesterone causes within a day a profound change in the amount and characteristics of the mucus. If present at all it resembles the thick, sticky and tacky postmenstrual type. The peak mucus day can hence be identified. Allowing 2–3 days for ovulation to be completed and 1 day for ovum fertilizability, the second infertile phase is defined as beginning on the evening of the fourth day after the peak mucus symptom.

Changes in the cervix itself can be used to check on the other indicators, though this is not essential. They were described above (see Q 1.5).

1.25 What practical problems can confuse mucus assessment?

1 The most serious is the effect of intercourse, and of sexual excitement without intercourse. Both the fluid of sexual arousal

and semen can mimic the sensations and the features of ovulatory mucus. This is another problem if use of the *first infertile phase* is attempted. Unprotected intercourse is then only allowed on alternate days to allow mucus assessment. To identify the first potentially fertile day, *the calculation at Q 1.18 (shortest cycle less 20) must have priority* over mucus observations: since WHO (1983) has reported that in almost 20% of cycles no mucus at all was observed at the vulva until 3 days or less before the peak day (PD). And sticky mucus is certainly not reliably 'infertile' (see Q 1.4) unless it occurs 6 or preferably more days before PD – a fact which can only be determined in retrospect.

2 Spermicidal jellies and lubricants can similarly cause confusion, particularly if the diaphragm is used in the fertile phase.

3 Mucus assessment is impossible during bleeding – a problem in some menstrual cycles.

4 Vaginal infections and discharges: these can cause difficulty, notably thrush and its treatments which tend to 'dry' the mucus.

1.26 What are the minor clinical indicators of fertility?

These tend to be specific to individual women, or only occur in some ovulatory cycles. When present they can be helpful in confirming the major signals. Among them are:

1 Ovulation pain (Mittelschmerz). Ultrasound scan studies show that this occurs 24–48 hours preovulation.

2 A midcycle 'show' of blood.

3 The onset of breast symptoms, acne and other skin changes, and variations in mood.

Recent research suggests that the pain of ovulation is usually caused by stretching of the ovarian capsule. If noted the woman may consider that her second infertile phase commences 5 days later, provided this matches the findings on her temperature/mucus chart (see Q 1.27).

1.27 What should be done if the different clinical indicators being used by the woman give slightly variable results?

Assuming – as here recommended – use only of the second phase, the woman should be instructed to act only on the latest of the signals being used. For example, if peak mucus plus 4 days would suggest that intercourse was safe on a Thursday evening, but only two higher temperatures had been recorded, intercourse would be deferred until the third higher temperature was recorded the following (Friday) morning.

EFFECTIVENESS

1.28 What is the efficacy of multiple-index natural family planning (NFP)?

If the second phase only is used, highly acceptable method-failure rates of 1–3/100 woman-years are obtainable, with user failure-rates under 10/100 woman-years. Higher rates should not necessarily be blamed on the NFP approach, if the couple have used a barrier method during the part of the fertile phase, since it may well be the latter that has failed.

In fairness, it should be reported that excellent method-failure rates have sometimes been reported for the use of multiple-index methods even where intercourse has been permitted in the first, preovulatory, phase. For example, the method-related failure rate in the WHO study was 2.2/100 woman-years. However as Trussell (see Q 0.12) has pointed out, this is not a relevant rate to quote to *average* potential users of the method; there is no doubt that it is extremely unforgiving of less-than-perfect use, which let us face it, is *normal* use of any method for most normal people. (Contrast the pill: most people forget pills from time to time, but the difference is that they are much more likely to get away with it.) In the same study the combined method-plus-user failure rate was reported as 22.3 but Trussell reassesses it at as over 80/100 woman-years!.

ADVANTAGES AND INDICATIONS

1.29 What are the advantages of methods based on fertility awareness?

1 First and foremost, they are completely free from any known physical side-effects for the user (but see Q 1.30).

2 They are acceptable to many with certain religious and cultural views, not only Roman Catholics. According to strict interpretations, they are used rightly when the intention is family spacing rather than family limitation.

3 The methods are under the couple's personal control (and abstinence is always available!)

4 The methods readily lend themselves, if the couple's scruples permit, to use as part of a package: i.e. along with an artificial method such as a barrier at the potentially fertile times.

5 Once established as an efficient user (after proper teaching), no further follow-up or expense is necessary.

6 Understanding of the methods can help subfertile couples to achieve a pregnancy.

PROBLEMS AND DISADVANTAGES

1.30 What are the problems of natural family planning methods?

1 Interestingly enough, the majority of *established* users believe the method to be helpful to their marriage/relationship rather than causing stress – but conflicts and frustrations are also reported.

2 A worrying potential hazard is the possibility of fetal abnormalities due to conceptions resulting from fertilization involving ageing gametes. Animal work and a couple of retrospective human studies have suggested this. However, several others including the WHO study mentioned above have shown no hint of an increase in the incidence of birth defects. The risk if real must clearly be very small.

3 A small increase in the risk of spontaneous abortion and ectopic pregnancy has also been suggested – but never proven.

1.31 Can fertility awareness predict the return of fertility after lactation?

Full breastfeeding, in which the baby takes no fluids other than from its mother, is a highly efficient natural contraceptive. The most important factor is the frequency and duration of suckling. In practice therefore the return of fertility is a prolonged process, during which many spurious attempts at follicular growth and ovulation occur over weeks or months before actual ovulation. Moreover the first ovulation often antedates the first vaginal bleed. The cervical mucus pattern at this time is not sufficient to help the woman distinguish false alarms from genuine ovulation. If artificial contraception is acceptable to her, she will simply have to play safe and begin to use it from the very first mucus sign of ovarian follicular activity.

For those who wish to continue the natural methods, workers in Birmingham have found that marked changes in the cervix (i.e. softening in consistency, widening of the external os and elevation of position) occur only in the days immediately preceding the first true ovulation. The reliability of the cervix as an indicator at this time requires further testing. (See Q 1.5.)

See Q 8.54 for the problems of identifying the infrequent ovulations of women approaching the menopause.

BREASTFEEDING AS NATURAL BIRTH CONTROL

1.32 Is there not a scheme for using breastfeeding as a satisfactory method of birth control?

Very much so, and no method could be more natural. A consensus statement from a conference in Bellagio, Italy, is summarized in the algorithm of Figure 1.3. If all three facts apply – amenorrhoea since the lochia ceased, baby no more than 6 months old, and breast-feeding total or very nearly so – the risk of conception by 6 months is only 2%. This compares favourably with other accepted methods of birth control. Hence it may be presented just like any other method to a woman provided there is the usual caveat, that there is no promise that she will not be one of those in whom the method fails.

However for even greater efficacy many women will prefer to use the progestogen-only pill in addition to their breastfeeding – see Qs 5.54 and 5.55.

THE (NEAR) FUTURE

1.33 What of the future? Are there any developments which may make fertility awareness methods more acceptable?

Some of these are suggested in Figure 1.2.

1   Already there are devices available like *'Bio–self'* which some-
    times give a direct read-out of the temperature (thereby assisting

Ask the mother:

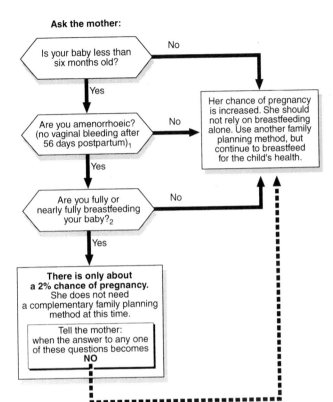

Is your baby less than six months old?

No →

Yes ↓

Are you amenorrhoeic? (no vaginal bleeding after 56 days postpartum)₁

No →

Yes ↓

Her chance of pregnancy is increased. She should not rely on breastfeeding alone. Use another family planning method, but continue to breastfeed for the child's health.

Are you fully or nearly fully breastfeeding your baby?₂

No →

Yes ↓

There is only about a 2% chance of pregnancy. She does not need a complementary family planning method at this time.

Tell the mother: when the answer to any one of these questions becomes **NO**

Figure 1.3 Use of the lactational amenorrhoea method during the first 6 postpartum months. Q 1.32.

Notes: 1. Spotting that occurs during the first 56 days is not considered to be menses.
  2. 'Nearly full' breast feeding means that occasional non-breastfeeds are given

many women who find mercury thermometers difficult to use), but primarily use microprocessors to give the woman a visual indication when the requirements of the BBT method have been fulfilled (see Q 1.22). When the instrument signals that she is safe, she knows that the second infertile phase has commenced. Refinements of this approach can be expected, and the price of the instruments is likely to fall.

2 Ultimately, the relative price of *ultrasound* machines may fall so low, and their user-friendliness may increase to such a degree, that women could simply plug them in to their television sets.

Follicular growth rupture and corpus luteum formation could then be monitored by the woman and her partner themselves!

3 More realistically, a number of *home kits* are being devised based on the cyclic changes in the hormones of the menstrual cycle, or their metabolites and other substances in body fluids. The most useful fluids are urine, saliva and breast milk; but biochemical changes in the mucus are also being studied. Detection of the LH surge is already possible using a dipstick. A kit designed to predict as well as detect ovulation, based on the ratio of the main oestrogen and progesterone metabolites in urine, is also at an advanced state of development.

4 Other approaches include:
  (a) The *Rovumeter*. This is a device which simply measures the daily amount of cervicovaginal fluid aspirated from the posterior vaginal fornix by the woman into a sterile, disposable, calibrated, plastic aspirator. Volume changes are more objective than the usual mucus awareness approach, and can apparently be used to predict and detect ovulation sufficiently reliably for family planning purposes.
  (b) An example of how new possibilities may arise by seren-dipity is some research at King's College Medical School in London into Raynaud's phenomenon. In normal women (as well as those with Raynaud's phenomenon) the findings are different at different phases of the menstrual cycle. It appears that oestrogen tends to increase the reactivity of the arteries of the hand. Progesterone tends to relax the vessels producing an overall increase in blood volume. Appropriate daily measurements could in theory therefore be used both to predict and to detect the woman's fertile period. A device for possible home use is already being tested.

QUESTIONS ASKED BY USERS/POTENTIAL USERS

These are so varied and numerous that space does not permit their consideration here. Referral to a trained teacher of fertility aware-ness may be helpful; but all the more important myths can be disposed of by reference to the answers above.

2

Male methods

2.1 What is coitus interruptus?

This is well described by its commonest euphemism, 'withdrawal' (in time, before ejaculation, ensuring that all sperms are deposited outside the vagina). There are many other terms, notably 'being careful' and also local idioms such as 'getting off at Cottingham instead of going through to Beverley' (used in North Humberside, but having many regional equivalents). These have often misled interviewers into thinking that no contraceptive method is being used.

2.2 What is the history of the method?

It is doubtless the earliest form of birth control. It is mentioned in Genesis, the only explicit mention of contraception in the Bible:

> Then Judah said to Er's brother Onan, 'Go and sleep with your brother's widow. Fulfil your obligation to her as her husband's brother, so that your brother may have descendants.' But Onan knew that the children would not belong to him, so whenever he had intercourse with his brother's widow he let the semen spill on the ground, so that there would be no children for his brother. What he did displeased the Lord and the Lord killed him also.

Although this text is widely quoted as implying that withdrawal is itself sinful, according to most commentators the sin was not in the method but in the failure to comply with the Levirate Law and perform his family duty.

Though Islamic societies and numerous Imams are basically pronatalist, the Koran describes a more liberal attitude to withdrawal and by inference to other methods of contraception. In the Tradition of the Prophet we find:

> A man said, O Prophet of God! I have a slave girl and I practise coitus interruptus with her. I dislike her becoming pregnant, yet I have the desires of men. The Jews believe that coitus interruptus constitutes killing a life in miniature form.

The Prophet (Mohammed) replied,

> The Jews are liars. If God wishes to create it, you can never change it.

Right up to the second half of the twentieth century, withdrawal remained a major and often the primary method of contraception. As late as 1947 the Royal Commission on Population in England found that amongst recently married couples with contraceptive experience, 43% used withdrawal as the sole method of birth control, the proportion rising to 65% in social class V. Studies in developing countries have shown its use, at least on some occasions, by more than half of all couples in Jamaica, Puerto Rico, and Hungary in the 1960s.

2.3 What is the effectiveness of coitus interruptus?

High failure rates alleged by the early family planners have been quoted and requoted by subsequent generations of writers. Yet the evidence contradicts that view. In 1949 the Royal Commission (see above) reported that 'no difference has been found between users of appliance and users of non-appliance methods as regards the average number of children'. Withdrawal was by far the most popular of the non-appliance methods, and the pregnancy rate was found to be a creditable 8/100 woman-years of exposure. A study in Indianapolis revealed a failure rate of only 10, compared with an average rate of 12 for all other methods, and amongst high-income couples the rate was precisely the same as for the diaphragm.

2.4 What are the advantages of coitus interruptus?

Chiefly that the method is free of charge, requires no prescription, and cannot be left at home when the couple go on holiday. Moreover it does not cause weight gain or pelvic infection! Its use has been associated with some of the lowest birth rates in history, for example in eastern Europe after the Second World War. It is obviously acceptable to many users.

2.5 What are the disadvantages?

Obviously intercourse is incomplete, and many find the method unsatisfying to both partners. Yet no significant adverse effects have ever been demonstrated among those who do choose to use it. It seems to be assumed without discussion that there would be an inevitable lack of satisfaction of the woman, compounded by anxiety that her partner would not withdraw 'in time'. Psychological problems are assumed to follow. Yet in a survey of nearly 2000 British women questioned in 1967–68 by Cartwright, only 31% of 311 who had discontinued use of the method did so because they found it unpleasant, and only 4% because they believed it harmful to health. In contrast, 54% of 381 former condom users gave up the method because they found it unpleasant to use.

Even among those professionally engaged in family planning, this method is too often overlooked, condemned or ridiculed. Marie Stopes stated that it was 'harmful to the nerves as well as unsafe'.

2.6 Why has the method been so neglected, except perhaps by Germaine Greer?

One reason perhaps is that it has no manufacturers to advertise its virtues. It has the reputation of being unsatisfying and ineffective. It should certainly not be *promoted*. But it is unfortunate that many unplanned pregnancies among young people having intercourse unexpectedly are probably caused by the conventional teaching of doctors and nurses. Withdrawal is often not attempted when it might have been, because the message that it is 'ineffective' has been so well conveyed. We must remember the old slogan: 'Any method of family planning is better than no method, though some methods are better than others.' While encouraging the use of more modern methods, we should remember that for many this one works; and that it is a very great deal better than nothing 'in an emergency'.

2.7 Aren't there sperm in the pre-ejaculate?

Yes there are, sometimes. Abraham Stone in 1931 asked several medical friends to examine preorgasmic secretions for sperm. He finally collected 24 slides from 18 individuals. Two showed many sperm, two contained few, and one an occasional sperm. Stone correctly reported that the figures were 'insignificant for a definite conclusion'. The chances of such sperm causing fertilization must be low – though not negligible (see Q 1.9).

A much more probable cause of failure results from partial ejaculation of a larger quantity of semen sometimes occuring a short while before the final male orgasm; or withdrawal during the latter rather than before it starts. Hence the suggestion that a spermicide or a sponge might be used as well (see Q 2.9).

2.8 Should a couple always be discouraged from using coitus interruptus?

The answer has to be no. It is a free country, and we must remember the basic teaching of psychosexual medicine, that there are innumerable methods of giving and receiving sexual pleasure, which the couple should feel free to devise for themselves. If they love one another, why should they not be able to have a sexually satisfying life and use coitus interruptus if that is their choice?

2.9 How do you counsel a couple who volunteer that coitus interruptus is their usual method?

Clearly there are better options, and these should always be discussed. If, however, they find the alternatives unacceptable, then I always suggest the additional use of spermicide (a pessary, or perhaps the sponge, see Q 3.55). This should cope satisfactorily with any small deposit of sperm before withdrawal.

2.10 Your conclusion?

Malcolm Potts, to whom I am indebted for much of this section, concludes in his book with Peter Diggory, *Textbook of Contraception Practice* (see Further Reading):

> Coitus interruptus is like a bicycle or a buffalo cart; there are better methods of transport and better methods of contraception, but for a great many people it represents a practical solution to an every day problem.

The condom

BACKGROUND AND MECHANISM

2.11 What is the definition of a male sheath/condom?

This is a closed-ended, expansile, tubular device designed to cover the erect penis and physically prevent the transmission of semen into the vagina. It is generally made of vulcanized latex rubber which is as thin as possible while maintaining adequate strength and often lubricated – to minimize 'loss of sensitivity' during intercourse, which is perhaps the method's chief disadvantage. It is also a method for use by (often) the least well-motivated of the partners: hence the renewed interest in female-controlled condoms, as well as more effective spermicide/viricides (see Qs 3.67–3.69 and 3.72)

2.12 What is the method's history?

This apparently dates back to Roman times, when animal bladders were used chiefly to prevent the spread of sexually transmitted disease. In folklore, the invention was much later, by Dr Condom, reputedly a physician at the court of Charles II. It is doubtful whether Dr C. even existed. Much more probably, the word condom was derived from the Latin (*condus*: a receptacle), as a euphemism for an item already well known. The earliest published description is that of the Italian anatomist Gabriel Fallopio, who in 1564 recommended a linen sheath moistened with lotion – again in order to protect veneral infection. Only in the eighteenth century do we find described the use of condoms specifically to prevent pregnancy. Condoms were then made from the caeca of sheep or other animals. Similar 'skin condoms' are still available but they have always been expensive and hence beyond the means of ordinary couples. They are also not recommended for safer sex to prevent virus transmission.

It was the process of vulcanization of rubber, first carried out by Hancock and Goodyear in 1844, which revolutionized the world's contraception as well as its transport.

2.13 How acceptable and how frequently used is the condom method?

An estimated 40 million couples use the condom worldwide, but with striking geographical differences. Japan accounts for more than a quarter of all condom users in the world. Seventy-five percent of couples who use any contraceptive in that country use this method, generally purchased by the woman. This may change if the pill should ever become a realistic option in Japan. By contrast, and despite the massive problem of the acquired immune deficiency syndrome (AIDS), condom use is unusually low in Africa, the Middle East and Latin America, which together account for much less than 10% of worldwide use.

2.14 What is the acceptability and usage of the condom in the UK?

For many, 'spoilt' by modern non-intercourse-related alternatives, it must be admitted the method remains completely unacceptable for sustained use. There is an undeniable change of sensations reported especially by men, though this sometimes has the benefit of prolonging intercourse.

In 1989 a survey for Durex by the Henley Centre indicated that 20% of all couples use the condom. This is really only a reversal of the preceding decline. Estimates are always approximate as many couples use the sheath as an occasional alternative if not addition to other methods; but it continues to be the second most prevalent method within each 10-year cohort, during the reproductive years. It is of concern that so few (estimated in 1991 as 3%) follow modern advice in situations of high infection risk, by using a combination of condom for protection with another method for contraception.

2.15 What is the image of the condom as a method and how can it be improved?

In the past condoms have been very much ignored by both the medical profession and consumers. They had a poor image. AIDS has changed all that – or has it? There are still widespread misconceptions about efficacy and reduced sensitivity. For centuries, condoms were associated with prostitution and extramarital intercourse. Even today as he purchases his condoms a married man may sense that the retailer assumes they surely cannot be for intercourse with his wife. Removal of this unfortunate image is unlikely so long as the media maintains double standards: there is widespread portrayal of intercourse on television, for example, yet it is perceived as against morality or good taste to mention the condom in the storyline.

Contrast this slogan from California: 'Use a condom and you will learn, no deposit, no return.'

EFFECTIVENESS

2.16 How effective is the condom method?

Method-failure rates can be less than 1 pregnancy/100 couple-years. These are based on selected populations where there has been no sexual contact whatever without the rubber intervening, the only failures being caused by condoms bursting due to a manufacturing defect (some bursts and most cases of condoms slipping off are user errors, see Q 2.19 below). These could be said to be 'not normal people'. Since successful use depends so very much on the motivation and care taken by the couple, failure rates do vary widely: from a low of 0.4/100 woman-years in the north of England, 1973, to a high of no less than 32/100 woman-years in Puerto Rico in 1961. A large population-based US study of the 1980s documented between eight and 11 failures at 1 year for single women. In four recent UK studies the range was more relevant to the *careful user*, from 3.1 to 4.8/100 woman-years.

As usual, failures are more frequent with the young and inexperienced, and among couples who wish to delay rather than prevent pregnancy. Among such, *average* use leads to at least 10% conceptions in the course of 1 year, a one in ten chance (and we do such couples a disservice if this information is withheld from them). Older couples use the method better, perhaps because of diminished fertility and a lower frequency of intercourse, as well as more careful use. For example, in the Oxford/Family Planning Association (FPA) study a pregnancy rate of only 0.7/100 couple-years was reported among women aged 35 and older as compared with a rate of 3.6/100 couple-years for women aged 25–34 (in both cases the husband having been before recruitment a condom-user for more than 4 years).

2.17 How important is additional spermicide use to condom effectiveness?

This theoretically should increase contraceptive protection. However:

1 Since the pregnancy rate among consistent users is already very low, it would be difficult to prove the extra degree of protection.

2 Spermicides alone tend to be rather inefficient at preventing pregnancy when the whole ejaculate is spilled, though they may be more effective if there are leaks of small amounts of semen.

3 The requirement to use a separate spermicide may be perceived as a messy additional intrusion during intercourse, and so might actually cause more pregnancies because of irregular use of the condom (or occasional reliance on the spermicidal pessary alone).

Note: There is also now a possible problem that the commonest spermicide (nonoxynol-9 or -11) causes apparent damage to the vaginal epithelium in *very* frequent use. This affects recommendations about virus transmission prevention but *not* those about routine contraception, see Q 3.78.

2.18 Are spermicidally lubricated condoms therefore preferred?

Because of doubts about interference with regular use (see Q 2.17) and some other anxieties (see Qs 3.78 and 3.79), the UK FPA has not for some years considered spermicides mandatory. All the same, the best protection in the event of spillage is probably provided by separate pessaries or foam; followed by a brand with an adequate additional spermicidal dose within the teat of the condom; and then by brands which are simply spermicidally lubricated. This would be almost impossible to prove because controlled trials are so difficult to mount and would necessarily involve a vast number of volunteers.

In my view, the highest priority should be given to making things as easy as possible for the variably motivated couples who choose to use this method.

2.19 What are the common errors in condom use that may lead to pregnancy?

Particularly when the Combined Oral Contraceptive (COC) has to be stopped on medical grounds after many years, most couples have no idea just how 'dangerous' a fluid semen will now become. It is important to stress that the 4–5 ml of an average man's ejaculate can easily contain 300 million sperm, and hence a minute proportion of this volume in a fertile man might cause a pregnancy. Common unrecognized errors include:

1 Genital contact, with the condom put on just before ejaculation – but often not in time to catch the first fraction of sperm.

2 Loss of erection, perhaps due to overexcitement or anxiety, so condom slips off unnoticed before ejaculation. Another cause of slippage is mentioned at Q 2.21.

3 Leakage on withdrawal, when the penis is flaccid.

4 Later genital contact with sperm already on glans and in urethra of the penis – from earlier intercourse – before a new condom is applied.

5 *Damage to the sheath* – see Q 2.20.

2.20 What may cause condom breakage, aside from manufacturing defects?

1 *Mechanical damage*, e.g. by sharp fingernails especially during attempts to force it on the wrong way, rolling it up tighter rather than unrolling it (an easy mistake while excited!).

2 *Chemical action*. It is not widely enough known that vegetable and mineral oil-based lubricants, and the bases for many prescribable vaginal products, can seriously damage and lead to rupture of rubber. Baby oil for example, often suggested as part of sex play, destroys over 90% of a condom's strength after only

15 minutes contact! The Durex Information Service (1991) has produced a useful leaflet listing 20 common vaginal preparations which should be regarded as unsafe to use with condoms and diaphragms, and there may be others. See Table 2.1.

Table 2.1. Vaginal and rectal preparations which should be regarded as unsafe to use with condoms or diaphragms:

Arachis oil enema	Nizoral
Baby oil	Nystan cream (pessaries OK)
Cyclogest	Ortho Dienoestrol
Ecostatin	Ortho-Gynest (Ovestin OK)
Fungilin	Petroleum jelly (Vaseline)
Gyno-Daktarin	Premarin cream
Gyno-Pevaryl (Pevaryl OK)	Sultrin
Monistat	Vaseline

Note: Some suntan oils and creams are similarly not 'condom-friendly'. But water-based products such as 'KY jelly', also ethylene glycol, glycerol and silicones are not suspect.

2.21 What instructions should be given to couples planning to use this method?

1 Avoid any chemical or physical damage: do not use oil-based lubricants such as Vaseline or baby oil. Use jelly such as KY, or a spermicidal product. See Qs 2.19 and 2.20.

2 Put the condom on the penis before any genital contact whatever. If there is no teat, make room for the semen by pinching the end of the sheath as it is applied. (Otherwise there is the risk of semen tracking up the shaft of the penis and either escaping or causing the condom to slip off.)

3 After intercourse, withdraw the penis before it becomes too soft, holding the base of the condom during withdrawal and taking care not to spill any semen.

4 Use only good-quality condoms (in the UK this means those which are kite-marked).

5 Use each condom once only. Inspect it for damage/possible leaks before disposal.

6 For maximum effectiveness, your partner should use a spermicide (e.g. foam, pessary or sponge).

7 *Most importantly, if the condom ruptures or slips off, on any potentially fertile day, obtain EMERGENCY (POSTCOITAL) CONTRACEPTION (see Q 7.5) within 72 hours.*

2.22 What are the advantages of the condom method?

The advantages are many and can be listed as follows:

1 easily obtainable, relatively cheap or free from NHS clinics;

2 free from medical risks;

3 highly effective if used consistently and correctly;

4 no medical supervision required;

5 protection against most sexually transmitted diseases including viruses;

6 possible protection against cervical neoplasia and invasive carcinoma;

7 offers visible evidence of use (particularly to the woman, who has the greatest motivation to avoid pregnancy);

8 involves the male in sharing contraceptive responsibility – though with 'unreliable' men this can be a disadvantage;

9 may increase the woman's pleasure by prolonging intercourse – this applies where the man's orgasm tends otherwise to precede that of his partner, as well as in cases of frank premature ejaculation;

10 minimizes post-intercourse odour and the messiness of semen, for those who perceive these as problems.

2.23 In what situations may the condom be particularly indicated?

1 Where couples are unable or unwilling to make use of formal family planning services.

2 During short-term contraception (e.g. while waiting to start oral contraceptives).

3 Where intercourse takes place only infrequently and unpredictably.

4 For protection against sexually transmitted infections, notably HIV.

5 With the agreement of the man (not always obtainable), for the prevention of cervical neoplasia, particularly when that has already been treated.

Items 4 and 5 are indications which may often apply even if the main birth control method being used is an IUD, a hormone or sterilization (either sex).

2.24 Against which sexually transmitted diseases does the condom provide protection?

A major benefit from the woman's point of view is the reduced risk of upper genital tract disease (pelvic infection with its serious threat to her future fertility). Consistent condom use is definitely protective against gonorrhoea and *Trichomonas vaginitis*; and probably also against the spirochaete of syphilis, chlamydia, and similar bacterial and protozoal organisms. It obviously provides little or no protection against infestations such as scabies and lice.

Most importantly, the rubber or plastic of which male or female condoms are made is an effective barrier when intact to viruses, including HIV, the far more infectious hepatitis B virus, herpes simplex types I and II and the wart viruses.

Whereas fertilization is possible only during about 8 days per cycle, viruses can be transfered at any time. As we have seen, condom conceptions are not uncommon. So the method can only provide relative protection ('safer sex'). Bilateral monogamy has much going for it! (see pp. 23–31 of my handbook for women, *The Pill*).

2.25 What evidence is there that the condom may be protective or even therapeutic against cervical cell abnormalities?

In a UK case-control study, for example, the relative risk of developing severe cervical dysplasia decreased with duration of condom or diaphragm use while it increased with duration of Oral Contraceptive (OC) use. After 10 years the relative risk for women using any barrier method was 0.2 compared to 4.0 for the pill-users.

In an American study, as many as 136 out of 139 women with cervical cell abnormalities who received no treatment apart from their partners adopting use of the condom showed complete reversal of the condition. Unfortunately there was no control group, and these findings need confirmation. The evidence, however, justifies enthusiasm for the method for certain categories at high risk for cervical neoplasia, or after it has been treated (see Q 2.23).

PROBLEMS AND DISADVANTAGES

2.26 What are the possible disadvantages of the method?

There are few:

1 coitus-related and interrupts spontaneity of intercourse;
2 decreased 'sensitivity', especially for the male (much less with modern products);
3 perceived as acting as a barrier in psychological as well as physical terms;
4 perceived to be messy, and may slip off or rupture;
5 few users appreciate how very small leaks of semen may yet cause a pregnancy (see Q 1.7);
6 hence a very high degree of motivation and extremely meticulous use required for long-term avoidance of pregnancy – these characteristics are regrettably possessed by relatively few men, in the heat of the sexual moment!

2.27 What are the possible side-effects of the condom?

Whatever else, it is difficult to imagine how death might occur – perhaps by inhalation?

1 *Allergy.* Most 'allergies' are excuses (especially by men). But irritation is not uncommon. Like true allergy, in either partner, this may often be solved by use of special *allergy* sheaths with bland lubricant but no spermicide, and reduced allergenic residues (left in the rubber after the manufacturing processes).
2 Of course the method fails to protect against disorders linked to the normal/abnormal menstrual cycle, such as menorrhagia, premenstrual syndrome, functional ovarian cysts, endometriosis, and carcinoma of the ovary and endometrium: which I describe as in a sense 'side effects of not using the pill' (see Q 4.49).

2.28 How can the disadvantages be minimized?

By using ultra-thin, and lubricated, condoms, and perhaps by involving the female more in the selection of specific brands and in their actual use. For example, if a condom (perhaps brightly coloured or ribbed) is applied by the woman as part of foreplay, this can counter the first and foremost disadvantage above, and even heighten eroticism.

2.29 Are there any condoms which are not recommended?

So-called American Tips which are designed to fit only over the glans penis, have a bad reputation for slipping off during use. Also not approved are some 'fun' condoms available from sex shops which do not conform to BSI specifications.

2.30 How are condoms manufactured?

In a highly automated process, condom-shaped metal or glass moulds are dipped into latex solution, from where they pass to a drying oven. After a second immersion in latex, the moulds pass into another heated air chamber for drying and vulcanization. The finished product is usually rolled off the mould by nylon brushes and then subjected to quality control testing. Each of the millions produced is tested electronically for pin-holes; and samples are put through a water test for holes and (increasingly) an air inflation test to bursting point. The international standard (ISO 4074) permits only seven samples out of 200 to rupture after inflation with 15 litres of air.

2.31 Are any future advances to be expected?

Trials are being conducted with plastic condoms which are good heat conductors, more loosely fitted and more lubricated on the inner surface over the major part of their length. If a method of holding these securely to the base of the penis can be perfected, these features may improve male acceptance.

See Q 3.67–9 for the female condom.

QUESTIONS ASKED BY USERS ABOUT THE CONDOM/SHEATH

2.32 The condoms keep breaking – why is this?

There are several possible explanations (see Q 2.20). Are you allowing any chemicals to come into contact with them? Sometimes you or your partner may be causing damage with fingernails while it is being put on. Waiting until she is more aroused and lubricated before penetration may help, or the use of KY jelly. Otherwise you could try a different brand – discuss with your chemist (see also Qs 2.33 and 2.35).

2.33 Do I have to use a spermicide with the condom?

This is no longer an absolute requirement. However, if you have ever had a sheath slip off or break it is more secure if your partner inserts a dose of spermicide first. And certainly if you ever 'cheat' – if there is some penetration before you actually put the condom on – a spermicide is extremely important in case of an early leak of sperm. Spermicidally lubricated sheaths will not help this problem but may otherwise be slightly more effective.

2.34 Some condoms have ribs and bumps etc. – are these contraceptives safe?

If they are kite-marked (BSI tested), the answer is yes. Beware of those that are not so approved.

2.35 If a condom breaks or slips off, is there anything you can do to avoid a possible pregnancy?

Yes, this is most important. Go at the next convenient moment to your clinic or family doctor and ask about *Emergency contraception* (postcoital treatment, see Ch. 7).

2.36 I seem to be developing an allergic rash from the condom – is there one specially made which overcomes this problem?

It is best for a doctor to examine your penis in case for example your 'allergy' is caused by something else such as thrush. If you are using a spermicidally lubricated condom, you could try one without the spermicide. There are also special sheaths which are made of rubber specially purified from additives and known as allergy sheaths. They are a bit dry, so careful use of a small amount of a water-based jelly lubricant such as KY may help. You could also try natural skin condoms which are available by mail order.

2.37   Do condoms have a shelf-life?

Yes; it is usually a long one of at least 5 years, but they can deteriorate more rapidly in abnormal conditions, such as in the tropics, and especially on exposure to ultraviolet light. See also Q 2.20.

2.38   Can I use the condom more than once?

This is definitely not recommended – it was only feasible with the old-style reusable types.

2.39   Why can't you easily get condoms free from your family doctor?

Why indeed? This is an excellent method which in my view should certainly be available from GPs, as it is from clinics.

2.40   Can you throw a condom away down the toilet?

From the environmental point of view it is better to use a dustbin.

2.41   My partner feels very dry, is there a lubricant you can safely use with the condom?

Some of this dryness may be removable by better sex technique – particularly by more foreplay, so that she is more aroused. If she has any soreness or itching she should be checked for thrush, irritation or allergy. Otherwise use a water-based lubricant (Q 2.20) sparingly, or better still a jelly which is also contraceptive (see also Q 3.52–3.53).

3 Vaginal methods of contraception

3.1 Why should we avoid the terms 'female or vaginal barriers'?

Although these are convenient, ideally I wish we could find better terms to use. They should preferably be avoided in discussions with prospective users, since sexual intercourse has to do with closeness, and one can reinforce wrong feelings and fantasies about the method being a 'barrier'.

3.2 What terminology will you be using? What types are available?

See Figure 3.1. To avoid confusion, I shall use the term occlusive caps for all the standard female barriers. This has two subgroups, namely the diaphragm and the cervical/vault caps, with the vimule being here considered as a modified vault cap. The sponge is in a different category. It is a carrier for spermicide: it does not perform as an occlusive cervical barrier.

3.3 What is the method's history?

It is a very ancient method, with descriptions dating back to 1850 BC; the Petri papyrus describes a spermicidal pessary made partly of crocodile dung. A section of the Talmud from the second century AD recommended a moistened sponge in the vagina before coitus. Rubber occlusive pessaries did not appear until the nineteenth century, in Germany, and the first diaphragm was popularized by

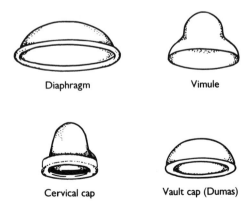

Diaphragm   Vimule

Cervical cap   Vault cap (Dumas)

Figure 3.1 Diaphragm and cervical vault caps. Q 3.2. (Reproduced courtesy of Mrs Walli Bounds)

Mensinga, the pseudonym of a German physician Dr C. Hasse. The development of vulcanized rubber enabled him to produce a thinner and more pliable device incorporating a flat watch spring in the rim. It became known as the Dutch cap through publicity given to it by the Dutch neo-Malthusians.

The occlusive pessary was referred to in the famous manual *The Wife's Handbook*, published in 1887 – for this action its author Arthur Allbutt was struck off the British Medical Register. Because of this kind of opposition, occlusive pessaries became readily available only in the 1920s. Then, to quote Malcolm Potts, 'diaphragms and caps were to Family Planning what the steam locomotive was to transportation; they were the first in the field, brought emancipation to millions, and for a long time had no rivals'. Ultimately they were overtaken by a new technology; yet the methods only have two major problems. Were these – lack of independence from intercourse and relative lack of effectiveness – to be overcome, there could be a large-scale return to vaginal methods.

3.4 How popular are vaginal methods worldwide?

The diaphragm reached the peak of its popularity around 1959, when it was reported that the method was used by about 12% of British couples practising contraception. Usage declined rapidly with the advent of the pill, and in 1986 only about 2% of contracepting women used the method in the UK. In most developing countries prevalence of use is too low to measure; and is likely to remain so until vaginal barriers are devised that do not require medical fitting or special training in use, and do not pose storage and supply problems.

3.5 How important is medical attitude and training to the acceptability of vaginal methods?

Crucially: it has been well said that often the biggest 'barrier to the barriers' is the medical profession, and sometimes (though less so) the nursing profession. Many women introduced for the first time to the diaphragm at the age of 35–40 express surprise at its ease and convenience. Often they complain that doctors and nurses had earlier damned the method with exceedingly faint praise.

This is a highly practical subject. The right attitude and skills can only be acquired by observing and being taught by experienced professionals. In my view one of these should be a family planning nurse (see Qs 3.33–3.40).

3.6 What is the mode of action of the diaphragm and cervical/vault caps?

The *diaphragm* lies diagonally across the cervix, the vaginal vault and much of the anterior vaginal wall. Since the vagina is known to 'balloon' during intercourse (see Q 1.3), a sperm-tight fit between the diaphragm and the vaginal wall is impossible. On a theoretical basis, the main functions of the diaphragm are:

1 to act as a carrier of the spermicide to the most important site, namely the external os, and prevent the spreading effect of intercourse (see Q 1.3);

2 holding sperm away as a barrier from the receptive alkaline cervical mucus, long enough for them to die in the acid vagina;

3 preventing this mucus from entering the acid vagina and thereby providing a film within which the sperm can swim to the external os, and possibly;

4 preventing physical aspiration of sperm into the cervix and uterus.

Some authorities question the importance of the spermicide (see Q 3.7).

Cervical/vault caps are meant to stay in place by suction, which makes it possible that the barrier effect is more important to their contraceptive action than is the case with the diaphragm.

3.7 How important is the use of spermicide with occlusive caps?

This is questioned, particularly by the Australian Family Planning Association, and especially for the cervical/vault caps which act by suction. It is a fact that with no type of occlusive cap has there ever been a proper controlled trial. This should compare (preferably by random allocation) women who follow the full routine of instructions concerning the use of spermicide (see Q 3.44), in every detail, with women who use exactly the same method carefully and after the same fitting routine but without any spermicide at all. Such a study has been attempted at the Margaret Pyke Centre. Pending further data, the bad results (an overall use-effectiveness of less than 75/100 woman-years) of a Marie Stopes Centre study into use of a small (60 mm) arcing diaphragm without spermicide, lead most authorities in this country to feel that spermicide use should definitely be recommended.

3.8 How effective is the diaphragm?

Table 0.2 (see Q 0.14) quotes an overall failure rate for the diaphragm of 2–15. As usual the lower failure rate relates to the older woman. Her conscientiousness in regularly using the method efficiently is of greatest importance. Table 3.1 relates the failure rates to an indicator of motivation recorded in the Oxford/FPA study, namely whether or not the woman considered her family to be complete. As clearly shown, the failure rate tended to be higher when the family was not felt to be complete, implying less careful use of the diaphragm when another baby would be acceptable.

3.9 Are the diaphragm failure rates of the Oxford/FPA study a good indication of the rates to be expected in routine family planning practice?

No.

1 At recruitment, every woman was aged 25–39 years, married, a white British subject, and had to be already a current user of the diaphragm of at least 5 months standing.

2 The women were basically 'middle class' and were probably unusually well motivated and careful.

3 Younger and more fertile women having intercourse more frequently must be expected to have a higher failure rate, even if the method were properly fitted and always used.

The most important factor is the recruitment in the Oxford/FPA study only of established users. By 5 months the most fertile and least careful women, along with those with anatomical problems interfering with the effectiveness of the method, would not have been available for recruitment – by virtue of already becoming

Table 3.1 Diaphragm failure rates per 100 woman-years according to age, duration of use and completeness of family.

Duration of use	Age 25–34:			Age 35+:		
	≤ 2 years	2–4 years	4 years+	≤ 2 years	2–4 years	4 years +
Family complete	6.1	3.5	2.3	2.1	1.6	0.7
Family not complete	5.3	4.3	2.4	4.5	2.0	1.3

Source: Oxford/FPA Study, 1982

pregnant! All studies show the highest failure rates in the first few months of use. Even using the data of Table 3.1, faced with an 'Oxford/FPA type' woman under 35 one can only quote a failure rate of around 5–6/100 woman-years for the first year of use. This is about the best to be expected, with a rate of around 10 for most young unmarried women of average motivation. (All these rates include user failures.)

3.10 What failure rates can be given for cervical/vault caps?

These are considered later (Qs 3.27–3.32). Available effectiveness data are sparse, but in a large multicentre study in the USA the pregnancy rate was 11% at 1 year of use.

3.11 In summary, what factors promote the effectiveness of the diaphragm and similar vaginal methods?

The following questions need to be asked:

1 Is she an established user or starting the method from scratch?

2 What is her age?

3 What is her frequency of intercourse?

4 What is her motivation for obsessionally careful and regular use? In particular is she really trying to avoid a pregnancy or just to delay one?

5 Is she at all uncomfortable about handling her own genitalia? This important factor is not at all linked with intelligence.

6 Are there any anatomical problems on examination? (see Qs 3.22, 3.30, 3.31 and 3.35).

7 During initial training, is she good at inserting the device and particularly at checking that the cervix is covered?

3.12 What common errors in the use of occlusive caps may lead to pregnancy?

The commonest clearly is failure to use, at intercourse on one or more occasions in the cycle of conception. Women often report minor errors in use of the spermicide. It is not at all clear how important these are, especially as they are frequently reported also in non-conception cycles.

During use, the most important error is failure to make a secondary check after insertion that the cervix is correctly covered.

Clinicians' errors include: wrong selection of users, poor fitting (with regard to size, choice of flat spring, coil or arcing diaphragm or other cap) and poor teaching.

ADVANTAGES AND BENEFICIAL EFFECTS

3.13 What are the advantages of occlusive caps?

1 Effective if used with care.
2 Much more independent of intercourse than the sheath (see Q 3.14).
3 In general, neither partner suffers any loss of feeling.
4 The method is under a woman's control and needs only to be used when required.
5 Aesthetically useful for intercourse during uterine bleeding.
6 No proven systemic effects.
7 Some definite non-contraceptive benefits (see Q 3.15).

3.14 Are occlusive caps necessarily intercourse-related methods?

No. In counselling, this is a most important point to explain. It is perfectly in order to insert a diaphragm several hours ahead of intercourse. Opinions differ as to how soon it becomes necessary to add extra spermicide just before intercourse (see Qs 3.44 and 3.49). But certainly removal of the requirement to put the cap itself in just before is beneficial to compliance. Since keeping the cervical mucus out of the vagina may be one of the most important mechanisms (see Q 3.6), it could even be that insertion well ahead of intercourse actually increases effectiveness, though this has not been established.

3.15 What are the beneficial medical effects?

1 Protection against most sexually transmitted diseases (STDs), including the agents causing pelvic inflammatory disease. (However the method is not believed to give adequate protection against HIV and other sexually transmitted *viruses*.)
2 Reduction in the risk of cervical neoplasia.
These are most important benefits in the modern world.

3.16   How are occlusive caps protective against STDs?

In two ways:

1   Partly by providing a mechanical barrier which reduces the chance of organisms reaching the cervix and upper genital tract. This will not be enough protection against the viruses including herpes; or non-viral diseases like syphilis which can form lesions of the vagina, vulva and elsewhere.

2   The associated spermicide is also relevant. Spermicides tend also to be 'germicides' (see Q 3.77, but also Q 3.78).

3.17   What is the evidence for at least some protective effect against cervical neoplasia?

In the Oxford/FPA study, the rate per 100 woman-years for Oral Contraceptive (OC) users was 0.95 and for intrauterine device (IUD) users 0.87. For diaphragm users, however, the rate was 0.23 after adjustment for age at first coitus, number of partners and smoking patterns. Another Oxford study showed a steady decline in the relative risk of severe cervical neoplasia for users of all types of barrier method from 1 down to 0.2 after 10 years. However diaphragm users may also be protected from this condition by their own sexual lifestyle and that of their partners.

MAIN PROBLEMS AND DISADVANTAGES

3.18   What are the disadvantages of occlusive caps?

1   Though not necessarily coitus related, they involve a woman handling her genitalia, some forward planning, and a slight loss of spontaneity.

2   Loss of cervical and some vaginal sensation (unnoticed by most).

3   May be felt in use by the woman's partner, though not by her if properly fitted.

4   Require fitting by trained personnel and a period of training in use, usually 1 week, during which another method must be used.

5   In practice less effective than hormonal contraception, or the IUD.

6   Perceived as being 'messy' due to the spermicide.

7   Capable of producing some local adverse effects (see Q 3.19).

3.19 What are the possible adverse medical effects?

1 Increased risk of urinary tract infections and symptoms. This problem seems to apply only to the diaphragm. See Q 3.51.

2 A small minority of women develop vaginal irritation and allergy due either to the rubber or more commonly to the spermicide.

3 Pressure effects due to the rim of the occlusive cap itself, leading rarely to vaginal abrasions or ulcers (see Q 3.54).

4 A significant increase in hospital referrals for the treatment of haemorrhoids was found in the Oxford/FPA study – no other researchers appear to have studied this possible effect.

There are also a few unresolved safety issues, considered later (see Qs 3.78–3.85).

Note: an excipient used in Cyclogest (progesterone) pessaries can damage rubber. If a cap-user is given this unproven form of treatment for the premenstrual syndrome, she should therefore be advised to use the rectal route of administration. (See also Q 2.20 for other substances which may damage rubber.)

SELECTION OF USERS AND DEVICES

3.20 What are the conditions for the successful use of occlusive caps?

In the main, the answer depends on favourable answers to the questions about the woman herself, listed at Q 3.11 above. In addition, experience plus a positive attitude by the providers, ideally both a doctor and a nurse, are of paramount importance. Skilful fitting, knowledge of when to suggest a cervical/vault cap instead, and above all really satisfactory teaching of the woman, are vital factors. The diaphragm is the first-choice medically fitted vaginal method for most women.

3.21 What are the indications for use of occlusive caps?

1 At the woman's choice.

2 As an alternative to medical methods (hormones, IUDs) for a woman who can accept reduced efficacy as traded off against side-effects of the medical method.

3 The need for contraception on an intermittent yet predictable basis.

4 For protection against pelvic infection or recurrence of cervical neoplasia. This possibility may be rejected, but can be worth suggesting even if another method is in use as the main contraceptive.

3.22 What are the contraindications to the diaphragm?

These include:

1 aversion to touching the genital area;

2 congenital abnormalities such as a septate vagina;

3 most forms of uterovaginal prolapse;

4 inadequate retropubic ledge on examination;

5 poor vagina or perineal muscle tone;

6 inability to learn the insertion technique;

7 lack of hygiene or privacy for insertion, removal and care of the cap;

8 acute vaginitis – treat first;

9 recurrent urinary infections – indication for vault or cervical cap;

10 past history of cap-induced vaginal trauma;

11 true allergy to rubber;

12 past history of toxic shock syndrome – though this not proved related to occlusive caps;

13 *virgo intacta* – sheath use is commonly advised first, until the vagina is 'ready'. But well-motivated tampon-users can receive a small diaphragm, with refitting planned to follow 1 month's regular use.

Items 3, 4, 5 and 9 do not always contraindicate cervical/vault caps (see Q 3.32), and an arcing diaphragm may solve 6.

3.23 What is the structure of a diaphragm?

See Figure 3.2. This is the most commonly used occlusive cap. It consists of a thin latex rubber hemisphere, the rim of which is reinforced by a flexible flat or coiled metal spring. The sizes, measuring the external diameter, range from 50 to 100 mm in steps of 5 mm.

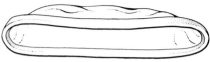

Flat spring

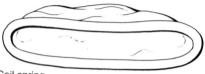

Coil spring

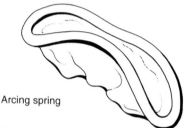

Arcing spring

Figure. 3.2 Types of diaphragm. Q 3.23 and following.
(Reproduced courtesy of Mrs Walli Bounds)

3.24 What types of diaphragm are available?

1 *The flat–spring diaphragm.* This has a firm watch spring and is easily fitted, remaining in the horizontal plane on compression. It is suitable for the normal vagina, and is often tried first.

2 *The coil–spring diaphragm* has a spiral coiled spring. This makes it softer than the flat-spring.

3 *The arcing–spring diaphragm* combines features of both the above and consists of a rubber dome with a firm double metal spring. It exerts strong pressure on the vaginal walls, but its main characteristic is that when compressed it forms an arc, directing the posterior part of the diaphragm downwards and away from the cervix during insertion. This can be an advantage, see Q 3.26.

3.25 What are the indications for the coil-spring diaphragm?

1 Because it exerts less pressure, it can be more comfortable for some women than the flat-spring.

2 The reduced pressure makes it seem to the woman like a half-size smaller than the equivalent flat-spring diaphragm. This can be useful since half-sizes (2.5 mm increments) are no longer available.

3.26 For whom might the arcing-spring diaphragm be indicated?

This is the most widely used type of diaphragm in some countries. Its main disadvantages are:

1 Its greater price in the UK.

2 Some women find it more difficult to handle during insertion because of its non-horizontal shape when squeezed.

Its main positive indication is in cases where the length or direction of the cervix, or the woman's own technique, are leading to a tendency to squeeze the diaphragm into the anterior fornix. See Q 3.40 (7).

3.27 What types of cervical/vault caps are available?

1 *The cervical cap.* This is shaped like a thimble (Fig. 3.1) and is designed to fit snugly over the cervix. The commonest variety is the cavity rim cap with an integral thickened rim incorporating a small groove. This is intended to increase suction to the sides of the cervix. The available internal diameters of the upper rim are: 22, 25, 28 and 31 mm. Other varieties are available abroad.

2 *The vault cap.* This rubber cap is shaped like a bowl with a thinner dome through which the cervix can be palpated. It covers but does not fit closely to the cervix. Five sizes are available ranging from 55 to 75 mm in 5 mm steps.

3 *The vimule.* This is a variation of the vault cap with a hat-shaped prolongation of the dome to accommodate longer cervices. There are three sizes: small (45 mm), medium (48 mm) and large (51 mm).

3.28 What is the mode of action of cervical/vault caps?

They all operate by suction, not by spring tension as the diaphragm. Otherwise the mode of action – and the uncertainties about the importance of spermicides – are the same as for the diaphragm, see Qs 3.6 and 3.7.

3.29 What indications and advantages do the cervical/vault caps share?

1 They share the advantages of the diaphragm but are suitable for patients with poorer muscle tone and some cases of uterovaginal prolapse.

2 They are generally not felt by the male partner.

3 There is no reduction of vaginal sensation.

4 They are unlikely to produce urinary symptoms.

5 Fitting is unaffected by the changes in the size of the vagina, either during intercourse or as a result of changes in body weight.

3.30 What are the conditions necessary to fit a cervical cap?

1 The cervix must be easily felt.

2 The cervix must be healthy, not torn.

3 The cervix must not point backwards, and ideally should point down the axis of the vagina.

4 The cervix must be straight sided.

3.31 What conditions are necessary for fitting a vault cap?

1 The cervix must be easily felt.

2 The cervix must be fairly short, but it may be quite bulky if it does not protrude too much into the vaginal vault.

3.32 In what circumstances would you recommend a trial of the vault or vimule caps?

The vault cap is under-used. It can be very useful where there are contraindications to the diaphragm (see Q 3.22), particularly absence of the retropubic ledge, poor muscle tone and a history of recurrent cystitis. It is a little easier for the woman to fit and remove than the cervical cap, and the precise contour and direction of the cervix are much less important.

Where there is a choice I would recommend a trial of the vault cap before the cervical cap. The vimule is rarely used – its sole indication is to accommodate a cervix which is so long that it prevents suction being exerted in a woman for whom a vault cap would otherwise be selected.

INITIAL FITTING, TRAINING AND FOLLOW-UP ARRANGEMENTS

3.33 What aspects are important in the initial counselling?

The factors in Qs 3.9 and 3.11 above should be very carefully explored with the woman, particularly determining that the method is socially and psychologically acceptable to her, that she is not being 'pressurized by circumstances' into using it, and in particular that she will be a regular conscientious user. She must also be told that the method can still fail despite ideal fitting, *and compliance* with every detail of the instructions as to use.

3.34 How is the fitting performed?

In a sensitive and unhurried way.

The practical aspects cannot be learnt from books. Apprenticeship is necessary in two aspects: fitting technique, and instruction of the patient.

3.35 What points are noted in the initial examination?

1 The apparent health and direction of the uterus and cervix. Tenderness must be absent.
2 The type of retropubic ledge. This can be more fully assessed with a practice diaphragm in position.
3 Assessment of the vaginal musculature and tone, including the perineal muscles.
4 If the diaphragm is chosen the distance from the posterior fornix to the posterior aspect of the symphysis is measured as shown in Figure 3.3.

Cervical cytology and other screening procedures are performed according to local practice.

3.36 Successful fitting of the diaphragm – what are the steps?

1 The woman should have emptied her bladder and an initial choice of practice diaphragm is made based on the distance

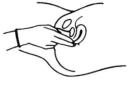

1. To measure for diaphragm size

Hold index and middle fingers together and insert into vagina up to the posterior fornix.
Raise hand to bring surface of index finger to contact with pubic arch.
Use tip of thumb to mark the point directly beneath the inferior margin of the pubic bone and withdraw fingers in this position.

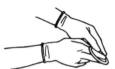

2. To determine diaphragm size

Place one end of rim of fitting diaphragm or ring on tip of middle finger. The opposite end should lie just in front of the thumb tip.
This is the approximate diameter of the diaphragm needed.

Figure. 3.3 Diaphragm – procedure for estimating the size of practice diaphragm to be tried. Q 3.36.
(Reproduced courtesy of Ortho-Cilag Pharmaceutical Ltd, Diaphragm Teaching Aid)

measured at the first examination (Fig. 3.3). A fitting ring can be used at this stage.

2 With the index inside the rim, compress the practice diaphragm between thumb and the remaining fingers. The labia are separated and the diaphragm inserted downwards and backwards to the posterior fornix, tucking the anterior rim behind the symphysis pubis.

3 Check that the cervix is covered.

4 Insert a finger tip between the anterior rim of the cap and the symphysis:
   (a) if the cap is too small, a wider gap will be felt or it may be found that the whole diaphragm is in the anterior fornix;
   (b) if the cap is too large it projects anteriorly/inferiorly and may cause immediate discomfort (or become uncomfortable or distorted later, after wearing).

5 The woman should be asked to stand and walk a few steps. On re-examination anterior protrusion may be due to a small cystocele or a poor retropubic ledge. In this event a vault or possibly a cervical cap should be tried.

3.37 Which way up should diaphragms be fitted?

This really does not matter. It may be slightly easier to remove a flat-spring type if it is inserted dome upwards and the patient is instructed to hook her index finger under the anterior rim. However, this is a non-problem anyway if she simply uses both index and middle fingers to grasp the rim. The arcing diaphragm forms the correct shape (with its leading edge pointing downwards) more readily if it is initially held dome upwards. This requires careful demonstration.

3.38 What are the important points when teaching the prospective user?

Thorough teaching which generates confidence in the user is essential for success. A three-dimensional plastic model helps but a short video is better still. Unless the doctor is a woman the nurse usually takes over at this stage (if she did not do the initial fitting). She must be very encouraging and able, without embarrassment on either side, and in secure privacy, to supervise closely all aspects of the learning process.

3.39 Successful teaching – how important is the position the woman should adopt?

This important aspect is often overlooked by the trainer. Unless instructed to the contrary, many women automatically adopt a half-standing, half-squatting position when inserting the diaphragm or when checking that it is correctly located over the cervix. This should be discouraged, as it makes it almost impossible for the fingers to reach the cervix. It may explain some so-called 'cap failures', caused solely because the woman was unable to check that the device was correctly positioned. The two best positions are:

1 Standing with one foot resting on a chair – a right-handed woman should raise her left leg and vice versa (Fig. 3.4).

2 Squatting right down on the ground.

Other positions are possible at the woman's choice.

3.40 Successful teaching (diaphragm) – what are the steps?

1 In her own preferred position as just described, teach the woman to locate her cervix. Most women prefer to use one finger, but it is an error to insist on this. Even 'short-fingered' women can learn to feel their cervix if taught to use both index and middle fingers.

2 The instructor then inserts the cap for the patient, allowing her to feel her cervix covered with thin rubber.

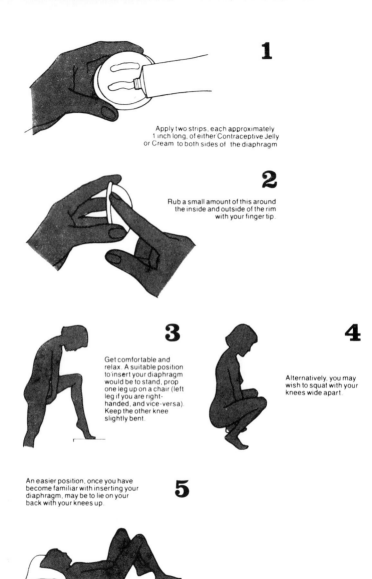

1

Apply two strips, each approximately 1 inch long, of either Contraceptive Jelly or Cream to both sides of the diaphragm

2

Rub a small amount of this around the inside and outside of the rim with your finger tip.

3

Get comfortable and relax. A suitable position to insert your diaphragm would be to stand, prop one leg up on a chair (left leg if you are right-handed, and vice-versa). Keep the other knee slightly bent.

4

Alternatively, you may wish to squat with your knees wide apart.

5

An easier position, once you have become familiar with inserting your diaphragm, may be to lie on your back with your knees up.

Figure. 3.4 Instructions for prospective user of the diaphragm. Q 3.39. (Reproduced courtesy of Ortho-Cilag Pharmaceutical Ltd, Diaphragm Patient Teaching Aid)

68

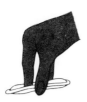

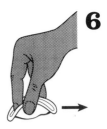

6

To insert your diaphragm fold it in half by pressing the middle of the opposite sides together between the thumb and forefinger of one hand. You may find it helpful to place your index finger in the dome between your thumb and fingers to help prevent it springing away.

If you have been given an arcing spring diaphragm hold it with the arc pointing downwards to ensure that the cervix will be covered.

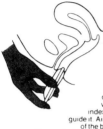

7

8

Hold the lips of your vagina apart with your other hand. Gently slide the folded diaphragm into your vagina, placing your index finger on the rim to guide it. Aim towards the small of the back as if inserting a tampon. You may feel the rim pass over the cervix.

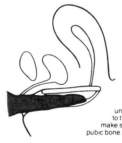

Use the index finger to push the front rim up behind the pubic bone.

9

To check if the diaphragm is in place insert your index finger into your vagina and touch the dome. You should feel the cervix underneath. Move your index finger to the front rim of the diaphragm and make sure it is firmly in place behind the pubic bone. Finally check that the back rim is behind the cervix.

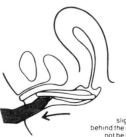

10

Do not remove your diaphragm for 6 hours after intercourse. Put your index finger in your vagina and hook it behind the rim of the diaphragm under your pubic bone. Gently pull the diaphragm down and out. You may find it useful to bear down slightly especially if it is well tucked up behind the pubic bone. The diaphragm should not be left in place for more than 24 hours.

3 The patient then removes the diaphragm for herself, either by hooking it out or (and this needs stressing) the use of two fingers each side of the anterior rim. If this is found difficult, practising with a slightly too large diaphragm may be all that is necessary to boost confidence.

4 She should feel again for the cervix to emphasize the different feel when it is uncovered.

5 She should then be taught to insert the diaphragm as described above and shown in steps 6–8 of Figure 3.4. Emphasis is placed on the fact that the direction of insertion is similar to that for a tampon – primarily backwards.

6 *She should then examine herself to check that the cervix is covered by the soft rubber dome.* It is absolutely vital to explain that the fact that a diaphragm fits snugly behind the symphysis and feels comfortable is no guarantee of correct insertion.

7 If the woman repeatedly inserts the diaphragm into her anterior fornix, the following may be tried:
    (a) two useful tips from the Sister-in-Charge at the Margaret Pyke Centre (MPC). First, the woman lies on her back and holds the diaphragm in her left hand (if right-handed). She then uses her right hand to separate the labia and guide insertion, vertically. Alternatively, and in any convenient position (see Q 3.39), she inserts the diaphragm halfway only, then the half which is still outside is pressed towards the symphysis while completing the insertion.
    (b) the use of an *arcing diaphragm*. When held dome down, compression between middle finger and thumb, with the index finger between to steady it, produces a downward bend (Fig. 3.2 and Q 3.26). This helps the posterior rim to pass below the cervix and so into the posterior rather than the anterior fornix. Occasionally:
    (c) with either diaphragm design, the woman's partner may be able to learn to insert it for her.

The use of an introducer is rarely much help, in our experience at MPC.

3.41 How are cervical and vault caps fitted?

1 The correct size allows the rim of the chosen cap to touch the fornices with no gap, comfortably to accommodate the cervix (the cervical cap being the only one that truly fits it), and to show evidence of a suction effect.

2 To insert the chosen cap, the rim is compressed between thumb and first two fingers and guided along the posterior vaginal wall towards the cervix. The cap is allowed to open by removing the thumb, and then is pushed over the cervix with the fingertips. A final check is made to ensure that the cervix is palpable through the cap and that there is no gap above the rim.

3 Cervical and vault caps are removed by inserting a fingertip above the rim and then easing the cap downwards, before removal with the index and middle fingers.

3.42 Successful teaching – what instructions for vault and cervical caps?

Feeling for the cervix, insertion and removal are taught as just described for the fitting. The important point is that if the right sort of woman has been chosen for these caps (which are a little more tricky to use than the diaphragm), she rapidly develops her own technique both for insertion and removal. Provided this is shown to lead to correct location, she should be encouraged to continue.

The correct size for vault and vimule caps is that which fits snugly into the vaginal vault and covers the cervix without exerting pressure upon it.

Further practical details about fitting these smaller suction caps are best learnt in the practical, clinical situation.

3.43 Successful teaching – what is the training 'timetable' for any type of occlusive cap?

It is usual and preferable to provide the woman with a practice cap for the first week, during which she should use an alternative contraceptive. This enables her to increase her confidence in the techniques of insertion and removal, and to test whether the method is comfortable during all normal activities. She should be informed of the full Family Planning Association (FPA) rules as below before she leaves after the first visit, but they should also be revised at the return visit before she starts to rely on the method.

3.44 Successful teaching – what actual instructions are given at the first visit? See Figure 3.4.

The wording that follows is addressed to a particular woman and relates specifically to the diaphragm (see also Q 3.49):

1 Always use the recommended spermicidal cream or jelly. Apply two strips, each of 1 in (2.5 cm), to each side. It is unnecessary

to smear the surfaces too much, but you may want to put some on the leading part of the rim. Or you could use C-film (Q 3.49).

2 Put your cap in place, using the position and technique you found most comfortable when you were fitted. This could be at any convenient time before lovemaking.

3 If you are having a bath, you should put your diaphragm in after rather than before it. (See also Q 3.97).

4 Most important: check the position of your diaphragm with either your index finger, or with index and middle finger as you prefer. The important thing is that you check that the diaphragm covers your cervix. This feels a bit like a rounded nose with a single nostril, upwards and backwards somewhere near the top of your vagina. You should get used to the particular way your cervix points, which may be forwards, backwards or straight downwards. Check that the rubber on your diaphragm actually covers the cervix – do not rely just on it feeling comfortable.

5 Should lovemaking take place more than 3 hours after you put the cap in, either insert more cream or jelly or foam with an applicator, or use a spermicidal pessary or film pushed well up with the finger. You need to allow about 10 minutes for pessaries to disperse in the vagina before your partner actually deposits semen there.

6 If you have intercourse more than once, more spermicide should be added beforehand, leaving the diaphragm in place.

7 You should leave your cap in place for at least 6 hours after the last intercourse. It can be kept in longer, but should be removed once a day for cleaning.

8 It is no problem if your period starts while the cap is in place. Also it is quite possible to get pregnant during your period. So continue to use your cap for any intercourse, especially towards the end or just after a period, when many people think they can get away without using it.

9 After removal the cap can be washed in warm water with mild toilet soap. It should then be dried and stored in its box in a cool dry place. Do not use disinfectants, detergents or any mineral or vegetable oil-containing oils or lubricants (see Q 2.20), as these may spoil the rubber.

10 Inspect your cap regularly for holes by holding it up to the light.

> **Note: Although you have been given the cap with spermicide, everything is just for practice during the first week. Wear it during the day to make sure it stays in place. You should not be able to feel it if it is the right size and in the right position. Report any discomfort or other problems when, after 1 week, you return to the clinic or surgery. You should come with it in position so that the doctor or nurse can do a proper check.**

3.45 What should take place at the second visit?

1 Any discomfort or problems should be identified.

2 If there are problems a change in the size of the cap or use of a different spermicide (e.g. C-film, Q 3.49(2)) may be recommended.

3 Repetition of the instructions above is important before the woman actually begins to rely on her method.

4 A final warning about the danger of risk-taking may be salutary, coupled with a reminder about *the availability if ever needed of postcoital contraception* (see Ch. 7).

3.46 What extra instructions are given for users of cervical/vault caps?

1 A usual recommendation is to one-third fill the bowl of either cervical, vault or vimule caps. None is used on the rim for fear of impairing suction.

2 With these caps, an extra measure of spermicidal jelly or a pessary should be added on the vaginal side before the first as well as subsequent acts of intercourse after insertion.

3.47 What arrangements are made for routine subsequent follow-up?

1 After the first two visits it is usual to see the patients at 3 months and then at least annually. (6 monthly visits used to be recommended but this is probably unnecessarily frequent.) The most important thing is:

2 The woman should feel free to return more frequently if difficulties occur.

3 Reassessment of the fitting is particularly required:
   (a) after full-term delivery;
   (b) after any unplanned pregnancy whether ending in a termination or miscarriage (chiefly to assess possible improvements in fitting or the user's technique);

(c) after having vaginal surgery;

(d) after the woman loses or gains more than 3 kg in weight

3.48 What is the scientific basis for the rules and regulations about use of occlusive caps, as in Qs 3.44–3.47 above?

Extremely weak: many assumptions, some of them fundamental ones, have never been tested in proper controlled trials, namely:

1 that spermicides add significantly to the effectiveness of occlusive caps;

2 that fitting the largest diaphragm that the woman finds comfortable will improve its effectiveness;

3 that extra spermicide should be used at each intercourse;

4 that extra spermicide should be used if intercourse is delayed for more than 3 hours after placement of the cap;

5 that the spermicide should be applied both to the top and under surface of the diaphragm;

6 that the shortest safe time after intercourse that any occlusive cap can be removed is 6 hours;

7 that gain or loss of as little as 3 kg in weight would influence the effectiveness of occlusive caps.

Basic research to establish the truth or otherwise of some of these points is at last being undertaken.

3.49 What variations in the instructions given to patients are worth considering?

Numerous variations are accepted practice in different countries around the world. As already noted, in Australia use of spermicide at all with occlusive caps is left to patient's choice. The rationale for this is the high rate of user-failure in that country and the belief that increased compliance is likely when 'messy' spermicides are avoided. This Australian view, however, is a minority view. Pending more data most authorities feel that spermicides should be used; but all possible efforts should be made to reduce the problems of non-contraceptive with which they are associated. For example, newer spermicidal jellies with a far better appearance, texture and smell are being marketed. In addition three variants seem reasonable:

1 Application of spermicide to the superior surface only of the diaphragm. This is the norm in America, and is becoming more

usual also in this country (about an 8 cm (3 in) strip of cream or jelly from the tube being applied).

2 Use of C-Film, one placed in the hollow of the diaphragm inserted dome down. A study from Scotland was not big enough to prove but strongly suggested that this method would give sufficient protection, and it was highly acceptable.

3 Increasing to 6 hours the interval after placement of the diaphragm and before intercourse after which further spermicide is advised.

Other minor variations are also permitted by various family planning authorities.

MANAGEMENT OF SIDE-EFFECTS AND COMPLICATIONS

3.50 What should be done if the partner can feel the diaphragm during intercourse?

1 Check the size – a bigger or smaller variety may be needed.

2 Re-teach the patient. The couple may have already decided not to use certain positions (e.g. for rear entry vaginal intercourse they might use the condom instead).

3 Change from a flat- to a coiled-spring diaphragm.

4 Change to a vault or perhaps a cervical cap.

5 Change the method.

3.51 Why are urinary tract infections commoner in diaphragm users, and how should they be managed?

1 The fact that urinary tract infections develop more frequently is believed to be caused mainly by the pressure of the rim on the urethra and bladder base, predisposing to urethritis and cystitis.

2 Some work has also suggested that use of the diaphragm and other occlusive caps may alter the vaginal flora so as to promote infections. Vaginal cultures from cap-users grow *Escherichia coli* more often than those from relevant controls.

It would appear that the first explanation is the more important, since the following actions usually help (especially item 2):

1 change to a smaller size of diaphragm;

2 change to a vault cap (or cervical cap).

The woman is also advised to empty her bladder both before and just after intercourse.

3.52 What are the possible causes of the complaint of 'vaginal soreness'?

1 There may be an incidental infection such as trichomoniasis or thrush (or urethritis, see above).

2 Inflammatory reactions, abrasions or even frank ulcers can also be caused by local pressure.

3 Allergy is possible, either to the spermicide or to chemicals in the rubber of the occlusive cap.

3.53 How should vaginal soreness be managed?

1 First examine the patient: particularly her vulva and the whole vaginal surface. If there is widespread erythema and multiple vesicles or scaling suspect allergy. Allergy can be treated by change of spermicide (see Table 3.2), but in this country plastic caps are no longer sold.

2 Swabs should be taken for possible infections. If there is a discharge with a slightly fishy odour a useful test is the pH using test paper whose range is pH 4–6. A result which is >4.5 suggests either anaerobic vaginosis or trichomoniasis, both treatable with metronidazole.

3.54 What should be done if actual abrasions or ulcers are seen?

I have personally only seen one severe case, in an arcing diaphragm user, but they have been described in users of other diaphragms, vimules and cervical caps.

In our case the ulcers were posterolateral on each side, 2–3 cm long and about 0.5 cm wide and deep, and very indurated. At first a carcinoma of the vagina was suspected! However, complete recovery followed non-use of the diaphragm (which was size 85 and fitted correctly) and abstinence from intercourse for 3 weeks. No other treatment was required.

The woman concerned had met a new partner, and intercourse had been unusually vigorous and frequent with the diaphragm left in place for long periods of time. Cases reported from the USA had similarly worn the diaphragm or vimule cap for 3 or more days in succession. This rare complication is also said to be more likely if the diaphragm is too large, and may be related to variations in individual anatomy (see also Q 3.96).

3.55 What is the contraceptive sponge, as currently marketed?

It is a small round disposable sponge made of polyurethane foam, with a depression at its centre designed to locate it over the cervix, and a tape for removal (Fig. 3.5). It is impregnated with a widely used spermicide (nonoxynol-9). Benzalkonium chloride is used instead, or as well, in some countries.

3.56 How is the contraceptive sponge used?

It is designed as an over-the-counter method. The woman simply moistens it with tapwater and inserts it into the vagina, so that (notionally) it covers the cervix. It can be inserted from a few seconds to 24 hours in advance of intercourse. It should then be left in place for at least 6 hours after the last coitus.

3.57 What is the mode of action?

It was initially believed that there were three actions:

1 a barrier effect;

2 action as a carrier of spermicide;

3 action as a sponge to absorb and mop-up semen.

However, it is now believed that its main action is as a carrier of spermicide, since it so commonly becomes dislodged and then leaves the external cervical os unprotected. Its effectiveness is not

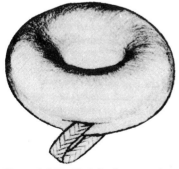

Figure. 3.5 The 'Today' collatex vaginal sponge. Q 3.55. (Reproduced courtesy of Mrs Walli Bounds)

proven to be different from that of spermicides used alone (see Table 0.2 and Q 0.14).

3.58 What is the effectiveness of the contraceptive sponge?

Use effectiveness appears to be in the range of 9–25/100 woman-years. Multicentre clinical trials have given varying results. The USA study yielded failure rates of about 17/100 women at 1 year for the sponge and 12.5 for the diaphragm, a difference which was significant. Unfortunately, about 20% of the women were lost to follow-up.

In the MPC study, 251 women were randomly allocated to the sponge and the diaphragm with 99% follow-up. The observed failure rates were around 25% for the sponge and 11% for the diaphragm (1-year life table rates). If apparent method-failures alone are considered, the sponge compares even more adversely with the diaphragm plus spermicide in both studies.

3.59 How might the effectiveness be improved?

Since in the USA and MPC studies the high method-failure rate occurred despite optimal teaching, there seems little room for improvement due to better teaching of compliant users. It would appear that improvements in device design are required: it should possibly be made larger and loaded with a new more effective spermicide, or combination of spermicides.

For the present, the best policy to achieve satisfactory failure rates with this product is to recommend its use only for those women who have from the outset a relatively reduced fertility (see Q 3.64).

3.60 What are the advantages of the sponge?

1 It is easy to use and does not require additional 'messy' spermicide.

2 It can be inserted from a few seconds to 24 hours in advance of intercourse, thereby allowing more spontaneous lovemaking than other barrier methods.

3 No special fitting is required.

4 It can be purchased without prescription.

5 It offers continuous protection during 24 hours, regardless of how often intercourse is repeated.

6 It cannot be felt by the male partner.

It also shares with the diaphragm plus spermicide the following:

7 No proven systemic effects.

8 Possible beneficial effects (see Q 3.61).

9 The method is under a woman's control and needs only to be used when required.

Most studies have shown its overall acceptability to be very high.

3.61 What are its beneficial medical effects?

Largely because of its spermicide content, the sponge appears to provide a measure of protection against sexually transmitted diseases and pelvic infection; though it is not recommended as sufficient protection against the viruses (i.e. for safer sex). Protection has now been demonstrated for *Chlamydia*, *Gonorrhoea* and *Trichomoniasis*. But see below for thrush.

3.62 What are the disadvantages of the sponge?

1 The main one is definitely its relative lack of efficacy.

2 A few women have difficulty removing the sponge and fragmentation has sometimes occurred.

3 There is some risk of adverse medical effects, see below.

But note that it does not have most of the disadvantages listed for the diaphragm at Qs 3.18 and 3.19.

3.63 What are the possible adverse medical effects?

1 Vaginal irritation has been reported. Epithelial irritation effects (see Q 3.78) with very frequent use and frank *allergy to the nonoxynol-9 spermicide* are also possible.

2 *Thrush is more common. There are no controlled data about other organisms like E.coli or those causing anaerobic vaginosis, but it is likely that the flora may be altered somewhat by the sponge's presence in the vagina*, as has been shown for the diaphragm (see Q. 3.51).

3 *Toxic shock syndrome* (TSS). There have been a number of reports in the USA. Unlike for the diaphragm (see Q 3.84), the Centers for Disease Control in Atlanta consider that the data do suggest a very slightly increased risk of TSS in sponge users. This rare possibility can be virtually eliminated by the instruction not to leave the sponge in situ during menstrual bleeding.

3.64 For whom might the sponge method be indicated?

1 Women whose natural fertility is less by virtue of:
   (a) *Age*. Fertility declines, most steeply after the age of 45, though less so in those with regular cycling (see Q 8.33–4). Hence the sponge *may* be very appropriate as well as acceptable from the age of 45 (more so after 50), through until 1 year after the menopause.
   (b) *Lactation*. The method could be used until uterine bleeding begins to return at weaning.
   (c) *Secondary amenorrhoea* (see Q 4.58).

2 It might be used, like spermicides, as an *adjunct* to other methods of birth control, such as the IUD or *coitus interruptus*.

3 It may also be used for those who are planning their first child fairly soon, or who are *spacing* their family.

4 It would certainly be better than nothing for women who are unable or unwilling to use any other more effective method.

3.65 For whom is the sponge not suitable, or contraindicated?

1 Primarily, it should *not be used by young and highly fertile women* who are not ready for a pregnancy. It is worth reminding them that its failure rate is more than 20 times higher than the contraceptive pill, which they may otherwise be abandoning.

2 Women of any age for whom, in their own view, a pregnancy would be disastrous.

3 Women who are reluctant to touch their genital area.

4 Women with *allergy* to the sponge itself or any of its constituents.

5 Those with a *past history of TSS* (see Q 3.63).

3.66 What is the place of the 'Today' contraceptive sponge in the range of contraceptives available?

A couple's choice of contraceptive is based on a variety of factors, of which efficacy is but one – and to some it may not be a prime consideration. Simplicity and great comfort in use, ease of obtainability (and hence privacy), and freedom from major health hazards, may outweigh the efficacy disadvantage for individual couples: though all should be reminded of the data at Qs 3.58 and 3.65. The method is welcomed, if used by the groups at Q 3.64.

3.67 What is the new female condom, first marketed during 1992?

Various designs have been proposed, including the *bikini condom* with its integral latex pouch, from America. The most promising is *Femidom*, first devised in Denmark, but now licensed by Chartex International in London (Fig. 3.6). Made of polyurethane and preloaded with an efficient silicone lubricant, it looks at first like an extra large male condom. The currently marketed version is 17 cm long. Both have a large (70-mm) diameter outer ring attached at the opening, designed to prevent it advancing beyond the vulva. A 60 mm diameter loose ring at the inner closed end aids its retention within the vagina and is also squeezed like a diaphragm for insertion. The whole device thus forms a well lubricated secondary vagina.

3.68 What advantages are claimed? Are there any problems?

Advantages:

1 over-the-counter method not requiring fitting by any outsider;

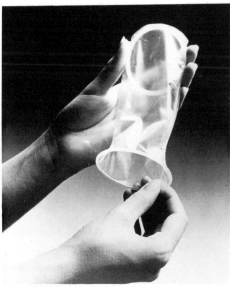

Figure 3.6 Femidom. Q 3.67.

2 under the woman's control;

3 insertable preintercourse, like sponge or diaphragm;

4 does not require erect penis at outset; male sensations more normal than intercourse with condom;

5 very complete barrier against STDs including viruses;

6 worth suggesting if local soreness makes sex uncomfortable or during menses or postpartum lochia.

Though users report several in-use problems, such as its prominence during foreplay and the potential for the penis to become wrongly positioned (between the sac and the vaginal wall), Femidom has been shown to be less likely than the male condom to rupture in use. At the time of writing (1993) there are no comprehensive efficacy data, but its use-effectiveness is expected to be broadly similar to the male condom.

3.69 What is the place of Femidom in the range of methods?

It is really too soon to say. Reports about its acceptability are mixed. It was given qualified approval as a method by about half the users in the first MPC study, who tried it up to 10 times but used a different method for contraception. Among 106 volunteers in MPC's trial of Femidom as sole contraceptive more than half found it unacceptable. However, nine of the 11 users who continued for 1 year, and most of 20 who had to stop using it solely because supplies ran out, would have wished to continue long term. As the first female-controlled method with high potential for preventing HIV transmission it must surely be welcomed to the range of contraceptive options. Further development of new variants will hopefully make it even more acceptable and use-effective.

Spermicides

3.70 What are spermicides?

These are a range of substances which chemically immobilize or destroy sperm. They are one of the oldest and simplest forms of fertility control and make a useful contribution, chiefly to increase the efficacy of other methods.

3.71 What is the mode of action of spermicides?

They have two main components: a relatively inert base and an active spermicidal agent. Hence they operate both physically and biochemically, forming a partial barrier and also immobilizing sperm. The base materials vary in their physical characteristics, the best being water soluble. The active ingredients are of five possible types:

1 surface-active agents, of which the most widely used is nonoxynol-9;

2 enzyme inhibitors;

3 bactericides;

4 acids;

5 local anaesthetics and other membrane-active agents.

3.72 What types are available?

All the spermicides currently used in the UK are listed in Table 3.2. Regrettably there is little real choice: they are all primarily in category 1 as just listed, and most use nonoxynol-9 or its almost identical longer chain variant, nonoxynol-11. This was probably

Table 3.2 Spermicides available in the UK

Name	Manufacturer	Active ingredients
Foams		
Delfen Foam	Ortho-Cilag Pharmaceutical Ltd	Nonoxynol–9 12.5%
Creams		
Duracreme	LRC Products Ltd	Nonoxynol–11 2%
Orthocreme	Ortho-Cilag Pharmaceutical Ltd	Nonoxynol–9 2%
Jellies		
Duragel	LRC Products Ltd	Nonoxynol–11 2%
Gynol II	Ortho-Cilag Pharmaceutical Ltd	Nonoxynol–9 2%
Ortho Gynol Gel	Ortho-Cilag Pharmaceutical Ltd	Di-isobutylphenoxy-polyethoxyethanol 1%
Staycept Jelly	Syntex Pharmaceuticals Ltd	Octoxynol 1%
Pessaries		
Double Check	FP Sales Ltd	Nonoxynol–9 6%
Norolen	WJ Rendell Ltd	Nonoxynol–9 6%
Ortho-Forms	Ortho-Cilag Pharmaceutical Ltd	Nonoxynol–9 5%
Staycept Pessaries	Syntex Pharmaceuticals Ltd	Nonoxynol–9 6%
Film		
C-Film	FP Sales Ltd	Nonoxynol–9 30%

All these products have vehicles which do not have adverse effects on rubber (see Q 2.20).

never the best choice: its main merit was that it had been marketed for years, so when drug regulatory authorities were set up they exempted it from detailed toxicology. It does not even penetrate cervical mucus! – unlike some alternatives which might have been much better choices.

With the arrival of the AIDS problem we are now suffering from neglect of this field by a generation of scientists: far too little research has been done to devise better substances, more effective and safer not only as spermicides but also as *viricides* (see Qs 3.77 and 3.78).

3.73 How are spermicides used?

To be effective the products should disperse quickly but yet remain in sufficient concentration at the cervix to exert their action at the end of intercourse. Aerosol foams such as Delfen seem to be preferable in this respect. The products listed can be inserted just before intercourse, with the important exception of the pessaries and foaming tablets. These should be inserted at least 10 minutes before ejaculation to allow sufficient time for dispersal.

3.74 How effective are spermicides used alone?

Spermicides are far more effective in vitro than they ever prove to be in vivo. This is fully discussed at Q 1.3. There are greater variations in reported effectiveness for spermicides than for almost any other birth control method. The limits range from less than 1 to over 30 pregnancies/100 woman-years! In a study of almost 3000 well-motivated women attending six family planning clinics in the USA with the proper instructions and follow-up, Bernstein documented a pregnancy rate of only 4/100 woman-years. More realistically, the normal use-effectiveness of spermicides used alone can be considered to be comparable with that of the contraceptive sponge.

3.75 Are spermicides recommended for use alone as contraceptives?

General teaching in this country has been that spermicides are not effective enough for use alone. However, they can be used in conditions of reduced fertility: for example, for the standard 1 year following an apparent menopause. They could equally be used as an adjunct when a couple refuses any alternative to coitus interruptus, or in the other circumstances for which the sponge is appropriate (see Q 3.64). But the latter is in general more popular, along with its main rival which is foam. (The other presentations are found to be more 'messy' by most.)

3.76 What are the advantages and disadvantages of spermicides?

These are summarized in Table 3.3. Many of the advantages are shared with the contraceptive sponge, but spermicides cannot be so well separated from coitus.

3.77 Do spermicides protect against sexually transmitted infections?

In vitro studies have shown that most of the common spermicides can kill sexually transmitted pathogens. Nonoxynol has activity against the organisms causing gonorrhoea, chlamydia, *Trichomonas vaginitis*, genital herpes and even AIDS (HIV). In vivo studies have mostly been small and uncontrolled, but in general they confirm a useful protective effect of nonoxynol, with one unwanted exception relating to the risk of virus transmission – see Q 3.78 below.

Table 3.3. Advantages and disadvantages of spermicides

Advantages	Disadvantages
1. Easy availability.	1. Perceived to be messy.
2. Freedom from major health risks.	2. Not highly effective in general use.
3. No medical intervention/ supervision necessary.	3. Are coitus-dependent and thus inconvenient to use.
4. Need only be used when required.	4. Waiting period of 10 minutes before some products effective.
5. Provide some protection against some sexually transmitted diseases.	5. Not effective if inserted more than 60 minutes ahead.
6. Allow the female to be in control of contraception.	6. Can cause local heat (foaming tablets), irritation or allergy.
7. Provide some genital lubrication.	7. Questions are now being asked about risks of spermicide absorption. See Q 3.74.
8. Are a valuable adjunct to other methods.	

VAGINAL CONTRACEPTION: UNRESOLVED SAFETY ISSUES

3.78 Is it true that nonoxynol seems capable of sometimes damaging the vaginal epithelium?

A study in Nairobi prostitutes of nonoxynol-containing spermicides as a possible aid to safer sex reported 'soreness' as a frequent complaint. This was at first thought to be linked in part with trauma from very frequent coitus, but further studies by Family Health International have shown that frequent use of the product itself is the main factor. When used four times a day for 14 days, nonoxynol-9 released from pessaries caused erythema and colposcopic evidence of minor damage to the vaginal skin. This might or might not cause irritation or other symptoms, but it has naturally led to concern that this adverse effect might actually increase the likelihood of transfer of HIV infection, even though nonoxynol does have virucidal activity in vitro. Coupled with the doubts about its effectiveness against intracellular virus, these data mean it should not be promoted as an anti-HIV virucide.

However, pending the development of more alternatives, for the time being it is considered good practice to continue to recommend nonoxynol and the similar surface-active agents listed in Table 3.2 for *normal contraceptive use* (less frequently than four times a day!), whether alone or with diaphragms or condoms. The Margaret Pyke Trust is actively involved with other bodies in urgent and previously neglected research into new and better substances for vaginal use as virucides and spermicides.

3.79 Are spermicides absorbed, and is there therefore a risk of systemic effects?

Yes, most substances in the vagina can be absorbed into the circulation. Hence it is impossible to say that any method that uses a spermicide is entirely free of the risk of systemic harmful effects. These could be by toxicity to vital organs, idiosyncrasy, or through carcinogenesis or teratogenesis. There have been some reports suggesting an association with unwanted effects (see Qs 3.80 and 3.81) following spermicide absorption, but the overall picture remains a reassuring one.

3.80 What is the evidence that standard spermicides might have toxic effects after absorption?

In 1979 it was suggested from animal experiments that nonoxynol-9 might have hepatotoxic effects and cause changes in serum lipids. However, controlled studies of the blood chemistry of women using spermicides have not demonstrated any significant changes, though long-term data are not available. Certainly no obvious harm has ever been reported among long-term users of vaginal contraceptives.

3.81 What is the evidence about teratogenesis?

Exposure to the spermicide early in pregnancy, or fertilization of an ovum by a sperm damaged by the spermicide, might in theory increase the rate of malformations. In 1981, one study reported an increase in various unrelated fetal abnormalities among the children of women who may have used spermicides around the time they became pregnant. This study has been criticized because of flaws in the study design. More recent studies have completely failed to show the risk. Present opinion is that spermicides do not have any teratogenic effect in ordinary use.

3.82 Are there reports of an increase of neoplasia in women using vaginal contraception?

No – neither as a consequence of systemic absorption, nor because of any effect of spermicide or rubber on the vaginal or cervical epithelium. A few women who are sensitive to spermicides may develop hyperkeratosis of the cervix or vagina. This has not been shown to result in neoplasia. Indeed, it is very likely that barrier methods are protective against cervical neoplasia (see Q 3.17).

3.83 Can vaginal contraception promote infection?

This may seem improbable, in view of the fact that both the barrier effect and the spermicide seem to protect against many STDs. Concern arises from evidence that *Staphylococcus aureus* and some streptococci, and *E. coli* can tend to proliferate in the presence of a diaphragm or a cervical cap. This has already been mentioned as a possible factor in the increased risk of urinary infections. It may also be relevant to TSS (see Q 3.84).

3.84 Can the diaphragm or other caps cause TSS?

Sporadic cases have been reported in the USA. However, the rate is so low that the risk is unlikely to be greater than that already existing from use of tampons by those diaphragm-users (compare Q 3.63 *re* the sponge).

3.85 What is the overall safety of vaginal contraceptives?

Even allowing for the unresolved safety issues above, potential users may be told that all these methods are still believed to be medically safer than the hormonal methods. However, honesty is necessary, and it would be wrong to say that any method that uses an absorbable spermicide is completely free from systemic effect.

In assessing safety it is also important to remember that unwanted pregnancies are overall more frequent among users of any of these methods. One then has to consider the potential health hazard of the resulting unwanted pregnancies.

THE (NEAR) FUTURE IN VAGINAL CONTRACEPTION

3.86 What innovative spermicides are being studied?

Inhibitors of the sperm's own enzymes, principally acrosin, show promise: and several surprising drugs (like propranolol), normally used for non-contraceptive indications, have aroused interest because of their effect on the sperm membrane and motility. Disinfectants are important because of their particular potential also as virucides: among these is chlorhexidine. Derivatives of natural products such as gossypol are also being screened. Another approach is to develop agents that directly alter cervical mucus both chemically and physically.

More research is also urgently required into better carrier (base) materials.

3.87 What is the state of research into occlusive caps?

1 *Disposable spermicide–coated diaphragms*. These are under study, designed to overcome the perceived 'messiness' of any vaginal contraceptive that requires separate application of the spermicide.

2 New sponges with different spermicides, or combinations of spermicide (see Q 3.86).

3 New cervical caps. There was great interest in the so-called custom-fitted cervical cap, made from a mould of the user's cervix. Trials of this *Contracap* gave a quite unacceptable failure

rate. However the objective remains attractive – of a non-coitally related appliance designed to be left in place in the upper vagina for long periods of time. *Leah's Shield* and *Femcap* are American inventions and there is also the *Gynaeseal diaphragm-tampon* devised by an Australian, Dr Cattanach.

4 *Intracervical devices.* Both medicated and non-medicated devices with some kind of flange or protruding arms to anchor them in the lower part of the uterus are possibilities which have been studied.

5 *Vaginal rings.* WHO did some preliminary work on a silicone rubber ring that releases nonoxynol-9 at a constant rate for at least 30 days. This seems a promising approach, preferably using a more advanced spermicide. However, nothing has been published so far.

QUESTIONS ASKED BY USERS ABOUT VAGINAL CONTRACEPTION

3.88 Can I use some kind of cap if my womb tilts backwards?

It is a myth that this makes it impossible to use the method. Some positions of your cervix (entrance to the womb) may make it preferable for you to be given an arcing diaphragm, and could lead to rejection of a cervical cap; but the method is not ruled out if you wish to use it.

3.89 In America they have inserters for diaphragms – are they available here?

Yes they are, but you need to ask yourself whether your wish to use one might be connected with some reluctance to touch yourself in the genital area. It may be that can be overcome by counselling, or perhaps you should think about using another method.

3.90 How do I know where my cervix is?

It is absolutely essential that you feel confident that you can find your cervix, whatever the kind of occlusive cap you are going to use. It is often helpful to ask your doctor or the nurse to tell you in which direction its little opening points. You may also find it much easier to feel if you use two fingers rather than one.

3.91 How much cream or jelly should I use with my diaphragm?

A common error is to use too much. See Q 3.44 for the standard instructions. If you find messiness a particular problem but still wish to use the method, ask your doctor or nurse about the possibility of following the American teaching, of putting spermicide only on the top of the cap when it is first inserted. (Continue to follow all the other rules you were taught.) Delfen foam may be preferred. Another possibility which has been successful in a Scottish trial is to obtain C-film from a chemist or clinic, for use on top of the cap.

3.92 Can the cap fall out when you go to the toilet?

Normally, this will not happen. If it does, soon after intercourse, consider postcoital contraception (see Ch. 7). Moreover, if your diaphragm or other cap comes out, it may be that you have a prolapse, or the wrong size, or are not inserting it correctly. So you should make an early appointment to discuss things with the doctor or nurse.

3.93 Can caps and diaphragms be fitted with strings to help removal? I have difficulty in getting mine out.

There are no longer any marketed with strings. You may have been taught to use just one finger to hook out the diaphragm but the solution to your problem may well be just to use two fingers, one each side of the front rim.

See Q 3.40 section 3 for another tip.

3.94 How do I check the diaphragm is in good condition? Its dome has become much softer and floppier and it has lost its new whiteness – do these changes matter?

You should hold your diaphragm up to the light and stretch it, being careful not to damage the rubber with your fingernails. If no holes are seen, and if the rim can readily be restored to a reasonable shape, then all is well. The change in colour and texture of the rubber is quite normal.

3.95 Can I leave the cap in during my periods?

The US FDA advises against this because of an unproven extra risk of the rare TSS. A better solution might be Femidom (see Q 3.67) to reduce messiness if you fancy lovemaking during any bleeding. Also, in the second half of a period there is the conception risk to consider (see Q 1.15).

3.96 I have heard you can leave the cap in all the time – is this right?

If you follow the rules, yes – almost! It can be in position most of the time if your love life is unpredictable and frequent. The important thing is to remove it at least once in 24 hours, 6 hours after the last intercourse, wash it in mild soap, rinse it thoroughly and then it can be reinserted. Continuous use without giving your vaginal wall an occasional rest seems a bad thing, however (see Q 3.54).

3.97 Can I have a bath or go swimming whilst the cap is in place?

Yes. However, it is ideally best if this is not until at least 2 hours after intercourse, in case it helps the sperm to escape the action of the spermicide. And if you make love after bathing with the diaphragm in, put in some extra spermicide first.

3.98 I have a baby – can I go back to using my old diaphragm or cap?

Quite possibly not. It is certainly important to get the fitting rechecked and have a full retraining in correct use (see also Q 3.47).

3.99 How often should I change the diaphragm or cap for a new one?

Only when your inspection at Q 3.94 shows damage, or as recommended by your clinic. Occlusive caps are quite expensive on the NHS and successful regular use of the same one for 2 years is very common. Remember too that if you lose your cap you can buy the right size over the counter at any chemist.

3.100 The contraceptive sponge seems a wonderful method – what is the drawback?

It is certainly a most comfortable and acceptable method for both partners. Its drawback is just that it is not effective enough to be recommended for most young fertile women.

3.101 If I buy the sponge from the chemist, can I ask a clinic or GP to show me how to use it?

Certainly. However, you may well find that they suggest you think again about using this method at all, if you must avoid pregnancy and do not come into one of the recommended categories in Q 3.64.

3.102 Won't the sponge fall out?

This can certainly happen, and dislodgement either outwards or up beside the cervix is one of the explanations for its highish failure rate.

3.103 Can I flush the sponge down the toilet?

It is more environmentally friendly to use the dustbin.

3.104 Is Femidom a recommended method?

Yes. Follow the instructions which come with it most carefully, every time. If you are careful to avoid wrong positioning of the penis (see Q 3.68), and the sperm are caught completely within the Femidom, it ought to be as good as a male condom both as a contraceptive and for safer sex.

3.105 Can I use a home-made barrier, 'in an emergency'?

Improvised barriers can be made. Probably the best is a suitable piece of sponge or plug of cloth, soaked either in vinegar solution diluted 1 in 20 with water, or in a soap solution.

3.106 Do you recommend the 'Honeycap', which my friend uses?

Definitely not. Available from some doctors in private practice in London, this is really only a size 60 arcing-spring diaphragm which is first soaked in honey for 7 days; and then used without spermicide for up to a week at a time. The honey is meant to reduce the risk of vaginal infection or odour, but this is unproven: and its effectiveness has also not been properly tested. It is highly likely to have the same failure rate as in the Marie Stopes Study above (see Q 3.7), which amounts to a risk, each year, that one woman would get pregnant out of every four users!

4 Oral contraception – the combined oral contraceptive (COC)

BACKGROUND: EFFICACY AND MECHANISMS

4.1 What is the definition of oral contraception?

An orally administered substance or combination which prevents pregnancy. Specifically at the present time such substances are only for use by women. Steroids and other potential systemic contraceptives may also be given by non-oral routes (see Chs. 5 and 8). In this chapter I shall consider only the combined oral contraceptive (COC), which is a combination of oestrogen and progestagen. Unless qualified, the word 'pill' refers to the COC. The progestagen-only pill (POP) is considered in Chapter 5.

4.2 What is the history of oral contraception?

This is discussed in more detail elsewhere (see my book *The Pill*, Further Reading). In brief, it was shown by the early 1900s that the corpus luteum of pregnancy stops further ovulation. In 1921 Haberlandt transplanted ovaries into female rabbits, and rendered them infertile for several months. He suggested that extracts from ovaries might be used as oral contraceptives. In 1941 Marker used diosgenin from the Mexican yam as the raw material for sex steroids. This led to the synthesis of norethisterone (known as norethindrone in the USA) by Djerassi and his colleagues in 1950. Frank Colton independently produced norethynodrel, which with mestranol was the first marketed oral contraceptive. Margaret Sanger, supported by her wealthy friend Catherine McCormack, financed the studies of the biologist Gregory Pincus and M. C. Chang together with the obstetrician John Rock. After systematic experiments in animals the first human trial was reported in 1956. The pill became available in the USA in June 1960 and in the UK during 1961. In 1963 the Wyeth Company achieved the total synthesis of norgestrel.

The first case report of venous thromboembolism was reported in *The Lancet* in 1961 by an astute British GP. Subsequently there have been numerous case-control studies, and three main prospective (cohort) studies, researching both the adverse and beneficial effects (see Q 4.47). Much more money has been spent on testing than on originally developing the method.

4.3 What is the usage of the pill, worldwide and in the UK?

There is enormous variation between countries, and within countries according to age groups. The differences have more to do with medical politics, religion, and the inertia of institutions, than with the acceptability or otherwise of the method to potential consumers. Estimated overall usage varies between less than 2% of married women in Japan through to about 40% in the Netherlands and Austria. According to the UK General Household Survey (1993, reporting data collected in 1991), the COC is used by 21% of the 13 million women aged 16–49, with the POP accounting for no more than an extra 2%. In the peak age group 20–24, 48% of all women (which is about 70% of contraception-users) take the COC.

In a 1986 survey for the RCGP, nearly 95% of sexually active UK women under the age of 30 reported use of oral contraceptives at some time.

4.4 What are the main mechanisms of contraceptive action of the combined pill?

These are summarized in Table 4.1. Without exception all steroidal methods operate by some combination of the mechanisms there described. The COC has a very similar primary action in most women, namely the prevention of ovulation: both by lack of follicular maturation and by abolition of oestrogen-mediated positive feedback which leads to the luteinizing hormone (LH) surge. The other mechanisms shown – reduction in sperm penetrability of cervical mucus (see Q 5.16) and of the receptivity to the blastocyst of the endometrium (see Q 5.17) – are primarily back-up mechanisms for the COC. They have greater relevance to the mechanisms of some of the oestrogen-free methods of Chapter 5. See also Q 5.33 for tubal effects.

4.5 What are the types of COC?

Current COCs are either fixed-dose or phasic. The latter are like the former in containing both oestrogen and progestagen. The ratio of the two is not fixed, however, but changed in a stepwise fashion, either once (biphasic pills) or twice (triphasic pills) in each 21-day course. They are discussed in more detail below (see Qs 4.158–4.164). We should note here, however, that like all COCs the phasic types remove the menstrual cycle; but they attempt to replace it with cyclical variations, chiefly in the progestagen dose.

Table 4.1 Various progestagen delivery systems (all except COC are oestrogen-free)

	Oral		Injectable		Implant Norplant	Vaginal ring LNG ring (WHO)
	COC	POP	NET-EN	DMPA		
Administration						
Frequency	Daily	Daily	2-monthly	3-monthly	5-yearly	3-monthly
Progestagen dose	Low	Ultra-low	High	High	Ultra-low	Ultra-low
Blood levels	Rapidly fluctuating		Initial peak then decline		Constant	Constant
First pass through liver	Yes	Yes	No	No	No	No
Major mechanisms						
Ovary: ↓ Ovulation*	+++	+	++	+++	++	+
Cervical mucus: ↓ sperm penetrability	Yes	Yes	Yes	Yes	Yes	Yes
Endometrium: ↓ receptivity to blastocyst	Yes	Yes	Yes	Yes	Yes	Yes
Use effectiveness	0.2–3	0.3–4	<2	0–1	0–1	3
Menstrual pattern	Regular	Often irregular	Irregular	Very irregular	Irregular	Irregular
Amenorrhoea during use	Rare	Occasional	Common	Very common	Common	Common
Reversibility						
Immediate termination possible?	Yes	Yes	No	No	Yes	Yes
By woman herself at anytime?	Yes	Yes	No	No	No	Yes
Time to first likely conception from first omitted dose/removal	3 months	c. 1 month	c. 3 months	6 months	c. 1 month	c. 1 month

* By two mechanisms – no preovulatory follicles formed, plus no LH surges occur.

There is yet no proof that this has important health benefits (aside that is from the giving of a low dose of each hormone).

4.6 What are 'everyday' (ED) varieties of COC? Do they have advantages?

These are regimens which include, usually, 7 days of placebo tablets. They have the advantage of a reduction in the risk that the user will forget to restart her next packet on time – a potent cause of pill failure (see Q 4.17). This system is also one way of removing the necessity for numbering, as opposed to putting the day of the week, against the pill blisters in phasic packets (compare Logynon ED with Logynon). A simpler solution, as in Trinovum, is the use of 7-day phases. 'Sunday start' schemes, with instructions for extra contraception in the first packet, are common in the USA.

4.7 What are the disadvantages of ED packaging?

This is often complicated by a starting routine involving a variable number of placebos, so extra contraception has to be advised for 14 days. Some women dislike the implication that they are too unintelligent to remember when to stop and restart treatment. It has even been suggested, thirdly, that some women think that the dummy lactose (sugar) pills might be bad for them!

For these reasons ED packaging has never been popular in the UK. However, in other countries well over half of all pill cycles are of this type – which I personally favour as an aid to compliance. There are ways of simplifying the starting routine so as always to start with an *active* tablet; and the placebos should perhaps be made of bran, as everyone knows that bran is good for you!

4.8 What modified regimens would you prefer to see marketed?

Since as will be described fully below the pill-free interval (PFI) is 'the Achilles' heel' of the COC's efficacy, there would be particular merit in returning to an earlier scheme of 22 active pills with six placebos. Indeed even without placebos this is good for compliance, since the 'finishing day' is then the same day of the week as the 'starting day'.

For special cases, optional 28-day ED packets of monophasic brands with only four or perhaps five placebo tablets would also be useful. Instead of or as well as tricycling (see Q. 4.28) these regimens with a much shortened pill-free time could be reserved for women taking interacting drugs (see Qs 4.33 and 4.188) or those with a history of past conception while taking the COC (Q 4.24).

4.9 What about other oestrogen–progestagen agents (especially sequential pills and regimens of hormone replacement therapy)?

Sequential pills have rightly been removed from the market in most countries (though not all). The older high-oestrogen varieties were shown to double the risk of endometrial carcinoma. They also were, surprisingly, less effective; probably because the oestrogenic first phase improved sperm penetrability when occasional women ovulated following the pill-free week (see Q 4.23).

Interestingly, however, older women are now frequently given a similar regimen of oestrogen alone, typically for 16 days, followed by oestrogen plus progestagen for 12 days. The oestrogen is, of course, a natural oestrogen, in doses which have a far smaller effect on the endometrium; and there is good evidence that these regimens do not increase the risk of endometrial cancer. But they are not safely contraceptive, the added progestagen may have disadvantages and for most fertile women a modified regimen which would be definitely contraceptive as well would be preferable. This whole matter is discussed further in Chapter 8.

4.10 What link is there between the COC cycle and the menstrual cycle?

Very little, but endless confusion is caused by the fact that women consider their hormone withdrawal bleeds as the same thing as 'periods'. In reality of course the normal menstrual cycle is removed during use of the COC. The ovaries show no follicular activity *during pill-taking* (contrast the situation between packets, see Q 4.15) and hence produce minimal endogenous oestrogen. Withdrawal bleeding (WTB) is an end-organ response to withdrawal of the artificial hormones, and is irrelevant to events elsewhere in the body and specifically at the pituitary and the ovaries. In physiological terms the pill causes secondary amenorrhoea for as long as the woman takes it – see Qs 4.49 and 4.50 for more about the benefits of the fact that the pill cycle and the menstrual cycle are so different.

Absence of WTB is totally irrelevant to future fertility, though a pregnancy test is indicated after two WTBs have been missed: sooner if there are good reasons to suspect pill-failure. Aside from pregnancy-testing, it is pointless to investigate this, by measuring prolactin for example (but not so if galactorrhoea present, Q 4.214).

Breakthrough bleeding (BTB) is likewise a purely endometrial response, but it may be heavy enough to simulate a 'period' to the woman. This also needs explaining in advance as a reason to continue taking her daily pills with extra diligence, rather than stopping.

Lack of adequate instruction about WTB and BTB commonly causes avoidable 'iatrogenic' pregnancies (see Q 8.16).

4.11 What is the importance of the pill-free interval (PFI)?

Enormous – yet it is still not explained in most pill leaflets or by many prescribers. It influences all the following issues:

1 the *efficacy* of the COC, in that lengthening of the PFI risks ovulation whereas mid-packet pill omissions are unimportant;

2 the improved *recommendations* once pills are omitted or vomited; short- or long-term use of *interacting drugs* or use of the pill if past 'breakthrough pregnancies' have occurred;

3 the minimizing of *health–risks*;

4 and, possibly, even the *reversibility* of the pill method.

All these points will be expanded in the next group of questions.

EFFECTIVENESS OF THE COC – CIRCUMSTANCES IN WHICH IT MAY BE REDUCED: INCLUDING DRUG INTERACTIONS

4.12 What is the efficacy of the COC?

The simple answer is in the range of 0.1–3/100 woman-years (see Fig. 0.2). The higher figure includes some degree of non-compliance (major degrees can boost the failure rate considerably – some studies range up to 7/100 woman-years); the lower figure may not be reducible (with present doses and regimens) because of individual variation in absorption and metabolism.

The theoretical effectiveness approaches 100%, partly because of the adjunctive mechanisms mentioned above (see Q 4.4). However it does appear that for some women the modern (less than 50 μg oestrogen) pills are only just sufficient for efficacy, particularly if omitted tablets lead to the slightest lengthening of the pill-free week. I argue below that in a few susceptible women this time may not be capable of lengthening by even a few hours with impunity. Minor errors of compliance are extremely common, and most women are uninformed about the critical importance of not lengthening the pill-free time. The slightly higher pregnancy rate with modern pills is thus explained chiefly in terms of 'reduced margin for error' plus, regrettably, lack of sufficient pill teaching by health care professionals who are often themselves poorly informed.

4.13 What is the effect of increasing age on efficacy?

The Oxford/Family Planning Association (FPA) study shows the (slight) expected decline in pregnancy rate with increasing age, due mainly to declining fertility and perhaps also some reduction in the frequency of intercourse (see Table 0.2 and Q 0.13).

4.14 Are overweight women more likely to conceive while taking modern ultra-low-dose COCs?

No. This has not been demonstrated, although it would be expected pharmacologically, since a 100-kg woman receives exactly the same dose in normal pill-taking as her 50-kg friend. Moreover *there is a definite weight influence on the efficacy of some progestagen-only methods* (see Q 5.13). My own belief is that the combined pill is so very strong as a contraceptive, for almost all women, that other factors like compliance errors produce too much 'noise' in an electronic sense for the expected effect of body mass to emerge. (The latter is more detectable perhaps if a systemic method has a method-failure rate above 1/100 woman-years.)

4.15 Since it is the contraceptive-free part of the pill-taking cycle, does not the PFI have efficacy implications?

Precisely. When you think about it, as few have since the pill was devised, we have here a bizarre contraceptive: one that we providers actually instruct the users *not* to use – for 25 % of the time. Any systemic contraceptive must be at its lowest ebb when it is longest since it was actually ingested (Fig. 4.1). Hardly surprisingly, biochemical and ultrasound data demonstrate varying degrees of return of pituitary and ovarian follicular activity during the pill-free time.

Figure 4.2 displays the findings from a 1979 study based on patients attending the Margaret Pyke Centre (MPC). It is the rapid

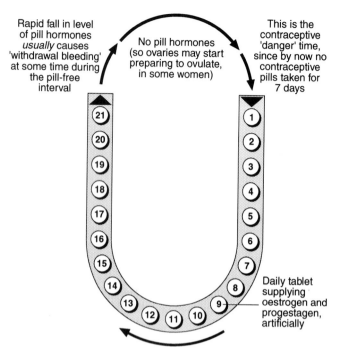

Figure 4.1 The pill cycle displayed as a horseshoe. Q 4.15.
Note: a horseshoe is a symmetrical object. Hence the pill-free interval can be lengthened, leading to the risk of conception, either side of the horseshoe, by forgetting pills either at the beginning or at the end of the packet

decline shown in the artificial hormones which leads to the withdrawal bleed (WTB). But the figure is mainly included to display the slight average increase in plasma oestradiol, implying regular return of ovarian follicular activity during the pill-free week. Wide standard deviations are also shown, meaning that in some women the levels are high – indeed as high as has been observed well into the follicular phase of spontaneous menstrual cycles. In a more recent MPC study, apparently preovulatory-type follicles of diameter 10 mm or more were present on the seventh pill-free day in 23% of 120 pill-takers; in three women the follicle was 16–19 mm in diameter (i.e. potentially only 2 or 3 days from fertile ovulation). In the other women there was no important change, suggesting continuing quiescence of their ovaries.

The pill-free week

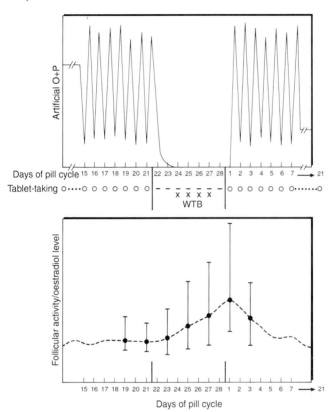

Days of pill cycle: 15 16 17 18 19 20 21 | 22 23 24 25 26 27 28 | 1 2 3 4 5 6 7 ⟶ 21

Tablet-taking: O····O O O O O O O | – – – – – – | O O O O O O O·······O
                                        x x x x
                                         WTB

Figure 4.2 The hormone changes of the pill-free week. Q 4.15 and following. Changes through the pill-taking cycle in the blood levels of both the ingested artificial hormones (oestrogen (O) and progestagen (P)), and in follicular activity as demonstrated by growth of the dominant follicle by ultrasound. WTB = withdrawal bleeding. Note the rapid return to low ovarian activity during the first 7 days of pill-taking. (From a study of patients attending the Margaret Pyke Centre)

However, for the purpose of maintaining contraception we have to be concerned about the extreme cases.* Among them, breakthrough ovulation is most likely to follow any lengthening of the

---

* Indeed in some women this may happen from time to time without any omitted pills lengthening the pill-free week, explaining rare failures of the COC despite perfect compliance. Women with such a past history should be told to eliminate/shorten the gap between the pill packets as described at Q 4.24.

PFI. Most important, such lengthening may result from omissions, malabsorption due to vomiting, and drug interaction involving pills *either at the start or at the end of a packet*. See the legend to Figure 4.1: pill-taking is depicted by a horseshoe because a horseshoe is a symmetrical object.

4.16 So what advice should we give when pills are missed for any reason?

Clearly the advice which is still given in some package inserts, to take extra precautions to the end of her packet, is wrong: it fails to allow for ovarian activity returning in the pill-free time. In a fascinating study of previously regular pill-takers, it was shown in 1986 that even if only 14 or even as few as seven pills had been taken since the last PFI, no women ovulated after seven pills were subsequently missed! (One in the seven pills group produced progesterone, however, albeit at non-fertile levels.) This and other work may be summarized by three propositions:

1 Seven consecutive pills are enough to 'put the ovaries to sleep'. (Therefore pills 8–21 in a packet simply 'keep them asleep'.)

2 Seven pills can be omitted without ovulation, as indeed is regularly the case in the pill-free week.

3 More than seven pills missed *in total* risks ovulation.

The 7-day 'Rule', as used by the UK FPA and also now agreed by the UK manufacturers, is based on this pharmacology and can be conveyed in a simple algorithm (Fig. 4.3). If 28-day packaging is used the woman must be carefully taught which are the dummy 'reminder' tablets, for omission if she misses any of the last seven active pills. All women should be asked to return for the exclusion of pregnancy if they have no bleeding in the *next* PFI.

How does the advice conveyed in Figure 4.3 apply in various categories of pill omissions?

4.17 It is easy to see from Figures 4.1 and 4.2 that missing pills at the start of a packet, lengthening the contraception-free time to more than 7 days, could well be 'bad news!' But what about omitted pills in the *middle* of a packet?

Tablets *omitted following on prior tablet-taking for 7 or more days*, and not followed by a PFI, are very low risk omissions for breakthrough ovulation. If we allow for the one woman who

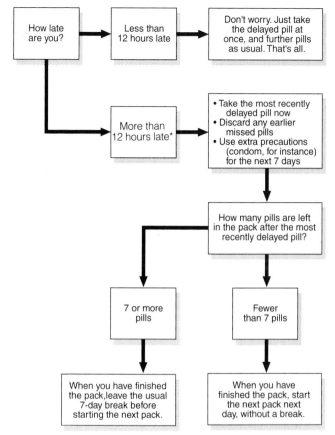

Figure 4.3 Management of missed pills. Q 4.16 (*with one pill or more)

The flowchart contains the following boxes:

How late are you?

Less than 12 hours late → Don't worry. Just take the delayed pill at once, and further pills as usual. That's all.

More than 12 hours late* →
- Take the most recently delayed pill now
- Discard any earlier missed pills
- Use extra precautions (condom, for instance) for the next 7 days

How many pills are left in the pack after the most recently delayed pill?

7 or more pills → When you have finished the pack, leave the usual 7-day break before starting the next pack.

Fewer than 7 pills → When you have finished the pack, start the next pack next day, without a break.

nearly ovulated and the small numbers in the study just quoted in Q 4.16: once seven tablets have been taken, at the very least up to four pills may be missed mid-packet with impunity!

Yet because of a wrong analogy with the normal menstrual cycle, *unless we prescribers re–educate them*, patients worry most about missed pills when it matters least, in mid-packet. They rarely even seek advice when pill omissions or a stomach upset have led to a lengthening of the pill-free time, or (at the end of a pack) will go on to do so. The former is the most serious situation of all but not seen as such: *'I just started my pack a bit late!'*

4.18 What are the implications of late-packet pill omissions?

If a woman omits two or three tablets at the end of her preceding packet and is allowed to recommence the next packet on her usual starting day (something she is sure to do, unless otherwise instructed), there will be an ovulation risk at the end of the thereby lengthened pill-free time, after what is a *falsely reassuring with-drawal bleed*. One consequence: any questioning later on about missed pills, perhaps in the antenatal clinic, must include asking about missed pills *before* the *last menstrual period* (LMP)!

A useful way of explaining the situation to an ordinary pill-taker is to say that missing pills at the end of a packet is like making her pill-free break early by mistake, so it would be a bit silly to add on the regular break on top. If instead she follows the scheme in Figure 4.3 and does go straight to the next packet, she will actually be more protected than usual – provided she has missed anything less than the usual seven tablets of the PFI!

4.19 How can the advice be simplified when faced with individual women who have missed two pills (a) near the end of a packet? or (b) after 7 pills have been taken mid-packet?

The recommendations of Figure 4.3 above are in my view still preferred for their general applicability and to avoid confusion *in the written word*. However, ideally the latter should also say something like: 'There are some situations in which your doctor may say that 7 days' condom use are not required.' This is because, face to face with the pill-takers mentioned: the first at (a) must start the next packet at once, but aside from that *neither* (a) nor (b) need actually take the 7 days of extra contraceptive precautions.

After all, having had only a 2-day PFI the first woman is actually less likely to conceive than in a normal pill-cycle!

4.20 What other 'rules' for missed pills are there which my patient may have read or been taught? Which are scientifically acceptable?

1 The 'take precautions to the end-of-packet rule' is probably commonest and is delightfully *simple*; but sadly (see Q 4.18) it is also 'dangerously' *wrong* for missed pills near the end of a pack!

2 The 'take precautions for the next 14 days, whatever happens' advice is acceptable; since the *second* 7 days of the fortnight does

cover the time of ovulation risk at the end of a PFI that has been lengthened by missed pills just before it (i.e. near the end of a pack). But, in practice, many men as well as women see use of the unpopular sheath method as pointless just after what they (falsely!) see as a reassuring 'period'!

We of course know that the ovary can easily be ovulating in synchrony with the endometrium bleeding, since that happens only because of exogenous hormone withdrawal....

3 In the USA, the FDA has in 1992 mandated a variation of the advice conveyed in Figure 4.3 for missed or not absorbed tablets from the last seven. This instructs: 'Throw out the rest of that pill pack and start a new packet with pill number one today.' This is scientifically valid. It also helps users of 'everyday' packaging, who can get muddled about the dummy pills to be omitted. They only have to be clearly instructed about which is their Day 1 pill. But this variant is slightly wasteful and leads to a (possibly muddling) change in that woman's start day for the future.

4.21 If a woman has missed several tablets, what are the indications for emergency (postcoital) contraception (see Q 7.5)?

Almost everything depends on *when* they were missed. The advice summarized in Figure 4.3 will be quite sufficient in every situation except when two or more tablets have been missed from the first seven at the start of packet: in such a manner as to *effectively* lengthen the PFI to 9 plus days. Then, and almost only then, postcoital contraception is justified (see Q 7.18), since the woman might happen to be one of the 23% described in Q 4.15.

For almost all mid-packet and late-packet (day 7–21) pill omissions postcoital treatment would be over-treatment. I suppose it might just be appropriate if intercourse took place after 4 or more had been forgotten or vomited....

4.22 What advice for vomiting and diarrhoea?

If the vomiting started less than 3 hours after a pill was swallowed and continues so a replacement tablet will not stay down, extra contraceptive precautions should start from the onset of the illness. They should continue for 7 days after it ends, along with elimination of the subsequent PFI as indicated above and by Figure 4.3.

Diarrhoea alone is not a problem, unless it is of cholera-like severity!

4.23 Surely the above discussion of the PFI takes too little account of the adjunctive contraceptive effects (see Q 4.4)?

Actually, these do not change the argument about the PFI. The most important extra effect is probably the progestagenic reduction in sperm penetrability of cervical mucus. But this too will be at its lowest ebb at the end of any PFI which has been lengthened: obviously, since it is then as long as is possible since progestagen was last ingested.

But the pills in the forthcoming pack should be able to operate usefully by their anti-implantation effect on the endometrium, despite a lengthening of the PFI.

4.24 Pending the marketing of packets with a shortened PFI, what is the best regimen for women who have had a previous combined pill failure?

Some of these may claim perfect compliance, others will admit to the complete omission of no more than one pill. Either way, since surveys show that most women miss tablets from time to time but very few conceive, the ability to do so *selects out those who are likely to have ovaries with above average return to activity in the PFI*. So all women in this group should in my view be advised to take three packets in a row, the so-called tricycle regimen (see Q 4.28 and Fig. 4.4), followed by a shortened pill-free gap. Often 6 days is a good choice in these cases since it is easy to remember, with each tricycle's start day now being identical to the finish-day – but the gap may be shortened even further in a 'high risk' case (see Q 4.33).

Tricycling is surely more logical than the reaction of many doctors after a woman conceives on the pill, a summary of which is 'read her the Riot Act about better pill-taking and give her the same one as before!' Even giving her a stronger formulation may be of less relevance.

4.25 Aren't there other disadvantages to taking a PFI?

Yes: in summary, *the 'cons' of the PFI are*:

1 Makes the COC method *less effective*.

2 The *withdrawal bleeds* can be heavy or perceived as a nuisance.

3 In some women *migraines* or other types of *headache* most often occur in the PFI, triggered by hormone withdrawal.

4 On theoretical grounds, compared with the normal cycle, it is 'unphysiological' to have a whole week with almost no oestrogen circulating (in the majority with quiescent ovaries, that is, not the one-quarter who start producing their own).

4.26 With all those snags, why do we continue to recommend the PFI to anyone?

Because one can list quite a few 'pros' as well:

1 Many women like monthly bleeds to reassure 'that all is normal', and that they are not pregnant, more frequently than every 10 weeks as in tricycling. Explaining pill physiology can overcome this objection in cases where tricycling is indicated.

2 Avoids the complaint of bloatedness and a premenstrual syndrome which some experience through the last weeks of a tricycle.

3 May avoid the breakthrough spotting which sometimes occurs, especially with low dose pills during the last packet of a tricycle sequence.

4 Tricycle regimens do entail taking more tablets per year: 15–16 packets rather than the 13 when a regular PFI is taken. This increase in the hormone dose taken runs counter to the general philosophy of giving the lowest dose of both hormones (see Q 4.140) for the desired effect.

5 One has to remember that all data generated from epidemiological studies about the (great) safety and the (remarkable) reversibility of the COC have been gained from women who *were* taking regular monthly breaks. So it might be best to stay with that concept for most pill-takers. In confirmation of that view:

6 In one study HDL-cholesterol suppression (see Q 4.92) by the COCs in use was restored to normal by the end of the PFI. In a major study now being analysed at MPC, if this phenomenon is duplicated for other important substances, then the PFI might prove to have a special value for homeostasis – allowing regularly some degree of recovery from systemic effects of the pill.

None of the above is strong argument against shortening the PFI, of course (see Q 4.8)

4.27 What do you conclude, given the advantages of the PFI?

A It can be useful to point out to a woman who wants to continue with the method but 'someone has suggested' that she ought to 'take a break' from the pill after 10 years' use, that she has already taken 130 breaks.... Or, put another way, she has really only taken it for 7$^{1}/_{2}$ years!

B With the above list of 'pros' it would seem wise only to cut out the gap between packets when there are good indications. In the short term this can be done upon request if the woman wishes to avoid a 'period' on special occasions like honeymoons – see Q 4.163 and Figure 4.12 for the procedure if a phasic brand is in use. In the long term there are several special indications as in Table 4.2 for eliminating the PFI, so the tricycling regimen is then preferred: see Q 4.28 and Figure 4.4.

4.28 Given all those pros and cons of the PFI, what is the tricycle pill regimen, and when is it indicated?

First, the regimen has nothing to do with triphasic pills. Indeed it necessitates use of *monophasic* pills – which are simply run together, three packets in a row, followed by a PFI of the selected length (either 7 days, or less if the indication is primarily to increase

Table 4.2 Indications for the tricycle regimen (using a monophasic pill)

1	*Headaches* including non-focal migraine, and other bothersome symptoms occurring regularly in the withdrawal week (see Q 4.25)
2	*Unacceptable* heavy or painful *withdrawal bleeds*
3	Paradoxically, to help women who are concerned about *absent withdrawal bleeds* (this concern and the nuisance of pregnancy testing therefore arising less often!)
4	*Epilepsy:* this benefits from relatively more sustained levels of the administered hormones (see also Q 4.33 for reason related to some antiepileptic treatments which are enzyme inducers).
5	*Endometriosis* – a progestogen-dominant monophasic pill may be tricycled, for maintenance treatment after primary therapy (see Q 4.99)
6	*Suspicion of decreased efficacy* (see Q 4.24)
7	*At the woman's choice.*

Note: In view of the possibility that the monthly pill-free interval has health benefits (see Q 4.26), one of these special indications should normally apply.

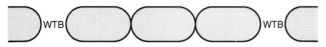

Figure 4.4 Tricycling a monophasic COC. Q 4.28
Note: must be monophasic packs. WTB = withdrawal bleeding

the method's efficacy, see below). See Figure 4.4. Three packets without a break, giving a 10-week cycle, is usually better tolerated than the four in a row which were previously advised. This will produce about five WTBs or, if the indication is headaches, only five bad headaches per year – instead of the usual 13!

Why tricycle? Table 4.2 summarizes the indications, some of which are discussed in more detail elsewhere.

4.29 What is the significance of BTB or spotting after the first pack during 'tricycling'?

If it occurs during the second or third packet in a woman who had no BTB problems with 21-day pill-taking, and *if none of the explanations in Table 4.12 (see Q 4.148) applies*, then it is most likely to be an 'end- organ' effect. In other words, the current formulation is proving to be incapable of maintaining this woman's endometrium beyond a certain duration of continuous pill-taking, i.e. without the 'physiological curettage' of a WTB. Though we lack data, it is my belief that this is less likely to be due to low blood levels of the contraceptive steroids than when BTB occurs in the other circumstances discussed at Qs 4.143–4.155. Therefore the first step, if this is a problem to the woman, is to try 'bicycling' (two packets in a row) rather than to use a stronger pill.

4.30 What is the enterohepatic cycle?

See Figure 4.5. After pill ingestion, the progestogens are 80–100% bioavailable from the upper small bowel, but ethinyloestradiol (EE) is subject to extensive 'first-pass' metabolism, chiefly by being conjugated with sulphate in the gut wall. After absorption the artificial oestrogen and progestagen are carried in the hepatic portal vein to the liver. Liver metabolism then, or later after the steroids have been transported around the body, creates metabolites of both steroids. The liver mostly forms glucuronides. Once these conjugates re-enter the lumen of the bowel, the bowel flora (chiefly *Clostridia* species) are able to remove the sulphate and glucuronide groups. This restores some EE for reabsorption and may help in some women to maintain its level in the circulation.

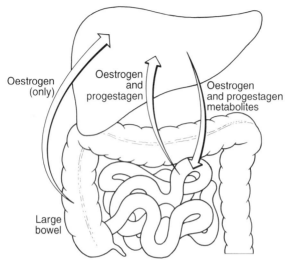

Figure 4.5 The enterohepatic circulation. Q 4.30 and following.
Note: the progestagen does not recirculate

However in the case of all the artificial progestagens in current use, the progestagenic metabolite which is reabsorbed after the action of the bowel organisms is biologically inactive. This has the important implication that *broad–spectrum antibiotics can have no effect on the efficacy of the POP* (see Q 5.10).

Moreover, according to the Liverpool workers, both studies in women with an ileostomy and formal studies with relevant antibiotics suggest that in the vast majority of COC-takers the recycling even of the oestrogen seems to be unimportant for maintaining efficacy. They agree however that, since we do not know which few individuals might be affected by antibiotics which destroy the relevant bowel flora, it is best to play safe as described at Q 4.32.

4.31 What is the effect on pill efficacy of DRUG INTERACTIONS linked with the enteroheratic cycle?

These may reduce the pill's efficacy mainly in two ways.

1 The first and by far the more important mechanism is by *induction of liver enzymes*, which leads to increased metabolism and thus elimination in the bile of both oestrogen and progestagen. (See Fig. 4.5 and Table 4.3.) Note that *valproate, clon-*

azepam, clobazam and, fortunately, the *newly marketed antiepileptics* (including vigabatrin, lamotrigine, but check the Data Sheets) *are not enzyme inducers.*

2   Alternatively, disturbance by certain *broad-spectrum antibiotics* (the clinically relevant ones are listed in Table 4.3) of the gut flora which normally split oestrogen metabolites arriving in the bowel can reduce the reabsorption of reactivated oestrogen, in a very small – but unknown – minority of women. Note that:

   (a) This problem does not relate to drugs used to prevent or treat *malaria*, to narrow-spectrum antibiotics like penicillin V nor to co-trimoxazole or erythromycin. In fact the last two products inhibit liver metabolism (see Table 4.3).

   (b) The effect only *applies to short-term antibiotic treatment*; or in long-term therapy *at the time of change to a new antibiotic.* This is because the bowel flora rapidly develop antibiotic resistance, within less than about 2 weeks.

Antibiotic-related *diarrhoea* is unlikely to be a problem, since any diarrhoea has to be 'cholera-like' before absorption is affected.

4.32 What should be advised during short-term use of any interacting drug – or the long term use of a broad-spectrum antibiotic?

If for example *griseofulvin* is to be used (up to say 6 weeks – if longer, see Q 4.33) in the treatment of a cutaneous fungal infection, extra contraceptive precautions are advised for the duration of the treatment. This should be followed by the '7-day rule' as Figure 4.3 above, with omission of the next PFI according to when in the pill packet the last potentially less effective pill was taken.

Rifampicin is such a powerful enzyme inducer that even if it be *given only for 2 days* (as for instance to eliminate carriage of the meningococcus), *increased elimination by the liver must be assumed for 4 weeks thereafter.* Extra contraception with elimination of the relevant one or two PFIs should be recommended to cover that time.

With *broad-spectrum antibiotics* there is that useful fact that the large bowel flora responsible for recycling oestrogens are reconstituted with resistant organisms in about 2 weeks. In practice therefore, if the COC is commenced in a woman who has been taking a tetracycline long term (e.g. for acne), there is no need to advise extra contraceptive precautions. There is a potential – but now believed to be small – problem only in the reverse situation, when the tetracycline is first introduced to treat a long-term

Table 4.3 The more important drug interactions with COCs

Class of drug	Approved names of important examples	Main action	Clinical implications for COC use
Drug which may reduce COC efficacy			
Anticonvulsants	Barbiturates (esp. phenobarbitone) Phenytoin Primidone Carbamazepine	Induction of liver enzymes, increasing their ability to metabolize *both* COC steroids	Tricycling preferred, using 50 µg oestrogen COCs, increasing to max 100 µg if BTB occurs. *Sodium valproate* and *clonazepam* are among anticonvulsants *without* this effect (Q 4.31)
Antibiotics (a) Antitubercle	Rifampicin	*Marked* induction of liver enzymes	Short term, see text. Long term, use of alternative contraception is preferred, e.g. DMPA with 8-week injection intervals (see Q 5.89)
(b) Antifungal (c) Broad spectrum	Griseofulvin Ampicillin and relatives Tetracyclines Cephalosporins	Enzyme inducer Change in bowel flora, reducing enterohepatic recirculation of ethinyloestradiol (EE) only, after hydrolysis of its conjugates	As for anticonvulsants Short courses – wisest to use additional contraception during illness and follow 7-day rule Long-term low-dose tetracycline for acne – no apparent problem, probably because resistant organisms develop, within about 2 weeks. POP is unaffected by this type of interaction
Diuretic Hypnotics Tranquillizers	Spironolactone Dichloralphenazone Meprobamate	Induction of liver enzymes probable	Avoid these drugs in COC-users (alternatives available)
Drugs which may increase COC efficacy			
	Ascorbic acid Paracetamol	Competition in bowel wall for conjugation to sulphate. If either of these drugs present, more EE available for absorption	No effect on the progestagen Advise: at least 2 hours separation of either drug from the time of pill taking (latest research suggests this may be unnecessary)
	Co-trimoxazole	Inhibits (weakly) EE metabolism in liver	None, if short course given to low-dose COC-user
	Erythromycin Ketoconazole	*Potent* inhibitors of EE metabolism	Beware! Cholestasis described with similar inhibitor–troleandomycin– could be due to hepatic accumulation of EE

pill-taker. Even then, extra precautions need to be sustained only for 2 weeks plus 7 days, with elimination of the next PFI if the first 2 weeks' antibiotic use extended into the last 7 days of a pack.

4.33 What if enzyme inducer(s) need to be prescribed long term?

1 *Rifampicin.* This is such a potent enzyme inducer that in some women a five-fold increase in the rate of metabolism of the COC was seen by the researchers in Liverpool. So they recommend alternative methods of contraception for long-term users of rifampicin and that the COC be avoided altogether, even in the higher dose tricycling regimen which is described below. Fortunately the main COC hormone affected is EE, so the injectable progestagen Depot medroxyprogesterone acetate (DMPA – see Q 5.80) is a good choice. Even then it is important to compensate for the enzyme induction by shortening the injection interval: 10 weeks would be usual but if rifampicin is the drug, 8 weeks is contraceptively safer (instead of the usual 12).

2 *Other long–term enzyme–inducers – mainly anticonvulsant thera-pies.* Here too an alternative method of contraception such as an intrauterine device (IUD) should first be seriously considered. DMPA may be a good choice (see Q 5.89), with a shortened injection interval, usually 10 weeks.

However, if the combined pill is preferred one may prescribe initially a 50 μg oestrogen-containing brand, of which only three remain on the market (Fig. 4.11, and see Q 4.34), and *also* recommend that the *tricycle regimen* described at Q 4.28 be used. This reduces the number of contraceptively 'risky' PFIs. It is particularly appropriate for epileptics since the frequency of attacks is often reduced by the maintenance of steady hormone levels. At the MPC we recommend that the woman also shortens the PFI at the end of each tricycle, arbitrarily to 4 days. A Diary card may help her in this, but the main thing is to explain that her 'period' (withdrawal bleed) will tend to continue into the start of the next pack.

4.34 What if it seems more appropriate to use one of the 'third-generation' progestagens (gestodene, desogestrel, norgestimate) for an epileptic pill-taker?

Since as yet (and regrettably) no 50 μg preparations are marketed, I consider it would be appropriate in selected cases to prescribe two sub 50 μg pills a day, e.g. one Marvelon plus one Mercilon 20 from the desogestrel 'ladder' (see Q 4.136 and Fig. 4.10). But if so the grounds must be good and record-keeping meticulous, since the manufacturer is unlikely to support this use of the product should a serious problem arise.

4.35 What may signal the need to consider an important drug interaction, or the need for a stronger pill?

Having excluded other causes (see Q 4.148), BTB may be the first clue to a drug interaction, and may also be used as an indication to *consider* increasing the dose or to advise a change of method. If the long-term user of an enzyme-inducing drug develops BTB on the COC, the first step is to give two or more tablets a day, if necessary to provide a combined oestrogen content of 80 or 100 μg (maximum), titrated against the BTB.

4.36 How can one explain all this to a woman, that she is not receiving a 'dangerously' strong pill regimen?

Explain that this is only the usual policy, described more fully at Qs 4.140–8, of giving the minimum dose of both hormones to finish just above the threshold for bleeding. Reassure her that she is metaphorically 'climbing a down escalator'. In other words her increased liver metabolism means that her system is still basically receiving a low-dose regimen while she is taking a 50 μg tablet (or even two per day as indicated). She is exposed to more metabolites, but this is not believed to be harmful.

4.37 Can a woman go straight back to the normal dose and regimen when enzyme inducers are stopped?

No: it may be 4 or more weeks before the liver's level of excretory function reverts to normal. Hence if any enzyme inducer has been used for a month or more (or *at all* in the case of rifampicin) it is therefore recommended by Professor Michael Orme of Liverpool that there is a delay of about 4 weeks before the woman returns to the standard low-dose pill regimen. This delay should be increased to 8 weeks after more prolonged use of established enzyme inducers. And logically there should then be no gap between the higher- and the low-dose packets (see Q 4.45 and Table 4.4).

4.38 What are the implications of long-term antibiotic treatment in women suffering from acne or (for example) cystic fibrosis?

On long-term antibiotics and when first starting oral contraception – no problem as discussed above (see Q 4.31–2). On oral contraception, when first starting antibiotics, or *when switching to a new broad–spectrum antibiotic* – here the counsel of perfection would be to use an additional method such as the sheath for the first 2 weeks to permit antibiotic resistance to develop (see Q 4.31). In practice these precautions are frequently not observed and breakthrough pregnancies resulting from this mechanism seem extremely uncommon.

4.39 What about anion-exchange resins like cholestyramine, or guar gum which is sometimes used to treat postprandial reactive hypoglycaemia? Might they impair absorption?

Yes, this is possible. It is therefore recommended that they are taken at least 2 hours after or 4 hours before the pill, or any other oral drug.

4.40 What effect does vitamin C have on pill absorption, and paracetamol?

Mega-dose *ascorbic acid* treatment (0.5–1 g daily) is of unproven value, though adequate amounts may be beneficial because of its antioxidant properties. The small problem here is that it competes with EE in the bowel wall for conjugation to sulphate. Hence less EE conjugation occurs and more is available for absorption. This could result in the woman receiving more oestrogen than planned, though a recent study suggests this may not occur with 30 µg pills (*cf* earlier 50 µg brands). The rebound ovulation risk on stopping the vitamin C is now also more theoretical than real.

Paracetamol similarly competes with EE metabolism in the gut. So *if a pill–taker takes either vitamin C or paracetamol on a regular basis the simple solution is to ensure each is always taken at least 2 hours earlier or later than the time of pill-taking.*

4.41 Are any of the interactions in which COCs affect the metabolism of other drugs of any clinical significance?

Oral contraceptive (OC) steroids are inhibitors of hepatic microsomal enzymes. So they may lower the clearance of diazepam, prednisolone, cyclosporin and some other drugs – including according to some reports (but not others), alcohol. Only the enhanced toxicity of cyclosporin is important clinically; the others are unlikely to be noticed.

Warfarin. COCs inhibit this drug's metabolism to a variable extent, and also and independently alter clotting factors. Thus the interaction is unpredictable. The combination would need very careful monitoring – and would usually be avoided.

As COCs tend to impair glucose tolerance, sometimes cause depression and may raise blood pressure, they naturally tend to oppose the (pharmacodynamic) actions of antidiabetic, antidepressant and antihypertensive treatments, respectively. This type of effect is easily compensated by monitoring dose/response of the other drug.

4.42 What else, apart from treating my patient well, should I do if I suspect a drug interaction of any type?

Practitioners who do detect possible drug interactions are asked to continue the practice of completing a yellow card for the Committee on Safety of Medicines.

4.43 Should women with an ileostomy or colostomy avoid hormonal contraception for fear of absorption problems, or be given a stronger brand than usual?

No, this is definitely unnecessary because the loose motions signify nothing about absorptive mechanisms in their upper small bowel, which ought to be unimpaired. Despite the interference in the enterohepatic cycle the bioavailability of EE as well as the progestogens was not detectably altered in studies by the Liverpool workers.

In reality, even when most of the rest of the bowel is absent, the jejunum is so efficient at absorbing sex steroid hormones that malabsorption and diarrhoea are very rarely the cause of reduced bioavailability. (See Q 4.44 and also Q 4.148 (*re* BTB).)

4.44 Does coeliac disease impair absorption of the COC?

No. Paradoxically, while this disease is active, the diminished function of the gut wall leads to less sulphation of absorbed EE (see Q 4.40 above). So more bioactive EE is absorbed than usual! Once coeliac disease is successfully treated absorption is normal.

4.45 What factors need consideration in devising starting routines for the COC?

1 First and foremost, some women with short cycles may ovulate early in the second week of the menstrual cycle. Hence the value of the Day 1 start. (First timers may usefully be warned that their first 'period' will come on after only about 23 days.)

2 After a first trimester pregnancy has ended, the earliest fertile ovulation seems to occur no earlier than at 12 days.

3 After a full-term pregnancy (in the absence of breastfeeding) the earliest possible fertile ovulation has been shown biochemically at around day 28. However, starting too early has to be avoided because of evidence that the oestrogen in the combined pill can increase the risk of puerperal thromboembolism. The coagulation factor changes of pregnancy are largely reversed by 2 weeks. So for most women a start date of Day 21 is appropriate. This should be further delayed in those at highest risk of any form of thrombosis, including the obese and after *severe pregnancy-related hypertension*, with alternative contraception for 7 days if the pill is therefore started beyond Day 21.

4 These and my other recommendations, which differ very slightly from those of the FPA, are summarized in Table 4.4.

Contraception after pregnancy. This important subject is discussed in much more detail at Qs 8.17–8.32: including, when there is amenorrhoea, how *not* to commence use of a new medical method (IUD, injectable or pill) when an implantation has already occurred (see Q 8.21).

A point to mention here is that, after excluding pregnancy during amenorrhoea, the COC may often best be started on the next Sunday (plus 7 days additional precautions); this avoids future bleeds at weekends. (See Q 4.46.)

4.46 Can I help my patients to avoid WTB at weekends?

Yes, but only if you think to discuss the point! With the above starting routines, depending on the weekday their first period happens to start and the length of their WTB, up to half of all menstruating women will bleed during part of one weekend in every four . . . . This is completely unnecessary!

Starting on the first Sunday of the next period is one option. This is popular in the USA, but must be combined with extra precautions for 7 days. Otherwise, at any time during follow-up

Table 4.4 Starting routines for the COC combined oral contraceptive

		Start when?	Extra precautions for 7 days?
1	Menstruating	Day 1 Day 2 Day 3 or later	No* No** YES**
2	Postpartum (a) No lactation	Day 21 (low risk of thrombosis by then, first ovulations reported day 28+)	No
	(b) Lactation	Not normally recommended at all (POP preferred)	
3	Post-induced early abortion/miscarriage	Same day or next day to avoid postoperative vomiting risk	No
4	Post-trophoblastic tumour	1 month after no hCG detected	As 1
5	Post-higher or same dose COC	Instant switch†	No
6	Post-lower dose COC	After usual 7-day break	No
7	Post-POP	First day of period	No
8	Post-POP with secondary amenorrhoea	Any day (Sunday? see Q 4.46)	No
9	Other secondary amenorrhoea (*pregnancy excluded,* see Q 8.21)	Any day (Sunday? see Q 4.46)	YES
10	First cycle after postcoital contraception (see Q 7.33)	1st day/or by day 2 when sure flow normal	No

* 14 days' extra precautions if Logynon ED or Femodene ED (see Q 4.7).

** Delay into day 2 may help, to be sure a period is normal. For later starts, up to the old routine day 5, I advise extra precautions for the 7 days which seemingly make any ovary quiescent (Q 4.16). The same can apply beyond day 5 (i.e. *not* waiting for that elusive next period) *if* the prescriber is sure there has been no risk of conception.

† This advice is because of reports of rebound ovulation occurring at the time of transfer.

you can simply advise up to five additional tablets from a spare pack to *shift the finishing day* to a Saturday or Sunday, thereby ensuring that the bleed will be completed during the next Monday–Friday.

4.47 Which studies have provided our present information about the wanted and unwanted effects of the COC?

There have been many case-control studies, but much of the most useful data has been generated by the cohort studies. Statements made in this book are based wherever possible on congruence of the findings of all the studies, by different investigators in different populations.

1 The Royal College of General Practitioners' (RCGP) Study. In brief 23 000 married pill users were recruited from the practices of 1400 GPs and matched (only for age) with a similar number of married control women not using the COC. The GPs informed the study coordinators of all subsequent medical effects, based on every surgery attendance or hospital referral for in- or outpatient care (including for pregnancy). Ex-users have been similarly followed up.

2 In the same year, 1968, Vessey launched the *Oxford/FPA Study*, which has similarly followed a total of over 17 000 clinic attenders since that time. In this study, users of different reversible methods of contraception act as controls for each other; 56% used oral contraceptives at the outset, compared with 25% who were diaphragm-users and 19% who were fitted with an IUD.

3 *The Walnut Creek Study*. This is a white middle-class area near San Franscisco, California, in which the Kaiser Permanente Health Insurance Scheme operates. Members of the scheme have an examination on entering, and all the health records are cross-linked and computerized. A total of 16 579 women were followed up over 12 years from 1968. As in the RCGP study the health of the COC users was compared with that of control subjects who were using other methods (unrecorded) or no method of birth control.

4 *The Nurses' Health Study*. In 1976, 121 700 female registered nurses in the USA completed a mailed questionnaire including items relevant primarily to risk of cancer and circulatory disease. Every 2 years follow-up questionnaires are sent, to update the risk factor data and to ascertain any major medical events.

The completeness of the follow-up in the last three of the above studies is exemplary: e.g. for fatal outcomes, ascertainment in the Nurses' study runs at about 98%.

4.48 What are the strengths and deficiencies of the main cohort studies?

They have the strengths of similar prospective epidemiological studies, particularly with regard to the completeness of data collection over the years, and the possibility of assessment of non-comparability between the groups compared, and of biases. However, they share obvious weaknesses:

1 Random allocation was impossible, so pill-users are different from non-users in many important ways: in the Walnut Creek Study COC-users tended to be on average taller, more physically active, more likely to smoke or drink in moderation (though not more likely to be heavy smokers or heavy drinkers), to sunbathe more frequently, to have initiated sex earlier and to have had more partners than non-users.

2 All the studies tended to include fewer young women than are now normally found amongst a pill-using population, because the unmarried are so difficult to follow in long-term prospective studies. Most relevantly – especially *re* breast cancer – use of the method by teenagers was unusual when the studies commenced.

3 By 1985 a large number of initially recruited women had been lost to follow-up, mostly because they moved house. However, checks on the characteristics of a sample of the latter have not shown them to differ in such a way as to significantly bias the results.

4 By the time the cohort studies report, they are invariably providing information about yesterday's contraceptives. Nearly all the data generated by the studies relates to brands containing at least 50 μg of oestrogen, and often also more progestagen than now recommended. The ultra-low-dose COCs now widely used are likely to cause even less morbidity and mortality than the very low rates emerging from these studies, but this will take many more years to prove and one must not forget that the rates of beneficial effects may also be different.

5 So far epidemiology has proved too insensitive as a research tool to distinguish effectively between different formulations of the COC. Questions about brands used were not even asked in the

Nurses' Health Study. This is a serious deficiency, as although there is only one artificial oestrogen in common use there are many different progestagens, which also produce different metabolites. The rates of both adverse and beneficial effects could be very different by formulation. Although there are good data to show that we should give formulations with the lowest acceptable dose of both the oestrogen and progestagen, we remain unable to choose the 'best buy' among such pills on epidemiological grounds. (We are forced instead to use metabolic criteria of relatively unproven value – see Q 4.92.)

6 Epidemiology is also weak when it comes to assessing risk ratios only slightly in excess of or less than unity. An increase in the risk ratio for breast cancer in ex-pill-takers over 50 to say 1.3 might never be statistically significant. Yet a 30% increase in the rate of such a prevalent condition would be highly significant clinically!

7 Because of the low prevalence of use, we are unlikely ever to have useful epidemiological data on the side-effects of the POP.

8 It is more difficult to study beneficial than adverse relationships; the death that does not take place as a result of some protective effect is far more difficult to recognize than the one that is associated with COC use. However, good data are available for Q 4.49.

ADVANTAGES AND BENEFICIAL EFFECTS

4.49 What are the beneficial effects of the COC?

These can be listed as follows:

Contraceptive

1 Highly effective – and the regular withdrawal bleeds give regular reassurance of that fact.

2 Highly convenient, non-intercourse-related.

3 Reversible – see Qs 4.54 and 4.55.

Non-contraceptive – Mainly gynaecological

4 A reduction in the rate of most disorders of the menstrual cycle:
   (a) less heavy bleeding; therefore
   (b) less anaemia;

(c) less dysmenorrhoea;

(d) regular bleeding, and timing can be controlled (see Qs 4.238 and 4.239);

(e) less symptoms of premenstrual tension overall (see Q 4.99);

(f) no ovulation pain.

5 Less pelvic inflammatory disease (PID) (see Q 4.52).

6 Less extrauterine pregnancies – since ovulation is inhibited: and as a long-term result of 5.

7 Less benign breast disease (see Q 4.82).

8 Less functional ovarian cysts (see Q 4.53).

9 Less need for hospital treatment due to bleeding from or size of fibroids (see Q 4.82)

10 A beneficial effect on some cancers, notably carcinoma of the endometrium and epithelial cancers of the ovary (see Qs 4.67 and 4.68).

Miscellaneous

11 Less sebaceous disorders (only with selected oestrogen-dominant COCs) (see Q 4.220).

12 No acute toxicity if overdose is taken: only vomiting, and in prepubertal girls the likelihood of WTB a week or so later.

13 Protection from osteoporosis and control of climacteric symptoms in older women (as a valid alternative to natural oestrogen replacement therapy, in risk-factor-free women needing contraception whose ovaries are beginning to function less well – see Q 8.37). The same can apply to younger women with premature ovarian failure, or oligomenorrhoea (see Q 4.58–60).

14 Obvious beneficial social effects.
Other possible benefits have been identified in one or two studies but have yet to be fully confirmed. They are listed in order according to my judgement of how likely it is that the protection is real:

15 Reduction in the rate of endometriosis (see Q 4.210).

16 ? less *Trichomonas vaginitis* (see Q 4.211).

17 ? less toxic-shock syndrome (TSS) (see Q 4.212).

18 ? less thyroid disease (both overactive and underactive syndromes according to RCGP study).

19 ? less rheumatoid arthritis (see Q 4.219). This has *not* been

confirmed for more modern pills in the latest studies from the USA. However pregnancy (which the COC to some extent imitates) usually does improves joint symptoms in this condition.

20 ?? less duodenal ulcers. This apparent effect could be due to anxious women avoiding COCs.

4.50 What is thought to be the unifying mechanism of the benefits, especially the gynaecological benefits? How can this be useful in counselling prospective pill-takers?

The removal of the normal menstrual cycle and its replacement by a situation which more closely resembles the physiological state of pregnancy. Women who, due to frequent pregnancies and prolonged lactation, have few menstrual cycles during their reproductive lives (say 50 rather than the 450 plus which would now be typical in developed countries) are less likely to get all the symptoms and conditions listed at items 4,7,8,9,10,15 and 19 in Q 4.49. The similarity of the protection that the COC gives against ovarian and endometrial cancers, for example, is probably because there is much less chromosome activity in the endometrium and ovaries than in cycling women. Less chromosome activity means less chance of harmful mutations during mitosis or meiosis.

So taking the pill is in some ways more 'normal' than using a barrier contraceptive and having numerous menstrual cycles, since the latter are in reality 'abnormal' and tend to promote gynaecological pathology: i.e. all the conditions at items 4, 7–10 and 15 above. In a real sense: *any woman who has been on the pill for 10 years has had iatrogenic amenorrhoea for 10 years* – but of a benign pregnancy-mimicking kind since oestrogen and progestagen are still available to the relevant tissues.

Some women find this story reassuring, that in summary the pill can be truly said to tend to 'restore normality'. It reduces the dangers of too many menstrual cycles among those many who now do the 'unnatural' thing, by not having huge families!

4.51 Do the latest ultra-low-dose formulations which reduce the risks also reduce the benefits to gynaecological pathology, in comparison with the older high-dose formulations?

There has to be some real doubt about this and it will take years to resolve. The protection against functional cysts (see Q 4.53) is definitely reduced by such pills, though there is certainly no proof that it no longer exists. The modern more oestrogenic pills may well also be less protective against benign breast disease, fibroids and endometriosis which are benefited by relatively more progestogen. My own concern is particularly about the triphasics (see Q 4.158), which imitate (albeit imperfectly) the normal cycle, yet eliminating this as we have just seen is likely to be relevant to the mechanism of the benefits.

There is no such thing as a free lunch! But one good thing: *any* oral contraceptive which regularly blocks ovulation ought to retain the protective effect against ovarian cancer.

4.52 By how much does the COC protect against PID and what is the mechanism?

The protective effect is large, a 50% or more reduction in the risk of hospitalization for PID. The disease is common in modern societies, and is such a major cause of subfertility (see Q 6.48), that in many parts of the world this is a significant non-contraceptive benefit of the pill. Although suggestions that the COC might facilitate transmission of HIV have been largely discounted (see Q 4.226), there is nothing to suggest *protection* against any of the sexually transmitted viruses. (Except: there are data that sexually transmitted diseases (STDs) are an important risk factor in promoting the sexual transmission of HIV. Hence the COC might reduce the risk of HIV infection *indirectly* through the reduced risk of PID.)

Mechanism

It seems likely that progestagens reduce not only the sperm penetrability of cervical mucus (see Q 4.4), but also its 'germ penetrability'. Indeed the two may even be connected, in that there is some evidence that sexually transmitted organisms such as the gonococcus may actually 'hitch a lift', i.e. use spermatozoa as their means of transport to the upper genital tract!

Note that infection and sexual transmission of organisms are probably not impeded at the level of the cervix/vagina: the effect is one of protection of the upper genital tract. Chlamydia infection of the cervix and lower tract appears commoner in pill-takers than controls (though appropriate controls are difficult to identify).

4.53 By how much does the COC protect against functional ovarian cysts, and what is the mechanism?

The reduction has been shown in practically all studies. In a Boston study, pill-users were one-fourteenth as likely to develop such cysts as non-users. Although benign, such cysts often lead to surgery.

Functional cysts are caused by abnormalities of ovulation. Most of the time the COC abolishes all kinds of ovulation (both normal and abnormal). On the other hand the POP increases the risk of cyst formation (see Q 5.34; and also Q 4.51 above *re* the lowest-dose combined pills).

REVERSIBILITY OF THE COC

4.54 Are COCs fully reversible as just stated (see Q 4.49)? Do they impair future fertility?

The short answers to these questions are yes to the first and no to the second. In the Oxford/Family Planning Association (FPA) study, for example, among previously fertile women who gave up contraception, by about 30 months over 90% of the ex-pill-users had delivered: a proportion which was indistinguishable from that for ex-users of the diaphragm and IUD. There was a definite delay of 2–3 months in the mean time taken to conceive, probably due in part to the advice pill-takers are often given (see Q 4.207). But a later analysis for *nulliparous* Oxford/FPA women stopping the pill *aged 30–35* showed a more marked delay of a year or so – though only affecting about half the population – in achieving delivery, relative to ex-diaphragm users. Despite this conception rates became almost identical after 72 months: hence no evidence of permanent infertility.

4.55 What then is 'post-pill amenorrhoea' (PPA)?

The term should be abolished (see Q 4.56). It is commonly used to mean secondary amenorrhoea of more than 6 months' duration following discontinuation of the COC. Most authorities now believe that the association is casual rather than causal. Of 1862 inhabitants of Uppsala County, Sweden, 3.3% reported a history of amenorrhoea of longer than 3 months. Amenorrhoea of more than 6 months' duration occurred in 1.8% of the population, most frequently in women under the age of 24. So this is quite a common condition. If a woman is predisposed but instead takes the

COC for many years, any episodes that would otherwise have been recognized will be masked by the regular withdrawal bleeds induced by her contraceptive. In such a woman, the pill could easily be unfairly blamed for her 'after pill' secondary amenorrhoea when it could after all only be revealed 'after pill'.

Moreover, studies show that the probability of PPA is not associated with formulation, nor in most studies with duration of use. Professor Jacobs of UCM School of Medicine in London has shown that the distribution of diagnoses was the same in cases of secondary amenorrhoea post-pill as in non-post-pill cases; and in the two groups the types of treatment needed, the frequency with which they were employed, and the excellent outcome in terms of cumulative conception rates were all the same. All this argues very strongly against a specific pill-induced syndrome causing secondary amenorrhoea.

4.56 What are the bad effects of continuing to use the term 'post-pill amenorrhoea' at all?

1 It leads to a tendency on the part of many doctors to defer investigation of patients with amenorrhoea which develops after the pill, thereby delaying the diagnosis and treatment of potentially serious conditions. Instead, since there is no specific syndrome, after 6 months without a period *all cases of secondary amenorrhoea should be referred* for investigation and appropriate treatment – whether they are 'post-pill' or 'post-condom'!

2 A second unfortunate result of accepting PPA as a real condition is that it deters doctors from prescribing oral contraceptives to women for whom they otherwise might be suitable. A past history of secondary amenorrhoea is good example (see Q 4.60). In some conditions, as we shall see, the COC can be positively beneficial and it is still frequently being needlessly withheld.

3 Thirdly, amenorrhoeic women often develop feelings of guilt that treatment with the pill has caused their amenorrhoea and has wrecked their chances of ever having a baby. In the first place it is most unlikely that the pill had anything to do with their problem; and secondly, even if it did, modern therapy of amenorrhoea is so effective that cumulative pregnancy rates approaching 100% can be confidently expected.

4.57 How are such cases investigated?

In the referral letter it is important to make clear to the specialist whether or not the women desires a pregnancy. It is crazy but not unheard of for high technology to be used to induce ovulation in a woman who promptly requests a termination when the resulting ovum is fertilized! (see Q 8.16).

It is beyond the scope of this book to go into details of hospital investigations; but three of the most helpful tests are simple and non-invasive, and may be appropriately arranged by an interested general practitioner.

1 Weight and height, from which can be calculated the Body Mass Index (BMI): namely, weight in kg/height in metres squared. This is easily derived on a pocket calculator in the surgery, and should be in the range 19–26.

2 The progestagen challenge test. This is usually performed by giving medroxyprogesterone acetate (MPA) 5 mg daily for 5 days. If this is followed by a WTB it means that the woman's oestrogen status is either normal or high. Absence of the WTB means subnormal oestrogen (see below). Plasma oestradiol may also be measured.

3 The third of this trio of essential tests is an ultrasound scan of the ovaries.

Other important tests are: plasma prolactin, thyroid function, FSH and LH.

4.58 What are the risks of prolonged amenorrhoea? How should the women be subsequently treated if they do not want a pregnancy?

The management depends very much on the diagnosis and particularly on oestrogen status, as well as whether the woman is ready yet for fertility enhancement.

Prolonged *amenorrhoea and oligomenorrhoea* (say less than four periods a year) are *not by any means always innocuous conditions*, according to Professor Jacobs. They should always be investigated, and management then depends on the diagnosis.

1 *Polycystic ovary syndrome* (PCO). First of all this is *not* the same as just the finding of polycystic ovaries on ultrasound scan, which is a very common finding in more than 20% of normal women, studied both on the pill and off it. So far as we know it is only clinically of importance if the ultrasound finding is linked with symptoms: irregular or absent menses and, usually, evidence of excessive androgen (acne or hirsutes). These symptoms with the scan findings do then add up to the 'syndrome'. Professor Jacobs is concerned that in the long term there would

be a risk of circulatory disease, because of abnormal lipid changes (low HDL-cholesterol, especially if it comprises less than 23% of total cholesterol). These get more marked the higher the woman's BMI, leading to higher insulin and therefore testosterone levels. It would be particularly bad news for her arteries if she was also a smoker. But PCO syndrome women are not at risk of osteoporosis.

The most important therapeutic point is to help her to lose weight, with more unrefined carbohydrate intake and exercise. If hirsutes is a problem she may require a consultant-led high-dose cyproterone acetate and oestrogen regimen, followed by Dianette for maintenance. If acne alone is the problem, perhaps with some irregular cycling, there is no need to refer. Dianette may be prescribed, usually followed by the pill – only the latter should be one of the modern 30–35 μg oestrogen varieties with a 'lipid friendly' progestogen.

2 *Secondary amenorrhoea in normal or underweight women.* This is often weight-related amenorrhoea and common in track athletes. The concern here is that they have no follicular oestrogen, little extraglandular oestrogen from peripheral conversion of androgen in fat depots, and moreover they have enhanced metabolism along the pathway which degrades oestrogens to antioestrogens. All these mechanisms lead to low oestrogen levels and a serious risk of osteoporosis. If the amenorrhoea has continued for more than 6 months, a progestagen challenge test (see Q 4.57) and an oestradiol measurement should be arranged, with ideally also a bone scan if it is low (less than 100 pmol/l).

These women would theoretically also be at risk of heart disease like women with a premature menopause if the hypo-oestrogen state were to continue for a very long time. They should certainly stop smoking which also lowers plasma oestrogen, and be encouraged to put on weight. Such women are usually very opposed to taking hormones. But they might be better off healthwise on a 'lipid friendly pill' or natural oestrogens than using say the diaphragm or contraceptive sponge. These would be no more than contraceptives, though perfectly adequate in view of the diminished fertility.

3 *Hyperprolactinaemia.* This may require specialist treatment with bromocriptine. Hypo-oestrogenism is not a problem in treated cases, if they are cycling and have normal libido. The COC is

relatively contraindicated, and the advice of the specialist in charge should be sought.

4 *Amenorrhoea but with normal oestrogenization* (positive progestagen challenge, ovaries show no ovulation but some follicular activity.). Here there is the contraceptive problem that at any time the woman might ovulate. There are no special grounds for using the COC, but neither is it contraindicated. The sheath or cap would be fine if acceptable. A reasonable approach would be to suggest the use of the sponge (see Q 3.64) until the first spontaneous period occurs. Since this suggests potential ovulation, the woman would then be advised to transfer to a more effective method – not excluding the COC as an option.

4.59 In summary, what is the place of the COC for women with amenorrhoea?

It is permissible to use the COC in a number of these cases. Its oestrogen content is of benefit where the oestrogen status is low, especially to prevent the long-term problems such as heart disease and osteoporosis. On the other hand the progestagen content of the COC can also be of value in women with oestrogen excess, to protect their uterus from carcinoma of the endometrium.

4.60 What advice should be given to a healthy woman who gives a past history of secondary amenorrhoea but is currently seeing normal periods?

All the evidence suggests that there is no reason to refuse the COC to such women, although they must understand that with or without the pill they might at some future time have difficulty in conceiving. Future fertility can never be proved in advance of becoming pregnant. Another important point is to *investigate* such a woman first if her current menses are in fact still erratic, for example, if she is experiencing *less than four periods per year*. She might well have the polycystic ovary syndrome (see above).

4.61 In order to preserve future fertility, should pill-users take regular breaks of say 6 months, every 2 or every 5 years?

The answer here is an unusually confident no. This follows from Qs 4.54 and 4.55: the pill is a reversible means of birth control, whose reversibility is not dependent on duration of use. Too often breaks demonstrate very well to the woman that her fertility is unimpaired – by an unplanned pregnancy! See also Qs 4.26 and 4.230 which add a health- rather than fertility-related perspective to this same issue, of duration of use/taking breaks.

4.62 Contrary to the common myth about its reversibility, doesn't the COC in fact much reduce the likelihood of infertility?

Yes. See Q 4.49. Many of the benefits of the pill relate to conditions which can readily impair fertility and childbearing, specifically:

1 less *pelvic infection*;

2 fewer *ectopics*;

3 less *endometriosis*;

4 less growth of *fibroids,* a cause of miscarriage;

5 less functional *ovarian cysts,* a cause of unnecessary surgery;

6 less surgery altogether, for all the conditions listed here, a frequent cause of *pelvic adhesions* and consequent infertility;

7 less unwanted *pregnancies*: which can lead in various ways to secondary infertility (e.g. by infected abortions of all kinds, or by puerperal infection).

For the same reasons there is no logic in pill-takers having a regular annual bimanual examination (see Q 4.167).

MAIN DISADVANTAGES AND PROBLEMS

4.63 What are the major established unwanted effects of COCs?

These can again be summarized before more detailed consideration. They are under four main headings:

Circulatory diseases (see Qs 4.83–4.88)

1 venous thromboembolism;

2 myocardial infarction;

3 strokes:
   (a) thrombotic;
   (b) haemorrhagic

4 hypertension;

5 other thrombotic events in the circulatory system (especially in solitary but vital vessels, e.g. the retinal artery or vein, see Q 4.190).

Liver disease

1 liver adenoma (see Q 4.82), or carcinoma (see Q 4.81);
2 cholestatic jaundice (see Q 4.196);
3 gallstones (see Q 4.198).

**Possible adverse effects on some cancers
(see Qs 4.64–4.81)**

Unwanted social effects (debatable, relates to whether removal of the fear of pregnancy has in some societies tended to promote intercourse with multiple partners, etc.).

> Note: There are many other possible adverse effects which are highly relevant but either less well established or less serious. They are considered below, either under 'Contraindications' or the section on 'Follow-up and monitoring'. See particularly Qs 4.112 and 4.113.

THE COC AND NEOPLASIA (BENIGN AND MALIGNANT)

4.64 Does the COC influence the rates of benign and malignant neoplasms?

It should not be surprising that artificial hormones can influence neoplasia; but recent research has confirmed the expectation that the effect of hormones would not be all in one direction. Some benign neoplastic conditions are benefited by OC use (e.g. benign breast disease), some are promoted (e.g. liver adenomas). Similarly two cancers are now clearly shown to be less frequent in pill-users (carcinoma of the ovary and endometrium); whereas the COC may possibly act as a co-carcinogen in the case of two other common cancers (see Q 4.71). The literature is complex and this story is still a long way from being fully told.

4.65 Why has it taken so long to begin to show associations between the pill and neoplasia?

1 The main reason is summarized in the word *latency*. There can be up to 30 years between first exposure to an agent and its manifestation in the incidence of tumours. Even the largest prospective studies tend to have too few numbers and take too

long to give an answer. Hence data have been obtained mainly from case-control studies, which are notoriously subject to bias. Other problems relate to:

2 The specificity of any co-carcinogen to the species, to the tissue and to tumour histology.

3 Time of life is relevant – in animal models chemicals can have contrary actions, promoting or inhibiting tumours according to when in the life of the individual exposure takes place.

4 Related to the last point is the fact that a chemical may have no effects in the generality of women, but may have a specific adverse (or beneficial) effect in certain at-risk groups. In the case of breast cancer, for example, interest is currently focused on young women, especially those who use the COC to delay their first full-term pregnancy since such delay, however caused, is a risk factor for the disease. Women with a family history of breast cancer or a personal history of benign breast disease are other important groups at special risk.

5 Finally there is the influence of formulation. Not only differing ratios of progestagen to oestrogen, but also different progesta-genic chemicals, are used around the world. It is particularly unfortunate that most studies cannot disentangle the effects of specific formulations (apart from generally showing that low oestrogen pills usually have a lesser effect). It is not impossible that some varieties might promote tumour growth whereas others could even have an opposite effect.

4.66 What is the benefit/risk balance sheet for neoplasia and the pill, so far as is currently known?

See Figure 4.6. The situation can best be explained to a patient in terms of 'swings and roundabouts'. Some cancers are definitely less frequent in pill-users (endometrium and ovary). Others may be more frequent (but in none of those shown is a causative link proven beyond doubt). For all remaining common malignancies (whether of the respiratory, gastrointestinal or renal tracts), there seems no association at all. A similar balance sheet can be struck for benign neoplasia (see Fig. 4.7).

The 'bottom line' in counselling is:

Populations using the pill may develop different benign or malignant neoplasms from non-users, but computer models using the best currently accepted data and assumptions do not

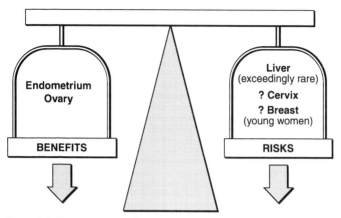

Figure 4.6 Cancer and the pill. Q 4.66.
Note: there is much more uncertainty about the adverse than the beneficial effects

so far indicate that the overall risk of either type of neoplasia is increased. (There is no proof of an overall reduction of risk either.)

Now let us consider some of the details.

4.67 What is the influence of COCs on carcinoma of the ovary?

At least 10 studies have yielded results pointing in the same direction, namely that epithelial ovarian tumours are less frequent in COC-users. Overall the risk is reduced by about 40%. There is increasing protection with increased duration of use amounting to a two-thirds reduction after more than 5 years, and the largest study now shows that the protective effect lasts for at least 15 years after pill-taking ceases. This is good news indeed as ovarian cancer carries a high mortality.

4.68 What is the influence of COC use on carcinoma of the endometrium?

In total contrast to the oestrogenic sequential pills, no longer available in this country, combined preparations are positively protective. This has been shown in seven studies to date, two others failing to show association (but none showing the opposite). The risk of this cancer in ever-users is reduced by about 50%. Four studies show increasing protection with increasing duration of use and three studies show some degree of persistence of the effect after stopping the method, lasting according to one of them for at least 15 years.

The similarity of the beneficial effects of the COC on these two cancers is striking, but not surprising (see Q 4.50).

4.69 What is the influence of the COC on trophoblastic disease (hydatidiform mole)?

There is no evidence that any form of this tumour of pregnancy occurs more frequently in recent pill-users.

However, workers at Charing Cross Hospital in London have shown that usage of the combined pill after this diagnosis and before human chorionic gonadotrophin (hCG) has reached undetectable blood levels, doubles the likelihood that the patient will require chemotherapy for incipient choriocarcinoma. Other researchers, notably from America, have failed to show this association: but their chemotherapy policy is far more aggressive.

The London team remains convinced of a causative link. Since it is not clear if the effect is due more to the progestagen than the oestrogen, they therefore continue to recommend that *all* hormonal methods are avoided until the hCG levels are undetectable, in urine at first, then confirmed in the blood. IUDs should also be avoided while hCG levels are high (in case an invasive cancer involving the uterine wall be present). Fortunately, in the vast majority of cases the hCG levels do become undetectable within 2 months of evacuation of the mole. The prohibition against hormonal methods, which is only precautionary (and in the USA only ever a relative contraindication), is therefore usually short-lived and *NOT* as long as until the next conception – which may anyway now be attempted 6 months after no hCG is detectable.

4.70 What is the influence of the COC on carcinoma of the cervix?

Studies on cervical cancer are complicated by confounding with the sexual variables: i.e. by the problem of getting accurate information about different patterns of sexual activity, both for women and their partners. The prime carcinogen is clearly sexually transmitted, probably a virus or combination of viruses.

Most studies, in different populations, do show an association between this cancer, plus its premalignant forms, and use of the COC – but is it causative or casual? The Oxford/FPA study (1983) supported the former view by demonstrating an effect of duration of pill-use among nearly 7000 parous women. No effect of duration of IUD-use was found among over 3000 users of that method with whom they were compared. The incidence of all forms of cervical neoplasia combined rose from 0.9/1000 woman-years in those with up to 2 years' pill-use to 2.2/1000 woman-years after 8 years. All 13 cases of invasive cancer occurred in women in the oral contraceptive group. The frequency of taking cervical cytology smears was similar but it was not possible to control for exposure to the sexually transmitted carcinogen.

In 1985 a WHO case-control study reported a 53% increase in the risk of invasive carcinoma of the cervix among women who had used the COC for more than 5 years. This was after controlling for seven relevant variables including the age at first sexual relations and number of sexual partners. However this study was again not able to assess the sexual practices of each woman's main or only partner, which may be the most important risk factor, nor the well-recognized effect of cigarette smoking.

4.71 What is your overall assessment of the association with neoplasia of the cervix?

It remains possible that the link with the COC is entirely caused by confounding with sexual activity. At worst, it may be a weak co-factor, certainly weaker than cigarette smoking: possibly speeding transition through the preinvasive stages.

The COC is not the true carcinogen for this cancer. Its influence is clearly many times less than the influence of sexual lifestyle. Users should have regular cervical smears. Three-yearly is still considered adequate to enable preventive action before invasive cancer develops (see also Q 4.72), unless there are other risk factors. (If resources were to permit, the first wider category to be offered more frequent smears should be all smokers, ahead of pill-takers unless they also smoke.)

4.72 Should women discontinue COC use once an abnormal cervical smear has been detected?

It is currently acceptable to continue COC use during the monitoring of a mildly abnormal cervical smear, during definitive treatment of cervical intraepithelial neoplasia (CIN), and subsequently. These are very weak, relative contraindications – though the recurrence risk for the problem would of course be minimized if the couple were prepared to use a barrier method instead or as well (see Qs 2.25 and 3.17).

4.73 What is the association between breast cancer and COC use?

Nowhere is the medical literature more copious, complex, confusing and contradictory. All the problems mentioned in Q 4.65 apply.

The life-time incidence of *breast cancer* is high (about 1 in 11), though many die of another condition. Therefore this disease must inevitably be expected to develop in women whether they take COCs or not. The risk factors include early menarche and late age of first birth, and prolonged lactation is probably protective; so use by young women before childbearing was rightly bound to receive scientific scrutiny.

The book edited by Mann (1990), which was the Proceedings of a meeting at the Royal Society of Medicine attended by almost all the researchers in this field, summarizes the literature to that date. A major cause of discrepancies may be the fact that long-term use of the COC by young women is a relatively recent and variable phenomenon between populations.

First, the good news. Cancer registration data show no increase at all in any of the age groups who have had access to the pill. And we can be confident that 'use of oral contraceptives in the middle of the fertile years (say between the ages of 25 and 39) has no effect whatsoever on breast cancer risk' (Vessey, writing in 1989).

The largest case-control study on this emotive subject (the Cancer and Sex Hormones or CASH study) based in Atlanta, USA, was repeatedly reported during the 1980s as not finding any excess risk of breast cancer, whenever in life the pill exposure occurred.

However, a reanalysis by Peto of CASH data reveals a significant excess risk, for all women aged 20–44 at diagnosis, if they used the COC before the first full-term pregnancy. Thus CASH now seems compatible with those other studies (references in Mann, 1990) which indicated some degree of excess risk in various young categories of women (under 25, or before the first full-term pregnancy).

To the latter must now be added what most people consider the 'lead' study, namely the UK National Case Control Study (NCCS), which reported in 1989. There was an excess of early pill-use among women developing breast cancer under age 36, the background risk of around 2/1000 users increasing to about 3/1000 after 4 years' use. The significant increased risk was duration dependent, whether exposure was before the first term pregnancy or after it, and reached 74% at 8 years. Sub-50 μg dose oestrogen pills seemed to have a lower risk. No clear difference between the progestogens available for study could be shown.

Yet, UK cancer registration data still show no increase among the under 40s. It is not yet clear whether this is because the register is seriously incomplete for young women, or whether the NCCS was wrong for some unexplained reason.

4.74 So what's the most likely scenario, based on the current epidemiology of breast cancer and the pill?

An authoritative interpretation of all the literature to date is that the risk is for breast cancer occurring at a young age, and that it diminishes or disappears at older ages. The RCGP found the risk only among pill-users aged 30–35 at diagnosis and not above 35, consistent with transient risk. The other prospective studies are also reassuring in this respect. *But it remains a matter of real concern that the risk could yet be found to persist into age groups where the disease is more prevalent.* We await the findings of a new study by NCCS on older women aged 36–45.

4.75 How might one explain to women the implications of the 1989 UK NCCS report, in context with the rest of the literature?

Among 1000 young COC-users for more than 4 years (sitting, say, in a large concert hall), three would be under treatment for breast cancer by age 36. Of these two could not blame the pill because the background rate is 2 : 1000. The third young woman represents the 1 : 1000 excess risk which may be pill related. It is likely that she was destined to develop the disease anyway, though at a later age.

4.76 What about COC use and breast cancer risk at the other end of reproductive life, nearing the menopause?

Most studies are reassuring, but some have suggested an increased breast cancer risk in COC-using women above the age of 40 or 45. At that age it may be more a matter of oestrogen-users not getting the usual breast cancer-protecting effect of diminished ovarian function, well established for those who have a premature menopause. The effect on breast cancer risk of prolonged oestrogen replacement therapy after the menopause is still a matter of controversy (see Q 8.38 and Table 8.2).

4.77 Are there clinically useful laboratory data about the pill hormones and breast cancer?

Laboratory data, yes, but clinically useful, not yet. A 1991 report of an in vitro study by Coletta from King's College Hospital showed a specific inhibitory effect of gestodene on some breast cancer cell lines in tissue culture. However this required a far higher tissue concentration than would be achieved in users of any current gestodene-containing pill. Also other in vitro studies from the Netherlands, in which oestrogen was given as well to one of the tissue cell lines (MCF 7) studied by Coletta – and after all some oestrogen is always present in vivo – failed to detect a growth-inhibiting effect of gestodene. Reassuringly, though, all of the progestogens studied (3-keto-desogestrel, levonorgestrel and gestodene) showed the same absence of growth-*promoting* effects, at levels comparable to those expected in vivo, and even in the presence of oestrogen.

There may yet prove to be something unique and valuable about gestodene in the prevention of breast cancer, but more in vivo work is necessary before prescribing practice changes solely on this account.

4.78 What are the clinical implications for routine pill-prescribing?

The British Committee on Safety of Medicines (CSM), in a statement in May 1989, declared that:

> The findings of studies that relate to the use of older oral contraceptives may not apply to their modern counterparts . . . . Taking into account both the benefits and potential risks of oral contraceptive use, *the CSM recommends that there is no need for a change in oral contraceptive prescribing practice on the evidence presently available.*

I would add today that the cancer issue should in future normally be addressed as part of routine pill counselling, and especially so as at Q 4.79 below if there are breast cancer risk factors. In summary:

1 Breast cancer should be discussed, in a sensitive way, as part of routine pill counselling for younger women, and well before 4 years' use – but *opportunely*. That word implies *judgement* by the counselling nurse or doctor, especially when faced by an anxious teenager. Unless raised by the woman, this is not an essential part of the very first visit, during which so much

practical information has to be conveyed. At the appropriate time, the discussion might well start with the 'concert hall' illustration at Q 4.75 above, but must also include the protective effects against malignancies of the ovary and endometrium.

The known contraceptive and non-contraceptive benefits of COCs seem so great to many – but not to all – well-counselled users as to compensate for almost any likely lifetime excess risk of breast cancer.

2 If the COC does truly increase breast cancer risk in certain categories of women, dose dependency has been shown at least for oestrogen and it is likely the risk will be minimized by the use of modern low-dose brands causing least metabolic disturbance. Fortunately, these are precisely the same pills which are recommended to reduce the risk of circulatory disease. It remains acceptable to prescribe such formulations for the young, including teenagers, without an arbitrary time limit.

3 Above age 30 prior to a new prescription for COCs (or HRT), and as indicated at any age, women's breasts should be checked, and breast awareness discussed — see Q 4.165. If a woman develops carcinoma of the breast, COCs should be discontinued if in constant use and, with very few exceptions as sometimes authorized by the oncologist, avoided in the future. See Qs 4.101, 4.103, 5.52.

4.79 What about COC use in high-risk groups for breast cancer, specifically (a) those with a *family history* of a young (under 40) first-degree relative with breast cancer? and (b) women with *benign breast disease (BBD)*?

No study has shown that COC-use materially increases the increased risk already present among such women, more than in the generality of women. In other words the current view is that there may be at worst the same *increment* of risk as among pill-users without either risk factor. But in my view both (despite the BBD pill-protection paradox of Q 4.82) should now be considered reasons for special caution. They are rather strong relative contraindications.

COUNSELLING may have two possible outcomes, so only the woman concerned can decide. One woman will choose the pill because there is *no greater increment* of risk caused by COC-use than there would be for a girlfriend without her breast cancer risk factor. Another will, contrariwise, request another method because the last thing she would like to do is run the risk of increasing her irreducible innate risk still further.

If the woman does choose the COC it should be a low oestrogen formulation for a limited duration, with specific counselling and extra surveillance. Some prescribers advise a COC using a modern progestagen in these circumstances, but the evidence that these would be safer than norethisterone or levonorgestrel is weak. There are some metabolic differences which might be advantageous. However, the fact that they are not implicated in the epidemiology of breast cancer is mainly because they have not yet been in use long enough for study.

4.80 What is the influence of COCs on the prognosis of breast cancer?

It has been reported that women who have never used COCs present with more advanced tumours that those who have used them during the year before detection of the cancer, and the latter group have a better prognosis. This could be due simply to 'surveillance bias' leading to earlier diagnosis among the COC-users; but some authorities think the COC does in reality have a beneficial effect on tumour growth and spread.

4.81 What is the influence of the COC on other cancers?

1 *Primary hepatocellular carcinoma*. Some case reports and three case-control studies have strongly suggested that COC-use may promote this rare cancer. The annual attributable risk must be very low, of the order of 3 or 4 per million users. The pill association is not established in hepatitis B-infected livers, fortunately since that is the main risk factor.

2 *Malignant melanoma of the skin*. An increased risk, particularly of the superfical spreading type of this cancer, has been suggested among COC-users. Most other studies show no link. It is becoming increasingly probable that the association is not causal, related to the pill itself, but to the confounding variable of exposure to ultraviolet light. (See Q 4.103 for COC-use in treated cases.)

3 No association has been shown with malignancy involving any other organ or tissue.

4.82 What is the influence of the COC on benign neoplasms?

See Figure 4.7.

1 *Benign breast disease (BBD).* A definite protective effect has been shown which increases with duration of use and is probably attributable to the progestagen component of the pill. The protection in some studies seems to be restricted to the commonest but less serious forms of the disease without epithelial atypia, the latter being considered the premalignant variety. This observation may possibly explain the paradox that COCs protect against BBD developing in the first place but have no demonstrable protective effect against breast cancer.

2 *Hepatocellular adenoma.* This tumour occurs 10–20 times more frequently in COC-users than in other women, but the background prevalence is so low that the incidence among OC-users is still tiny (around 1/100 000 users per year). The risk is greatest in older women using relatively high-dose pills for a long period of time (see Qs 4.86, 4.200 and 4.202).

3 *Other benign tumours showing no association.* These include benign trophoblastic disease (but see Q 4.69) and prolactinoma of the pituitary gland. For some years it was widely held that COC-use increased the risk of the latter, but two good case-control studies have provided strong evidence against the association.

4 *Fibroids.* While older high oestrogen OCs were believed to cause fibroids to increase in size, current more progestagen-dominant brands have been shown to reduce the risk of hospital referral for fibroids (see Q 4.99).

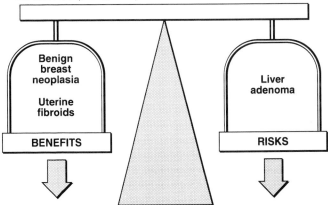

Figure 4.7 Benign neoplasia and the pill. Q 4.82

THE COC AND CIRCULATORY DISEASES

4.83 Which circulatory diseases have been shown to be commoner in COC-users?

1 Venous disease:
   (a) deep venous thrombosis;
   (b) pulmonary embolism;
   (c) rarely thrombosis in other veins, e.g. mesenteric, hepatic or retinal.

2 Arterial diseases. These include:
   (a) myocardial infarction;
   (b) thrombotic strokes;
   (c) haemorrhagic strokes, including subarachnoid haemorrhage (SAH). The data on SAH are much less convincing and probably relate secondarily, in studies showing the association, with hypertension in COC-users not always being recognized;
   (d) other arterial diseases such as thrombosis of mesenteric or retinal arteries and possibly some cases of Raynaud's disease (Q 4.217).

4.84 What effect does the COC have on blood pressure?

In the majority of combined pill-users there is a slight, measurable increase in both systolic and diastolic blood pressure, within the normotensive range. Early large studies showed a 1.5–3 times higher risk of clinical hypertension, but modern varieties with reduced oestrogen and progestagen (both are relevant since there is synergism once oestrogen is being taken) have lowered the rate.

Predisposing factors include strong family history, and a tendency to water retention and obesity. Past pregnancy-associated hypertension (toxaemia) does not predispose to hypertension during OC use, in controlled studies. But the RCGP study showed that *past toxaemia history* (which may be a 'marker' for essential hypertension, not diagnosed before the pregnancy) does strongly predispose to myocardial infarction, especially in smokers (see Q 4.103).

Hypertension is itself an important risk factor for the arterial diseases above, especially heart disease and both types of stroke. See Qs 4.168–4.171 for the clinical implications.

4.85 What is the overall relative risk of circulatory disease in COC-users?

The overall mortality risk ratio in the RCGP prospective study (mostly of 50-μg pills) was 4.0 for all vascular disease. Epidemiological estimates of the risk ratio for the individual conditions vary between about 1.5 (for myocardial infarction in non-smokers) and 6 (for venous thrombosis). Very few deaths or incidents of disease have been described under the age of 35, and most have had other risk factors (principally smoking). Indeed, recent analyses of all the good studies at Q 4.47 above can find *no statistically significant increased risk of myocardial infarction among users of modern sub–50-μg formulations unless the women also smoke!*

4.86 What is the difference between relative risk and attributable risk?

This is a most important distinction which is not often understood by either patients or journalists. A small relative risk may cause more attributable cases than a large one, if the background prevalence is low.

In Table 4.5 the data relate to older 50-μg pills, but make a general point. The first set of figures apply to the frequency of hepatocellular adenoma in controls as compared with COC-users. The second set (rounded), based on the RCGP report in 1981, refer to the circulatory disease mortality among controls who smoked as compared with COC-users who smoked, in the age group 35–44. The difference in the excess number of cases caused by the method explains why it is reasonable to accept a 20-fold increase in the risk of benign liver tumours, but a four-fold increase would be unacceptable for smokers above age 35.

The excess risk of myocardial infarction through COC use can now only be demonstrated in smokers, among whom a 21-fold increase as compared with non-smoking non-takers is shown by the RCGP study. *So although non–smokers may now use the COC well above age 35 (see Q 4.232) the teaching about smokers remains unchanged.*

Table 4.5 Attributable risk

Background prevalence	Relative risk	No. of cases	No. of cases attributable
(A) 1 in 10^6	× 20	20	19
(B) 150 in 10^6	× 4	600	450

4.87 Does the relative risk of circulatory disease increase with duration of use?

Venous disease is clearly unrelated to duration of COC use. It relates to current use, oestrogen dose, leg mobility, and various predisposing prothrombotic blood disorders in the woman (see Q 4.110). As to *arterial disease*, things seem clearer since the reports of the Nurses' Study. Provided those who develop sustained hypertension are identified and discontinue COCs, the relative risk of arterial disease does not appear to increase with increasing duration of pill-use. The key factors seem to be current COC-use and the age of the woman, plus predisposing proatherogenic *and* prothrombogenic risk factors.

4.88 What is the relative risk among ex-users of the COC?

There is no 'carry-over' effect for *venous thromboembolism* beyond about 1 month, and by 8 weeks the measured coagulation changes have all returned to normal.

The 1983 report of the RCGP showed an ex-use effect for cerebrovascular disease – with a lower risk ratio than for current users, but persisting for up to 6 years after stopping OCs. Another study (Slone and coworkers in 1981) suggested an ex-use effect for myocardial infarction. However a reanalysis suggested that the link with ex-use was really only true for smokers. More importantly, the Nurses' Health Study with no less than 921 960 person-years of follow-up between 1976 and 1984, and almost complete ascertainment of both fatal and non-fatal heart attacks and strokes, 'found no evidence to suggest an increase in the risk of cardiovascular diseases among past users of oral contraceptives, even with prolonged previous use'.

4.89 What is the main causation of circulatory disease problems in COC-users?

Mostly they are due to the 'soil' (the woman, including her smoking habits) rather than the 'seed' (the pill, *causing* specific predisposing changes). The answers to Qs 4.87 and 4.88 plus much other data put together convince me that when the COC is (rarely) involved in the causation of arterial diseases, it is primarily by *current* changes affecting platelets, coagulation, fibrinolysis and (probably) prostaglandins in a predisposed woman, i.e. one who already has arterial wall damage (atheroma). The absence in the best epidemiology of a duration of use or ex-use effect suggests that the COC on its own has little if any atherogenic effect.

Intriguingly, the Nurses' Health Study relates to US pill brands which at that time used only norethisterone prodrugs or levonorgestrel. Future epidemiology is expected to be even more reassuring about combinations with modern 'lipid friendly' progestagens (see Q 4.136), with even the hint of the possibility of a reduction in the risk of significant atherogenesis below that of non-users. In the mean time we may use the modern COC at a woman's request to age 50 or so, without age or duration of use causing significant concern *in non-smokers* (see Q 4.232).

4.90 What is the influence of the oestrogen content of the COC on metabolism, and risk?

1 Oestrogen induces alterations in clotting factor levels which may be thrombogenic. More important changes include reduced levels of antithrombin III, elevated fibrinogen and increased platelet aggregability. These changes explain the increased risk of *venous* thrombosis. However, it is important not to overlook the fact that if there is already arterial wall disease, oestrogen may also promote superimposed arterial thrombosis. There is evidence of a compensatory increased fibrinolytic activity, also an oestrogen effect. This may explain the relative rarity of overt disease in most pill-users.

> **Note: This protective fibrinolysis is impaired by heavy smoking.**

2 Hepatic secretion of many different proteins is stimulated by oestrogens. These proteins are involved in the transport of hormones, vitamins and minerals, the control of blood pressure and immunological processes. When oestrogen is given the stimulatory effect can sometimes be suppressed by concomitant administration of a progestagen. But the interactions are complex: there may also be synergism or independence of the effects, and differences between progestagens. See Tables 4.6 and 4.7.

3 Finally, oestrogens have been shown to raise arterial blood pressure both in short-term challenge experiments and in longer-term studies. When a norethisterone-levonorgestrel group progestogen is added there is synergism (see Q 4.91).

Table 4.6 Complexity of interaction of contraceptive steroids

	Oestrogen	NET or LNG progestagen	Remarks
1 Blood pressure	↑	↑	If given *with* oestrogen But no marketed progestagen-only method appears to have this effect on BP
2 Hepatic secretion of plasma proteins especially SHBG*	↑	↓	
3 HDL-cholesterol*	↑	↓	
4 Sperm penetrability of cervical mucus	↑	↓	

Note: there is not always interaction: for other variables the effects of oestrogens and progestogens may be independent.
* NET and LNG either reduce the oestrogen-mediated increase, or, in a high enough dose, may actually lower the levels. However, the new progestagens – desogestrel (DSG), gestodene (GSD) and norgestimate (NGM) – in the doses used appear only minimally to oppose the effects of the oestrogen. They therefore permit it to raise SHBG and HDL-cholesterol; and the synergism of NET and LNG with oestrogen in raising blood pressure has not been demonstrated with DSG, GSD or NGM. Yet like all progestagens they do antagonize oestrogen in its effect on cervical mucus.

4.91 What is the influence of the progestagen content on metabolism and risk?

1 First, the risk of venous thromboembolism seems minimally affected.

2 Secondly, provided oestrogen is also given, increasing the dose of progestagen leads to an increased rate of diagnosis of clinical hypertension. (On the other hand when given without oestrogen, as in the POP or DMPA, progestagens have no demonstrable effect on blood pressure.)

3 When oestrogen is kept constant, the incidence of arterial diseases, both as a group and individually, is correlated with the progestagen dose in some epidemiological studies. This has only been shown for norethisterone–levonorgestrel group progestagens, referred to from now on as the 'second generation'.

Table 4.7 Some metabolic effects of combined oral contraceptives

	Blood level	Remarks
Liver		
Liver functioning	Altered	These many changes cause no
(a) generally	in all users	apparent long-term damage to
(b) specifically		the liver itself. The liver is
Albumen	↓	involved, however, in the
Transaminases	↑	production of most of the
Amino acids	Altered	changes in blood levels of
Homocysteine	↑	substances shown elsewhere in
		this table, including the
		important changes in
		carbohydrate and lipid
		metabolism, and coagulation
		factors
Blood glucose after	↑	These changes, barely detectable
carbohydrate ingestion		with the latest pills, may partly
Blood lipids	Altered, mostly ↑	explain the increased risk of
HDL-cholesterol – in low		arterial disease with earlier
oestrogen/progestogen		preparations
-dominant COCs	↓	
Clotting factors		
(a) generally	Mostly ↑	Both the pill and smoking affect
(b) specifically		these interrelated systems.
Antithrombin III	↓	Fibrinolysis is enhanced by COC
(anti-clotting factor)		in the blood, but reduced in the
Fibrinolysis	↑	vessel walls
Tendency for platelet	↑	
aggregation		
Hormones		
Insulin	↑	These hormone changes are
Growth hormone	↑	related to those affecting blood
Adrenal steroids	↑	sugar and blood lipids (above)
Thyroid hormones	↑	
Prolactin	↑	
LH	↓	These effects are integral to
FSH	↓	contraceptive actions. However,
Endogenous oestrogen	↓	the first three tend to rise in
Endogenous progesterone	↓	some women during the pill-free
		week. Hence any effective
		lengthening of the pill-free time
		may lead to an LH surge and
		ovulation

Table 4.7 (contd)

	Blood level	Remarks
Minerals and vitamins		
Iron	↑	This is a good effect for women prone to iron deficiency
Copper	↑	
Zinc	↓	Effects unknown, but not believed to cause any health risk for most pill-users. Pyridoxine is discussed at Q 4.184
Vitamins A, K	↑	
Riboflavine, folic acid	↓	
Vitamin B$_6$ (pyridoxine)	↓	
Vitamin B$_{12}$ (cyanocobalamin)	↓	
Vitamin C (ascorbic acid)	↓	
Binding globulins (including SHBG)	↑	These globulins carry hormones and minerals in the blood. Because their levels increase in parallel with the latter, the effective blood levels of the hormones or minerals are usually not much altered.
Blood viscosity	↑	
Body water	↑	This retention of fluid explains some of the weight gain blamed on the pill
Factors affecting blood pressure	Altered	
Renin substrate		Changes do not correlate as well as expected with the incidence of frank hypertension
Renin activity	↑	
Angiotensin II		
Cardiac output		
Immunity/allergy		
Number of leucocytes	↑	See Qs 4.225 and 4.226
Immunogobulins	Altered	
Function of lymphocytes	Altered	

Notes:
1 In the table ↑ means the level usually goes up, ↓ down.
2 'Altered' means that the changes are known to be more complex, with both increases and decreases occurring within the system.
3 The changes are generally (a) within the normal range, (b) similiar to those of normal pregnancy
4 These effects are obviously highly relevant to the interpretation of many laboratory tests. See Q. 4.237.

4.92 Can known metabolic effects explain the epidemiology and point towards safer products?

To a limited degree, yes. As the dose of one of these 'second-generation' progestagens is increased in the presence of constant oestrogen, plasma insulin levels rise and high-density lipoprotein-cholesterol (HDL-C) levels fall, as do those of the even more important subfraction HDL_2-C. Since HDL-C and HDL_2-C are markers of centripetal movement of blood fats and reduced risk of (distal) atherogenesis, these metabolic changes are believed to be unfavourable.

Oestrogen alone raises HDL_2-C. Oestrogen combined with a *sufficiently small dose* of levonorgestrel or norethisterone as in the triphasic products causes less change to HDL_2-C. In combination with the less antioestrogenic more 'selective' 'third-generation' progestagens, namely desogestrel, gestodene, or norgestimate, this important lipid subfraction is usually unaltered or somewhat elevated. Even if the latter is not an improvement on nature, there is nothing to suggest it would be harmful. So such 'lipid friendly' products are now favoured for all women with circulatory risk factors (see Q 4.136). But because they are not free of thrombogenicity (Q 4.89), due mainly to their oestrogen content (Q 4.90), I remain to be convinced they may be safely used by women at high risk of circulatory disease (Q 4.101 (A)).

4.93 Surely lipid changes which are artificially (pill) induced do not mean the same as those occurring naturally?

This is a fair comment, but increasingly the correlation is being confirmed by epidemiology. For example, the RCGP study showed a higher incidence of arterial events in users of the self-same relatively progestagen-dominant brands which were shown to be associated with more HDL-C suppression in the large cross-sectional studies of Professor Victor Wynn in London. And oral oestrogen replacement with conjugated equine oestrogens (Premarin) is not entirely 'natural', yet has been convincingly shown to reduce the risk of arterial disease in postmenopausal women.

It will take time to prove conclusively that COCs which leave unaltered or increase HDL-C are truly 'even safer' with respect to atherogenesis than those which do. But in the meantime I am myself sufficiently convinced to recommend them for smokers and others with arterial disease risk factors.

4.94 If oestrogen raises HDL-C levels, is it disadvantageous to prescribe the lowest dose brands, especially those with only 20 μg?

No. Most importantly, it is well established that oestrogen is capable of promoting thrombosis, arterial as well as venous, and also hypertension (see Q 4.90). And thrombotic risk is not less important, quite the reverse. Current-use effects are probably much more important than any long-term effect on the arterial wall (see Qs 4.89, 4.90)

Actually the preferred 20 μg EE-containing desogestrel product, Mercilon (20), is still adequately oestrogenic, tending to elevate or at least not depress both HDL-C and sex hormone binding globulin (SHBG). It is a good choice for older women, smokers under 35 and also the relatively obese.

In summary, we try to follow the dictum of Wynn:

> If we can measure any substance in the pill-user, we would like it to be normal – or as near normal as possible.

And one's enthusiasm in this respect is the greater the more clinically relevant the substance appears to be. This is discussed further in relation to pill-prescribing (see Qs 4.133–40)

4.95 Patients are naturally anxious about the known adverse effects of the combined pill on cancer and circulatory disease. Assuming they otherwise wish to use the method, how may this anxiety be reduced?

See Figures 4.8 and 4.9. The media do the general public a disservice by tending to exaggerate the bad systemic effects, and by not pointing out the counterbalancing non-contraceptive benefits, aside from the advantages of efficacy, reversibility and convenience. Another form of counterbalancing is shown on the right-hand side of Figure 4.6, namely the comparison with the risks of pregnancy (so effectively avoided by the COC) and the avoidance of the risk and inconvenience of the alternative methods.

Potential users can be reminded that there are many other risks in life which, though greater than pill-taking, are readily tolerated; for example having babies or travelling by car (Fig. 4.9).

Finally the risks of OCs can be further reduced by more careful prescribing of lower-dose preparations, with good subsequent monitoring (see Qs 4.101, 4.103, 4.114, 4.133 and 4.165).

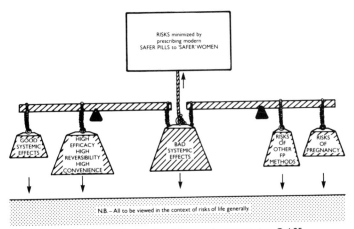

Figure 4.8 The risks versus the benefits of hormonal contraception. Q 4.95.
(See Fig. 4.9 for 'the risks of life generally')

4.96 How can a busy doctor ever convey enough information about COCs to enable worried women to make a fully informed decision?

So much is now known about the method that this is becoming ever more difficult to do. The advice of the Medical Defence Societies is

> A doctor has the duty to give such warnings and carry out such checks as are considered by his/her peers to be necessary having regard to the relevant circumstances of the case. There is no obligation to explain every risk but there is the need to be forthright in explaining risks.

In other words, you should be frank about what is known and honest about what is not yet known; communicate the main pros and cons of the method as in Qs 4.49–4.63; explain the practicalities, rules for missed pills, minor side effects most especially breakthrough bleeding; and allow time for questions to be asked and answered. Full records should be kept. A pretty tall order!

For most busy practitioners who wish to maintain high standards 'allow time' means more accurately 'make time', plus delegate. In the real world, how do they present? – in the middle of a busy surgery, as like as not needing postcoital contraception (see Ch. 7, a whole chapter to take account of there!) first, and then to start the COC before their follow-up visit . . . . Can all this ever be well done without the availability of counselling by a (family

Annual number of deaths
per 100 000 exposed

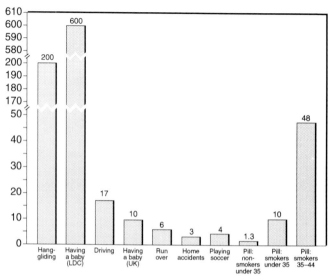

Figure 4.9 The risks of various activities (annual number of deaths per 100 000 exposed). Q 4.95.

The pill and smoking data come from the RCGP study (1981) and concern circulatory diseases alone. Though they are the best available prospective data, they apply to older pills with at least 50μg of oestrogen. The newer formulations are definitely safer: we are not able yet to say by how much. Modern studies can find no excess risk of arterial disease in pill-takers who are non-smokers. So although the overall circulatory disease estimate here for non-smokers under 35 is the best available, it could be too high. There are no good data for older non-smokers using modern pills whose excess risk is believed very low, and so acceptable to age 50. Q 4.232. With regard to cancer, the benefits tend to cancel the risks, so in this figure overall excess cancer mortality is assumed to be zero (see Fig. 4.6).

(Redrawn from Guillebaud J 1984 The pill. Oxford University Press, Oxford, Figure 1)

planning-trained) nurse, supplemented by you perhaps at the end of your surgery or during the next dedicated family planning session? See Q 8.15.

4.97 What else is important as an adjunct to good counselling?

The written word! In my view *counselling should always be supplemented by a leaflet,* and I think the best is still 'Choosing and using the combined pill', published by the UK FPA. Among other things this has advice for missed pills and a medicolegally important list of those side-effects which should lead the woman to seek urgent medical advice (see Q 4.176).

Finally, much medical time may be saved if those women who desire the impossible, a 2-hour consultation about oral contraception, are referred to my comprehensive paperback entitled *The Pill* (see Further Reading)!

SELECTION OF USERS AND FORMULATIONS: CHOOSING THE 'SAFER WOMEN'

4.98 For whom is the COC method particularly indicated?

At the patient's choice, where maximum protection from pregnancy and independence from intercourse are the most important features in her own view.

It is particularly valuable for the healthy young sexually active non-smoking woman who is sufficiently motivated to be a reliable pill-taker and not at risk of viral STDs. (When this applies she should be advised to use condoms, instead or as well.)

4.99 For what gynaecological conditions is the combined pill prescribed?

Because the extra requirement for treatment increases the benefit side of the benefit–risk equation, it may sometimes be acceptable to prescribe higher-dose pills or to give the COC to women with one or more relative contraindications. A specialist's advice should be sought where appropriate.

COCs can be used to:

1 Relieve spasmodic dysmenorrhoea.

2 'Regulate' menstrual cycles, especially in cases of prolonged bleeding with no demonstrable pathology. The reason for cycle irregularity or secondary amenorrhoea should always be determined first but then the pill may well be appropriate (see Q 4.58).

3 Relieve premenstrual tension. This is not always successful, and some women develop similar symptoms only when taking the COC.

Table 4.8 Risk factors for arterial CVS disease

Risk factor	Absolute contraindication	Relative contraindication	Remarks
Family history (FH) CVS disease (arterial or venous) in a first degree relative <45 years	Known atherogenic lipid profile or prothrombotic haemostatic profile – or tests not available	Normal blood profiles or first attack in relative >45	*Note: If FH of arterial disease should test BOTH for lipids and haemostasis*
Diabetes mellitus (DM)	Severe, or diabetic complications present (e.g. retinopathy, renal damage)	Not severe/labile, and no complications, young patient with short duration of DM	POP usually a better-choice hormonal method
Hypertension	BP >60/95 mmHg on repeated testing	Systolic BP 135–160 mmHg Diastolic BP 85–95 mmHg	POP often better See Q 4.168–4.172
Cigarette smoking	40+ cigarettes/day	5–40 cigarettes/day	Smokers are THE PROBLEM!
Increasing age	Above age 35 in all smokers BUT age alone is *not an absolute contraindication* (see Q 4.232)	Age 40–50 non-smokers	
Excess weight	>50% above ideal for height (BMI >35)	20–50 above ideal (BMI 30–35)	BMI is body mass index (see Q 4.57)
Migraine	Focal, crescendo or ergotamine treated	Uncomplicated/acceptable to the woman	Relates to stroke risk. Consider tricycling if non-focal type headaches mainly in pill-free interval (see Q 4.28)

Notes:
1 Some of the numbers are a little arbitrary and may be applied less restrictively in certain circumstances (e.g. the COC might be allowed reluctantly to a currently healthy 25 year old admitting to two packs of cigarettes a day). They also relate to use solely for contraception.
2 Use of COCs for medical indications often entails a different risk–benefit analysis, i.e. the extra therapeutic benefits may outweigh expected extra risks.

4 Control menorrhagia. If fibroids are present and surgery not indicated a relatively progestagen-dominant pill should be chosen with continued monitoring by the same observer.

5 Control endometriosis as maintenance after first-line treatment (progestagen-dominant brand, best using the tricycle regimen (see Qs 4.28 and 4.210)).

6 Control functional ovarian cysts (see Q 4.53).

7 Relieve oestrogen deficiency and control gynaecological/ menstrual cyclical symptoms in peri-menopausal women still requiring contraception.

Note: Triphasic pills are not appropriate for these indications.

4.100 What are the four questions to be asked when prescribing the COC?

1 Who never? (See absolute contraindications, Q 4.101.)

2 Who usually not? – the not-so-safe women. (See Table 4.8 and Qs 4.103.)

3 Which pill? (See Qs 4.133, 4.149 and 4.150.)

4 Which should be the second choice of pill? (See Qs 4.151 and 4.156.)

4.101 What are the absolute contraindications to COCs?

Any compilation of contraindications reflects the judgement of the compiler, as much as the available science at the relevant date. The answers to this and the next two questions are as assessed by me in 1993!

Certain important diseases are considered in more detail later.

A. Past or present circulatory disease

1 Any arterial or venous *thrombosis*. This normally includes any documented idiopathic thrombophlebitis in a varicose vein, but not as in Q 4.121.

2 *Ischaemic heart disease* or angina, and all *cardiomyopathies*.

3 *Severe* or *combined* risk factors for arterial disease (see Table 4.8 and below). Also **family history of a young close relative** (*age under 45 years) suffering arterial or venous thrombosis* if it is impossible to arrange adequate investigations. If it was an arterial event the tests should assess *both* lipids and haemosta-

sis, since congenital abnormalities of either could have caused the family member's problem – hence:

4 Specific *atherogenic lipid disorders* (which are known about), especially hereditary hypercholesterolaemia with cholesterol above 7.5 mmol/l (see Table 4.8).

5 Specific *prothrombotic abnormalities* of coagulation/fibrinolysis – including the congenital thrombophilias with abnormal levels of individual factors (see Q 4.110), presence of antiphospholipid antibody (the lupus 'anticoagulant'), and postsplenectomy for any indication if the platelet count is above 500×10^9/litre.

6 Other *known conditions predisposing to thrombosis* – including: blood dyscrasias; autoimmune and rheumatoid disorders with this risk, including polyarteritis nodosa, scleroderma and severe SLE (see Q 4.113); Klippel–Trenaunay syndrome; severe 1° or 2° polycythaemia; from 4 weeks before until 2 weeks following mobilization after elective major or leg surgery, during leg immobilization or varicose vein treatments (offer instead POP or injectable) (see Q 4.177–81); and climbing above 4000 m (details at Q 4.106). *Severe* inflammatory bowel disease, including Crohn's disease, also comes into this category – see Q 4.112.

7 *Focal and crescendo migraine*; migraine requiring ergotamine treatment (see Qs 4.124–6).

8 *Transient ischaemic attacks* even without headache.

9 Past *cerebral haemorrhage* – which is believed often secondary to *cerebral venous thrombosis*, also to avoid pill-induced BP increase if *past subarachnoid haemorrhage* (Q 4.109).

10 Most types of *valvular heart disease* (discuss with cardiologist, COC may be permitted if no disturbance of haemodynamics or risk of arterial embolism); pulmonary hypertension.

B. Disease of the liver

1 *Active liver disease* (i.e. whenever liver function tests currently abnormal, including infiltrations – such as the glycogen storage diseases – and cirrhosis).

2 History of *cholestatic jaundice* whether or not pill related, or of cholestatic jaundice in pregnancy. Dubin–Johnson and Rotor syndromes which are congenital deficiencies of hepatic excretion.

> **Note: after any viral hepatitis, severe infectious mononucleosis or other reversible hepatocellular damage; COC-taking may be resumed 3 months after liver function tests have returned to normal**.

3 Liver *adenoma, carcinoma* (see Q 4.82, 4.81)

4 *Symptomatic gallstones* (but COC may be used after chole-cystectomy, see Q 4.198).

5 The *porphyrias* (attacks may be precipitated).

C. History of serious condition affected by sex steroids or related to previous COC-use

The more important examples are:

1 the *porphyrias* already mentioned;

2 *chorea*;

3 COC-induced *hypertension*;

4 COC-associated *acute pancreatitis* (but see Q 4.199);

5 *pemphigoid gestationis* (formerly called herpes gestationis);

6 *haemolytic uraemic syndrome*;

7 *otosclerosis* (this can deteriorate in pregnancy, and the COC is to some degree pregnancy mimicking. However, some authorities permit supervised COC use, especially after definitive surgery);

8 *Stevens–Johnson syndrome* (erythema multiforme), if COC-associated;

9 *SLE* (see Q 4.113);

10 *trophoblastic disease – but only until βhCG levels are undetectable*. In the USA this is considered a relative contraindication even when hCG levels are high.

This is not necessarily a complete list – see Q 4.104.

D. Existing or possible pregnancy

E. Undiagnosed genital tract bleeding

F. Oestrogen–dependent neoplasms

Especially breast cancer (but some oncologists do permit COC in selected cases in prolonged remission). Past breast biopsy showing premalignant epithelial atypia is usually also considered an absolute contraindication. All other cancers are normally relative contraindications (see Q 4.103), supervised use being permitted.

G. Woman's own continuing anxiety re COC safety, unrelieved after counselling

Several of the above (e.g. D,E,F and G) are not necessarily permanent contraindications.

4.102 Relative contraindications – how assessed and how applied?

Here we have the impact not just of my judgement as compiler, but yours as prescriber! The art of medicine is nowhere better shown than in assessing how strong each of the contraindications at Q 4.103 is (and that differs within the list as well as in different individuals), and then balancing the risk of each against the benefits to each pill-taker; with allowance for synergism between risk factors and the general teaching that two or more relative contraindications equal one absolute contraindication; all in the light of everything relevant like her probable fertility and her other contraceptive choices; and *all, most emphatically, being discussed openly with the woman, so that she makes the final decision . . . .* Now see Q 4.103.

4.103 What are the relative contraindications to the COC?

1 First see Table 4.8, i.e. risk factors for arterial disease are all relative contraindications: provided normally that only one is present, and not to so marked a degree that it alone would absolutely contraindicate this method. This category includes essential hypertension controlled by treatment; also past tox- aemia of pregnancy which seems greatly to increase the risk of myocardial infarction in smokers (RCGP Study). But *age alone* is no longer seen as a risk factor for non-smokers (see Q 4.232).

2 Long-term partial immobilization (e.g. in a wheelchair). *Com- plete* paralysis of the lower limbs is viewed by some as an absolute contraindication.

3 Sex steroid-dependent cancers in remission. Seek the specialist's advice: most will (appropriately in my view) permit COC use for melanoma in remission after treatment (whether or not diag- nosed during pill-taking). But the history of breast cancer is almost invariably considered an absolute contraindication (Q 4.101).

4   Oligo-/amenorrhoea should be investigated but the pill may subsequently be prescribed (see Q 4.54–8)

5   Hyperprolactinaemia: this is now considered only a relative contraindication for patients under specialist supervision

6   Very severe depression, if likely to be exacerbated by COCs. But unwanted pregnancies can be very depressing!

7   *Chronic systemic diseases.* These are discussed further below (see Qs 4.104-13). In general they are *weak* relative contraindications, mainly signifying extra counselling and above average monitoring. In the stronger category which I describe as *'more strongly contraindicated/ so other methods usually preferred'* are: *sickle cell anaemia* (see Q 4.108); *Crohn's disease* in remission (see Q 4.112); *diabetes* (see Q 4.115–6); *chronic renal disease*; and mild (not steroid-treated) *systemic lupus erythematosis* (SLE), though presence of the antiphospholipid antibody absolutely contraindicates the COC (see Qs 4.110 and 4.113). In these the common reason for special caution is that the condition may lead in various ways to an increased risk of venous and/or arterial thrombosis. If that risk became established, as in a diabetic with evidence of arteriopathy, it would be an absolute contraindication, see Q 4.115 and above. In the case of SLE and Crohn's there is also the risk of sex hormones causing deterioration of the condition.

   Splenectomy, for whatever reason performed (e.g. in the treatment of sickle disease), is only a relative contraindication. However *the platelets should be monitored,* initially at least annually, and a count rising to above 500×10^9 per litre would absolutely contraindicate the oestrogen of the COC.

8   Diseases requiring long-term treatment with *enzyme-inducing drugs* which might reduce the efficacy of the pill (see Qs 4.31, 4.33): especially tuberculosis and epilepsy.

9   New *relative contraindications now include (see Qs 4.79 and 4.72):*
    (a)   if a young first-degree relative has had breast cancer;
    (b)   the presence of established BBD;
    (c)   during the monitoring of abnormal cervical smears;
    (d)   during and after definitive treatment for CIN.
Women in groups (a) and (b) need recounselling after about 4 years' use. CIN follow-up (i.e. groups (c) plus (d)) amounts to only a *weak* relative contraindication, so it would be usual to continue the COC with smear monitoring as advised by the laboratory.

4.104 On what criteria can one decide whether the COC may be used for patients with intercurrent disease?

First, there are some conditions which are positively benefited (see Qs 4.49, 4.99) or at least not affected. There are persistent medical myths (see Q 4.235), and it is unfortunate that women continue to be unnecessarily deprived of the pill for the wrong reasons, like thrush, uncomplicated varicose veins, past amenorrhoea or fibroids.

It is impossible to list every known disease or state which might have a bearing on pill-prescribing, but *here are some useful criteria*:

In general, discover first what the disease does in relation to known risks or effects of the COC. Does it cause *changes which summate with adverse effects of the COC*? Does it:

1 Increase the risk of arterial or venous thrombosis, anywhere? This includes consideration of restricted mobility (Qs 4.103, 4.105).

2 Predispose to arterial wall disease?

3 Adversely affect liver function?

4 Show a tendency to an important degree of hormone dependency, either by medical reputation (usually then a relative contraindication), or in that individual (absolute contraindication). If there was deterioration with previous administration of steroid hormones or during pregnancy, it means enough to be an absolute contraindication if the condition is serious.

5 Require treatment with an enzyme-inducing drug?

If 5 is true the pill can still be an option, but special conditions apply (see Q 4.33). If 1–4 apply there is the real problem of deciding whether the COC should be absolutely or (as at Q 4.103) relatively contraindicated. *The added risk obtaining in pregnancy may fully justify some increased risk due to the COC,* at least in young and hence more fertile women, primarily because it is so effective. Its other benefits may also be highly relevant in some conditions. This is not so, however, for the list at Q 4.76 (absolute contraindications). For them, remember injectables!

If none of the above criteria applies, then the condition could normally be added to the list in Q 4.105.

4.105 Can you list those medical conditions in which the COC may be used with caution since there is no evidence that deterioration may be caused?

According to current information, the following diseases all come

into this category (but there are many others): AIDS (see Q 4.226), asthma, Gilbert's disease, treated Hodgkin's disease (if fertility preserved), hereditary lymphoedema, multiple sclerosis, myasthenia gravis, Raynaud's disease (unless the phenomenon proves to be symptomatic of a contraindicating condition), renal dialysis, retinitis pigmentosa, rheumatoid arthritis, sarcoidosis, spherocytosis, thalassaemia major, thyrotoxicosis and Wolff-Parkinson-White syndrome. Also most cancers under treatment, if hormone dependency or an increase in the risk of thrombosis are not suspected.

In individual cases the prescriber should, nevertheless, first review the checklist at Q 4.104 above and, normally, consult with the hospital specialist(s) supervising treatment for the main disorder: to obtain their support and also to guard against unforeseen drug interactions, etc. Such women need extra supervision within primary care as well. But reliable protection from pregnancy is often particularly important when chronic diseases are present.

4.106 Is the combined pill best avoided at high altitude?

Yes. Acute mountain sickness can kill, through hypoxia leading to acute pulmonary oedema and cerebral oedema, and blood clots in the small arteries are a feature *post-mortem*. In milder attacks well short of that, when unacclimatized people climb above about 3000 m (*c.* 10 000 ft), there is an increasing risk of venous or arterial thromboembolism. Increased capillary permeability leads to shifts in body fluids, tissue oedema and haemoconcentration, leading to raised blood viscosity in the short term. Acetazolamide (Diamox), which has been shown to improve climbing performance and prevent acute mountain sickness, acts as a mild diuretic and might exacerbate the thrombotic risk. There is also pulmonary hypertension in the more severe cases, which would itself contraindicate the COC.

It would appear prudent for women climbing or trekking to high altitudes to consider the COC as *absolutely contraindicated* (at least above 4000 m) and use instead an injectable or the POP. In residents, after prolonged acclimatization there is a physiological polycythaemia which slightly increases blood viscosity; but this alone would be only a *relative contraindication* to oestrogen in the combined pill.

4.107 What about long-haul aeroplane flights and thrombosis risk?

Although all commercial flights are pressurized to the equivalent of about 2000 m, there are now numerous case reports of thrombotic events (with or without the pill). Some extracellular to interstitial fluid shift is common; mild ankle oedema results, but more important is the likelihood of haemoconcentration. Other important factors are the maintained sedentary position, coupled with a diuresis due to alcohol and caffeine, all perhaps superimposed on dehydration due to prolonged sunbathing on a Far Eastern beach just before boarding!

To quote my book *The Pill*:

> There is no necessity to come off the pill – many flight attendants use it all the time. But follow their example and take some exercise during the flight: such as a brief walk around the plane every hour or so.

4.108 May the combined pill be prescribed to patients with sickle-cell disorders?

Yes is the answer for those with sickle-cell trait. The situation with regard to homozygous sickle-cell disease (SS and SC genes) is more uncertain. There is an increased risk of thromboembolic disease especially strokes in such women, and pregnancy may precipitate a crisis. The COC imitates pregnancy, and the oestrogen of the pill might in theory lead to superimposed thrombosis during the arterial stasis of a crisis. Therefore, until recently most manufacturers and many authorities have included the frank sickling diseases among absolute contraindications to the COC. However studies in the West Indies and West Africa have shown that the COC ought now to be considered only a relative contraindication (especially when balanced against the great risks of pregnancy in sicklers). Injectables especially DMPA, are usually an even better choice (see Q 5.93).

4.109 May a woman who has made a complete recovery from a subarachnoid haemorrhage, and had her intracranial lesion treated, use the combined pill?

The COC is relatively contraindicated if there is a close subsequent watch for hypertension, but the POP or an injectable would be preferable. This is because almost all women on the combined pill have a detectable slight increase in systolic and diastolic blood pressure, and one can never be certain that such a woman would not have some other weakness of a cerebral artery or angeiomatous malformation.

4.110 What are the congenital thrombophilias? How does their frequency compare with congenital lipid disorders?

Hereditary disorders which increase the risk of thrombosis are uncommon, but becoming better characterized. The four most important are deficiencies of antithrombin III, protein C, protein S and plasminogen; with rarer ones like the dysfibrinoginaemias, fibrinolytic abnormalities, and heparin cofactor deficiency. Antiphospholipid antibodies (lupus anticoagulant) may be familial or acquired and occur in about 1 in 1500 of the population. Compare this with about 1 in 500 for familial hypercholesterolaemia.

Most of the few women who suffer thrombotic events on the COC are probably different from the generality of pill-takers, i.e. predisposed, though the detailed explanation is often not identifiable even after an event.

4.111 In view of Q 4.110, how can we identify the predisposed women in advance? Should there be routine blood screening of all prospective pill-takers?

In some countries this is the practice, but usually only in the private sector because of the expense of the tests and the very low incidence of positive results. Even there, any reassurance from this non-selective screening is largely false because the usual screening tests for haemostasis (like the activated partial thromboplastin time) are largely irrelevant to the congenital thrombophilias, which require tests of the specific factor for diagnosis.

So I recommend treating women rather than laboratory tests! In this country we normally rely on a *careful family history regarding close relatives under age 40–45 to provide the clinical clue to referral for further testing* (or less often, a past personal history of a minor possible thrombosis such as in a varicose vein) – as in Table 4.8. But testing should then be thorough, and if the correct tests of haemostasis – and in arterial cases also of lipids – are not available then the COC is best avoided. See Table 4.8 and Q 4.120.

4.112 Why are the inflammatory bowel diseases (Crohn's or ulcerative colitis (UC)) relative contraindications?

1 Both occur more commonly in COC-takers in some studies. Crohn's (but not UC) is also associated with smoking.

2 Non-granulomatous colonic Crohn's may improve if the COC is stopped (see Q 4.201).

3 In exacerbations of either illness there is a high risk of thrombosis, especially venous thromboembolism. Therefore if the COC is used it should be only in mild cases not prone to severe hospitalized exacerbations, and if such occur the pill should be stopped at once, and would be absolutely contraindicated so long as the disease remained severe.

Malabsorption. Since contraceptive steroids are so well absorbed mainly in the jejunum which is unaffected, malabsorption of the COC is usually not a problem in either condition.

4.113 May the COC be used by women with systemic lupus erythematosus (SLE)?

Increasingly, this is being seen as an *absolute contraindication, except in the mildest very stable fully investigated cases not on steroids, with close supervision.* This is because:

1 There are now numerous case reports and some comparative studies describing the onset or flaring up of symptomatic SLE when oestrogen was given, either in the COC or even, interestingly, as hormone replacement therapy postmenopausally. SLE may deteriorate seriously with renal involvement for the first time during use of COCs, but not with progestogen-only therapy.

2 There is a recurring theme of recovery or improvement once the artificial oestrogen was discontinued.

3 Cases may develop the lupus anticoagulant/antiphospholipid antibody and once this is detected the COC is definitely contraindicated for fear of thrombosis.

Obviously each patient has to be taken on her own merits. But since progestogen-only pills and injections have been tried in SLE women with no significant increase in episodes of active disease, these are usually *preferred to the COC.*

4.114 The pill is acceptably safe, but who are the 'dangerous women'?

These are all the women just considered with absolute and relative contraindications; but especially (in routine practice) they are those with a recognized risk factor for arterial disease. See Table 4.8, which also suggests appropriate action to be taken if one is present.

Note also the importance of *synergism*: as a rule the contraindication becomes absolute rather than relative if more than one of these risk factors should apply.

The issues of age and duration of use are considered further at Q 4.230–4.

4.115 May the combined pill be used by patients with established diabetes mellitus (DM)?

Arterial disease is more probable in diabetics; hence ideally they should avoid oestrogen with its prothrombotic risks. *A barrier method, or the POP, are much to be preferred (see Q 5.44).*

In practice, however, some young diabetics are permitted use of an ultra-low-oestrogen combined pill using a 'lipid friendly' progestogen. Mercilon with only 20 μg oestrogen would be a good choice (see Q 4.136). Necessary criteria are:

1 Young, ideally under age 25, and preferably with a short duration of the DM.

2 Free of *any* signs of complications of the disease, affecting arteries, nerves, kidneys or retina.

3 Free of the other conditions in Figure 4.9. It is vital that such a patient is not also a smoker or hypertensive.

4 Perceived to need maximum protection against pregnancy and there is no satisfactory alternative.

Diabetics occasionally need an increased dose of insulin, not in itself a problem. They should be on the COC for the shortest possible time, encouraged to have their family as young as their circumstances allow, and then be transferred to another method – possibly sterilization.

4.116 May potential or latent diabetics take the COC?

Yes: caution used to be advised, because the early pills did impair glucose tolerance and create hyperinsulinism. However the RCGP study and others have shown absolutely no increase in the incidence of late-onset-type DM among current or ex-pill-users. Moreover, the more recent lowest-dose COCs do not even raise plasma insulins significantly. None of the following need therefore be considered as contraindications: a strong family history of DM (maturity onset); gestational diabetes; birth of a baby weighing more than 4.5 kg (10 lb).

Such women are just supervised a little more closely than usual and need particular advice to avoid obesity.

4.117 Is it true that smoking a packet or more cigarettes per day makes the person at least a decade older as regards CVS risk?

This follows directly from the right side of Figure 4.9, which is derived from the RCGP report of 1981. The circulatory disease risk for smokers on the pill at age 35–44 is not distinguishable from that for non-smokers above 45. The precise risk is likely to be lower for each age with the use of modern pills, and indeed no excess caused by the modern COC without smoking is now detectable. But the differential of around 10 years between smokers and non-smokers in the 1981 RCGP Study may well have increased, bearing in mind that horrendously increased risk ratio of 21 for pill-takers who smoke, at any age! (See Q 4.86.)

4.118 What effect does smoking have on the mortality of arterial disease in pill-users?

The 1983 report of the RCGP showed that the pill-user who also smoked was not only more likely to suffer an arterial disease event (chiefly a heart attack or stroke) but was also much more likely to die as a consequence, i.e. a higher case-fatality rate was noted in smokers.

4.119 In Table 4.8, when there is a family history of arterial disease occurring in a young close relative, why are normal tests of both lipids and haemostasis required before the pill is acceptable?

Because the familial problem might be of either type (see Qs 4.101 and 4.110), and arteries are closable prematurely because of either accelerated atherogenesis or a thrombophilia. Haemostasis problems do usually show up by venous thrombosis, often at an even younger age, but that family history might have been overlooked as it is less fatal. Hereditary lipid abnormalities are of course more likely if the close family member involved was a non-smoker.

4.120 Of what relevance is a clear-cut family history of venous thromboembolism as opposed to arterial disease?

This is certainly relevant, especially if your patient tends to obesity or has an atherogenic risk factor (Table 4.8), promoting disease of an important *arterial* wall in which thrombosis might occur. (Cigarette smoking does not, interestingly, promote venous thrombosis.) Where available, appropriate blood screening should first be arranged, particularly to exclude the rare thrombophilias mentioned at Q 4.110. If such comprehensive tests cannot be done then it may be best to consider the family history as an absolute contraindication.

4.121 If a young woman suffers a thrombosis in an arm vein after an intravenous injection, does this mean a predisposition to thrombosis? Should she avoid the COC in future?

The answer is no to both questions. The episode would be due to a chemical thrombophlebitis. This is not associated with any tendency to venous thrombosis elsewhere in the body.

4.122 Why are varicose veins not a contraindication in Table 4.8?

Varicose veins are not relevant to pill-prescribing though they are often acting as a *marker* for another adverse factor such as obesity, or may have previously been involved in a definite thrombotic process (i.e. thrombophlebitis). In the latter case, like any past thrombosis, this history would be an absolute contraindication to an oestrogen-containing pill; unless detailed study of coagulation factors was possible and proved sufficiently reassuring. Thus this caution is worthwhile if it prevents the woman having an occlusive event somewhere much more important next time. In the absence of such a past history, the possession of varicose veins does not contraindicate the COC, provided the woman herself wishes to use the method (see also Q 4.179).

4.123 In what way does the possession of blood group O influence prescribing policy?

Women possessing blood group O have been shown to have a lower risk of thrombosis than those with other blood groups. The protective effect probably applies to arterial as well as venous disease. Knowledge of her blood group may therefore be helpful in a positive way, when prescribing to a woman who is otherwise not an ideal pill-user. For example, one would be happier to prescribe the COC to a 34-year-old smoker if she were known to be blood group O rather than A.

4.124 What is a working definition of migraine (Table 4.8), and what types of migraine contraindicate the combined pill?

In general, migraine headaches vary greatly between individuals and between attacks: but attacks share the features of a unilateral headache with nausea and usually other symptoms such as blurred vision or photophobia, often in a prodrome. There are four types which contraindicate oestrogen in the combined pill:

1 focal migraine (see Qs 4.126 and 4.127);

2 crescendo migraine – that is, any migraine sustained for days while becoming ever more severe (hence 'crescendo'), even without any of the focal symptoms;

3 occurrence of the woman's first-ever attack while taking the COC. This means the COC should be stopped; but if no further problems develop in that attack and there are no focal symptoms in any later attacks, this may be subsequently considered only a relative contraindication;

4 the concurrent use of ergotamine as therapy.

4.125 Why does treatment with ergometrine or sumatriptan contraindicate the COC?

Cerebral thrombosis can occur anyway as a rare complication of any type of migraine. Ergotamine is a cerebral vasoconstrictor. Since the circulating blood may be altered by the oestrogen of a prescribed COC in a prothrombotic direction, the concern is that the combination could lead to the tragedy of an avoidable stroke.

Since sumatriptan (Imigran) has similar vasoconstricting actions and is contraindicated in 'hemiplegic migraine', I would propose that the COC should also be avoided if treatment includes this drug – at least until there are more data.

4.126 What are the features of focal migraine?

Any migraine which is associated with a clear history of symptoms (however transitory), either during an aura or during the headache phase, which *can be interpreted* as being caused by transient impairment of cerebral blood flow, is a focal migraine. Such symptoms are the following:

1 *Eye symptoms*:
   (a) loss of any part of the field of vision;
   (b) tunnel vision;

(c) teichopsia – defined in my medical dictionary as 'the scintillating line of light along the boundary of a migrainous field defect'. (The word apparently comes from the Greek *teichos* meaning a city wall, hence the other name 'fortification spectra', because many sufferers describe 'battlements'). If 'flashing lights' are symmetrical with no field defect, I cautiously allow COC; but we need more data.

2 *Neurological symptoms and signs*:
   (a) weakness on one side of the body or affecting one limb;
   (b) loss of sensation or marked paraesthesiae on one side of the body or affecting a limb or one side of the tongue;
   (c) nominal dysphasia (cannot find the right word for things);
   (d) focal epilepsy.

Such attacks are termed *hemiplegic migraine* if severe and the condition may be familial. *However*, simple general blurring of vision, photophobia and phonophobia (intolerance of light and sound) would be only relative contraindications to starting, or cautiously continuing, the oestrogen-containing pill, along with appropriate warning advice for the future, as below.

Persistent blurred vision indicates fundoscopy (see Q 4.190).

Although the main feature of focal migraine is asymmetry, a one-sided headache has no special significance, being a standard feature of any migraine.

4.127 Why is focal or hemiplegic migraine so significant?

There is a reduction in blood flow measurable during migraines with the relevant aura. Many authorities believe that there is first of all a chemical change and the change in brain perfusion is secondary. However even so the concern about oestrogen is that it causes prothrombotic changes in the blood which might, at the margins, just be enough to turn transient ischaemia into permanent ischaemia (i.e. a stroke) – which does after all sometimes happen in migraine without the pill. So, with or without the headache in fact, focal symptoms have to mean: 'avoid the combined pill; or if it is currently in use, stop it today, and for ever'. This vigorous reaction is necessary because of reports by many neurologists (notably Bickerstaff, who wrote a monograph in 1975 on the subject) that a number of those very few, young pill-takers admitted with strokes gave such a history during the days or weeks leading up to their admission. Most of the remainder had either a crescendo headache beginning many hours before the event, or had developed migraine for the first time while taking the COC.

It is a very reasonable hypothesis that these women would not have suffered irreversible cerebral arterial insufficiency had the oestrogen in the combined pill been stopped sooner. This is never going to be proved by a controlled trial, but the philosophy 'better safe than sorry' explains my cautious approach above.

4.128 What other factors are important to reduce still further the risk of strokes in modern pill-prescribing?

1 *vasoconstrictive disease*, perhaps secondary to systemic illnesses like collagen disorders;

2 of special relevance, *hypertension* (see Qs 4.168–4.170);

3 other circulatory *risk factors* (especially diabetes, heavy smoking, also all blood dyscrasias known to be linked with thrombosis);

4 any *past history of a thrombotic event*.

4.129 Can women with symptoms or syndromes mentioned in the last few questions, whether occurring before or on the COC, use a POP or injectable?

Most neurologists with whom I have consulted give as their opinion that the critical hormone involved is oestrogen. Hence any oestrogen-free contraceptive may be used, after assessment of other risk factors. Even during a relevant attack the woman could be transferred immediately to the POP or perhaps DMPA (see Q 5.96). The woman should be warned of course that she may continue to get the migrainous headaches, even perhaps with focal symptoms. But there would now not be the added concern that her contraceptive treatment would amplify the small risk which always exists of a thrombotic stroke in any woman with bad migraines.

4.130 What about diffuse (non-focal) migraines which the woman can tolerate? Do these contraindicate the pill?

Sufferers from simple migraine without aura (formerly known as common migraine) or migraine with aura in which (so far in any woman's case) there are none of the asymmetrical symptoms listed above, may take the combined pill. It is only a relative contraindication, if they have a normal blood pressure and ideally do not smoke. But all such women *must be given a clear description of the relevant symptoms* which are listed at Q 4.176 and within the FPA Pill leaflet, with the instruction to *'stop the pill and immediately take professional advice'*.

4.131 Which COC brands or regimens are best for headaches and non-focal 'common' migraines?

Monophasic pills are generally preferred to triphasic pills (fully described below Q 4.158–64). The latter are not good for women with a tendency to headaches, since the extra fluctuations of the hormone levels may act as a trigger. In addition, in any woman whose headaches tend to happen in the PFI , it can be enormously helpful to prescribe the tricycle regimen, but with a monophasic pill (see Q 4.28). *Note*: this is provided such migraine headaches never have focal symptoms.

4.132 How well known is all this about the importance of enquiring about migraine, both when first prescribing and then during monitoring of the COC?

Not very. For example, without doubt the commonest prescribing error which emerges in my sterilization counselling clinic is the combined pill being given to women who have definite focal migraine. One reason is that in the past it has not been given prominence in most lists of contraindications.

Choice of formulation: the safer pills

4.133 Obviously we should choose to prescribe the pill so far as possible to 'safer women' – but what are the 'safer pills'?

The doses in the first brands marketed in the 1960s, on which indeed much of the epidemiology is based, were clearly too high. On the market then was a brand which gave more of the same oestrogen in a day than is now given in a week; and virtually the same daily dose of a progestagen as now covers a complete cycle! See Table 4.9.

In short, safer pills are 'smaller pills'. Both the constituent hormones are capable of unwanted metabolic effects and their epidemiological consequences.

Oestrogen: here 'smaller' is simply a matter of lower dose, and the dose of EE given should *normally* be no more than 20–35 μg.

Table 4.9 Reduction in doses since combined pills were first introduced

	Dose of sex steroid per tablet in 1962	Minimum of same as used in 1992
Ethinyloestradiol (EE)	150 μg in Enovid10	20 μg in Mercilon 20, Loestrin 20
Norethisterone (NET)	10 000 μg in Ortho-Novum 10	500 μg in Ovysmen/Brevinor

Progestagen: the 'metabolic impact' of the progestagen can be minimized in two ways:

1 The so-called 'third-generation' products do appear to cause less of what appear to be adverse metabolic changes while still retaining good activity as contraceptives and cycle controllers (see Q 4.136). So these can be considered 'smaller', but in a pharmacological rather than dose/quantity sense.

2 With *any* chosen progestagen there should obviously also still be a preference for the lowest acceptable dose.

Latest data suggest that a policy based on preferring 'smaller' pills as just described really does reduce the risk of *major side–effects*. Clinical experience also shows that, with one exception, *minor side–effects* (see Q 4.183) are less frequent and less severe. (The obvious exception is cycle control: but that can be handled, as part of the pill prescribing scheme to be described.)

4.134 What are the fundamental problems in applying a 'smaller pill' policy?

There are three:

1 The first is *knowing what really are the 'smaller'* presumed safer pills. Epidemiology is best, but so slow to give results that it tends only to tell us about 'yesterday's pills'. So in the here and now, prudence forces us to pay more attention than we would wish to metabolic changes, especially those which the available epidemiology suggests are important (see Q 4.94).

2 Then there is *individual variation*. A medium-dose pill for one woman could be in its biological effect a low-dose pill for another, or a high-dose pill for a third.

It is thus a false expectation that any single pill will suit all women. We return to this point below, see Figure 4.11 and Qs 4.140–8.

3   The third problem, linked with 2, is the *lack of provision by the manufacturers of a sufficient range of pills* in some of the 'ladders' (to be described).

4.135 Why is *d*-norgestrel called levonorgestrel? Please explain.

Norgestrel is a racemic mixture of a *d*-isomer and *l*-isomer. It is given the prefix '*d*' because it shares the same spacial orientation as other molecules which by the conventions of stereochemistry are all called the *d*-forms. However, when in solution it deviates light in the opposite direction (i.e. to the left) and is therefore known as levonorgestrel.

The opposite applies to *l*-norgestrel which rotates light to the right. It is also biologically inactive. Yet it has to be metabolized. Hence where there exists a choice (e.g. see Table 5.1) it is preferable to use the nearest equivalent brand which uses pure levonorgestrel.

4.136 If there are risk factors or in older women, why are the 'third-generation' progestagens desogestrel, gestodene and norgestimate normally preferred to levonorgestrel and the norethisterone group?

In oversimplified terms they are more 'selective', with greater relative affinity for the receptors for progesterone (wanted effect) than for androgens (unwanted, as it correlates with HDL_2-C reduction). This seems to explain why products using them are effective contraceptives, yet produce less potentially adverse changes than otherwise equivalent products with LNG or NET like Norimin/Neocon or Ovranette/Microgynon in lipid metabolism (see Qs 4.91 and 4.139). So in my view they are preferable, according to present data, for older women and all possessing the established arterial disease risk factors.

Mercilon with only 20 μg of oestrogen seems as effective as other COCs in compliant women, without a vastly greater risk of breakthrough bleeding. It is especially appropriate for use by the overweight or older woman (to reduce the risk of thrombosis in veins, or in arteries affected by early atheroma). See Q 8.17. A similar 20-μg product using gestodene as the progestagen would be welcomed.

4.137 What are the pill brands available, and how may they be classified?

The practitioner is faced with a bewildering variety of formulations (Tables 4.10, 4.11). As first proposed by Dr Barbara Law, former Chairman of the Joint Committee on Contraception, they may be grouped in ladders according to the particular progestagen they contain, each lower rung representing a lower hormone content than those above (Fig. 4.10). The philosophy behind this display

Table 4.10 Combined oral contraceptives (COCs) available in Britain (1993)

	Levonorgestrel (μg)	Ethinyloestradiol (μg)
Ovran (Wyeth)	250	50
Eugynon 30 (Schering)	250	30
Ovran 30 (Wyeth)	250	30
Ovranette (Wyeth)	150	30
Microgynon (Schering)	150	30
Trinordiol (Wyeth) (triphasic)	6 × 50	30
Logynon (Schering) (triphasic)	5 × 75	40
	10 × 125	30
Logynon ED = Logynon + 7 inert tablets		
	Norethisterone (μg)	Mestranol (μg)
Norinyl-I (Syntex)	1000	50
Ortho-Novin 1/50 (Ortho-Cilag)	1000	50
	Norethisterone (μg)	Ethinyloestradiol (μg)
Norimin (Syntex)	1000	35
Neocon (Ortho-Cilag)	1000	35
BiNovum (Ortho-Cilag)	7 × 500	35
	14 × 1000	35
TriNovum (Ortho-Cilag)	7 × 500	35
	7 × 750	35
	7 × 1000	35
TriNovum ED = Trinovum + 7 inert tablets		
Synphase (Syntex)	7 × 500	35
	9 × 1000	35
	5 × 500	35
Ovysmen (Ortho)	500	35
Brevinor (Syntex)	500	35
	Norethisterone acetate (μg)	Ethinyloestradiol oestradiol (μg)
Loestrin 30 (Parke Davis)	1500	30
Loestrin 20 (Parke Davis)	1000	20

Table 4.10 (contd)

	Ethynodiol diacetate (µg)	Ethinyloestradiol (µg)
Conova 30 (Searle)	2000	30
	Desogestrel (µg)	Ethinyloestradiol (µg)
Marvelon (Organon)	150	30
Mercilon (Organon)	150	20
	Gestodene (µg)	Ethinyloestradiol (µg)
Femodene (Schering)	75	30
Minulet (Wyeth)	75	30
Femodene ED = Femodene + 7 inert tablets		
Tri-Minulet (Wyeth)	6 × 50	30
Triadene (Schering)	5 × 70	40
	10 × 100	30
	Norgestimate (µg)	Ethinyloestradiol (µg)
Cilest (Ortho-Cilag)	250	35

is that the lower down a ladder one is, the less likely is injury if one falls off! The POPs are shown as being the least likely to cause side-effects – on ground level.

4.138 Why are there only five ladders in Figure 4.11, and how do they differ from each other?

1 Since norethisterone acetate and ethynodiol acetate are converted in vivo with better than 90% efficiency to norethisterone, all formulations with them are part of the norethisterone group.

2 Progestogens of the norethisterone group and levonorgestrel when given in other than the *lowest available doses*, at or near the bottom rung in Figure 4.10 (which *are* acceptable): these tend to lower HDL-C (specifically HDL_2-C). This effect is believed to signify an increased liability to arterial disease in long-term use, especially in smokers and others with the risk factors.

Though artificial oestrogen (EE) has the opposite effect, it has its own problems (see Q 4.90). The obvious prescribing aim is to reduce the biological effect of *both components* to the acceptable minimum.

4.139 Which COC brands are unacceptable for *normal* prescribing?

1 First, *the 50–µg oestrogen brands*, since the aim of effective contraception is achievable with less oestrogen in most cases.

Table 4.11 Preferred group of low-dose COCs available in Britain – associated with more acceptable blood lipid profiles

	Levonorgestrel (µg)	Ethinyloestradiol (µg)
Logynon/Trinordiol	6 x 50 5 x 75 10 x 125 [92]	6 x 30 5 x 40 10 x 30 [32]
	Norethisterone (µg)	**Ethinyloestradiol** (µg)
Binovum*	7 x 500 14 x 1000 [833]	7 x 35 14 x 35 [35]
Trinovum	7 x 500 7 x 750 7 x 1000 [750]	7 x 35 7 x 35 7 x 35 [35]
Synphase*	7 x 500 9 x 1000 5 x 500 [714]	7 x 35 9 x 35 5 x 35 [35]
Brevinor/Ovysmen	500	35
	Desogestrel (µg)	**Ethinyloestradiol** (µg)
Marvelon	150	30
Mercilon	150	20
	Gestodene (µg)	**Ethinyloestradiol** (µg)
Femodene/Minulet	75	30
Tri-Minulet Triphasic Triadene Triphasic	6 x 50 5 x 70 10 x 100 [79]	30 40 30 [32]
	Norgestimate (µg)	**Ethinyloestradiol** (µg)
Cilest	250	35

Note: Phasic pills as a group do have certain disadvantages which, unless there are special indications, tend to make them less 'preferred' than similar monophasics. Please read Qs 4.158–64.
[ ] Indicates mean daily dose of phased brands.
*Confusing to the user, so Trinovum usually preferred to these two.

Gracial is a new (1994) 22-day biphasic, giving desogestrel 25 µg + EE 40 µg for 6 days, then desogestrel 125 µg + EE 30 µg for 15 days. See Table 4.15, p. 215. However, there are very definite exceptions (Qs 4.150, 4.188).

It is now thought (see Q 4.89) that most of the rare *arterial* disasters occurring in pill-takers are caused by a *thrombotic event* superimposed on pre-existing arterial disease, itself caused for

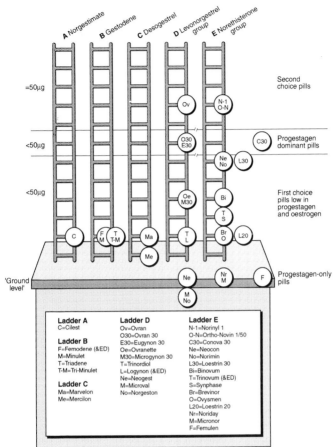

Figure 4.10 Pill ladders – arranged by progestagen. Q 4.137 and following. The two formulations labelled 'progestagen-dominant pills', should be avoided (Q 4.139) unless there are special indications

example by smoking. Thrombosis seems to be primarily oestrogen-dose dependent, though there are data showing that the progestogen can modify the effects of oestrogen on the clotting factors. Hence a little caution is even required with the 35-μg products, especially in the overweight.

2 Secondly, the brands giving 250 μg of levonorgestrel (*Eugynon 30, Ovran 30*) and 2000 μg of ethynodiol diacetate (*Conova 30*) are unbalanced, excessively HDL-C-lowering COCs. Their use

should be restricted to gynaecological indications, such as the maintenance treatment of endometriosis (see Q 4.99).

3 Note that the well-known 150/30 LNG pills (*Microgynon/ Ovranette*), and the NET-group products *Loestrin 30* and *Neocon/ Norimin* are under a slight cloud and no longer in the 'preferred' group (Table 4.10). This is because a clear majority of research studies now show statistically significant potentially adverse lipid changes (especially suppression of HDL_2-C).

So Microgynon 30/Ovranette remains entirely acceptable for younger women who are free of all known arterial disease risk. It has *not* 'become unsafe' for the remainder: only, there are now options which appear *on present evidence* to be metabolically 'even better'. This is the same principle which earlier led to reduced prescribing of previous pills (Minovlar and, later, Eugynon 30) which were the market leaders in their day.

Note: These policies must be interpreted flexibly: the changes are small. Individual women may only be suited by, say, Microgynon. Price is also a not unimportant consideration these days!

4.140 What are the recommendations of the National Association of Family Planning Doctors (NAFPD) and how should they be applied?

They are as follows (1984):

The pill of choice should be the one containing the lowest suitable dose of oestrogen and progestogen which:

(1) provides effective contraception,
(2) produces acceptable cycle control (a concept expanded below),
(3) is associated with fewest side effects and
(4) has the least known effect on carbohydrate and lipid metabolism and haemostatic parameters.

These guidelines assume individualization. Some women react unpredictably and several brands may have to be tried before a suitable one is found. Some are never suited. This is hardly surprising. Individual variation in motivation and tolerance of minor side-effects is well recognized. But as we shall see there is also marked individual variation in blood levels of the exogenous hormones and in responses at the end-organs, especially the endometrium.

To give a *brief summary of what follows*, prescribers should try to identify early in the use of the COC method, if necessary over a series of visits, the lowest dose for each woman which does not cause the annoying symptom of BTB (2). This should minimise adverse side-effects (3) – both serious and minor – and also reduce the measurable metabolic changes (4). This approach does not impair effectiveness (1).

4.141 What are the implications of individual variation in absorption and metabolism for the blood levels of the exogenous steroids in the average pill-user?

1　Blood levels, whether of EE or of all the progestagens which have been studied, vary at least ten-fold between women who are apparently similar, taking the same formulations and sampled exactly 12 hours after their last tablet was swallowed (see Fig. 4.11). The pharmacokinetic area under the curve (AUC) varies less, but still about threefold.

　　This is due to individual variation:

(a)　in absorption;

(b)　in metabolism, in the gut wall and in the liver, see Qs 4.30 and 4.31;

(c)　in degree of binding to transport proteins especially SHBG in the blood plasma, which themselves are variably altered by different pills;

(d)　in the efficiency with which normal EE is reformed and reabsorbed by the activity of the large bowel flora (see Q 4.31).

2　In addition to variable blood levels between women, there is a superimposed variation in target organ sensitivity. This is very difficult to assess and complicates matters further (see Q 4.156).

3　Then there is a further five- to ten-fold fluctuation in any woman between the peaks after absorption and the troughs when the next daily tablet is taken. This saw-tooth pattern is shown in Figures 4.2 and 5.3 (see Q 5.83). Figure 5.3 also conveys one of the presumed advantages of slow-release systems of administration: relatively constant daily blood levels.

4.142 What is the relevance to pill-prescribing of this great variation in blood levels and AUC between different women taking the same formulation, as in Figure 4.11?

First, as already discussed fully above (see Q 4.35), there is pretty good evidence from research on enzyme inducers that women whose blood levels are low tend to suffer problems with endometrial stability (chiefly BTB). They may even conceive (especially if they ever lengthen the PFI).

4.143 What about those women with relatively high circulating blood levels of artificial steroids? What evidence is there that side-effects can be correlated? correlated?

It is a very tenable hypothesis that metabolic changes and both major and minor side-effects of the COC are more common and more marked in those women whose blood levels are exceptionally high. In support, pill-takers in an American study who developed clinical hypertension were statistically more likely to have high blood levels of EE, than control takers of similar pills without any rise in blood

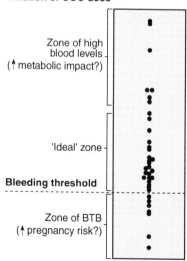

Titration of COC dose

Figure 4.11 Schematic representation of the approximately 10-fold variability in peak blood levels of both contraceptive steroids, and the rationale of suggested 'titration' against the bleeding threshold. Q 4.141 and following

pressure. Too few confirmatory studies of this hypothesis have been performed, though a major one is in progress at the MPC.

4.144 Is it feasible to measure the levels of either the oestrogen or progestagen in body fluids?

This is not yet practical as a clinic procedure, though a simple testing kit for levels in the saliva or urine would be a great asset.

4.145 Without blood level measurements, how might one attempt to 'tailor' the pill to the individual woman?

I believe that one can, to a degree (see below). But not by the approach which used to be recommended, namely attempting to base the choice on assessed features of that woman's normal menstrual cycle. This was, in my view, always illogical, when one recalls that all COCs remove the normal cycle and replace it with an artificial one. That being so it is surely preferable to make the replacement cycle as good as it can be for all. The aim is that it should, after adjustments during follow-up (see Qs 4.228–9 and Tables 4.14 and 4.15), eventually be 'better' than each woman's normal cycle, rather than a slavish imitation of it.

I therefore promote the 'tailoring' approach which follows, designed to discover with the woman's cooperation the 'smallest' pill (see Q 4.133) which gives her adequate control of her cycle.

4.146 In Figure 4.11, what does absence of BTB mean?

On the hypothesis of Q 4.143, it could mean two very different things. Absence of BTB means either that the woman has ideal blood levels of the artificial hormones, *or that they are higher than necessary for the desired effect of contraception* – with plausibly a greater risk than necessary of causing unwanted effects.

4.147 How then might we avoid giving the women who tend to the higher blood levels (or larger AUC) a stronger pill than they really need?

By attempting during follow-up to give each woman the 'smallest' (lowest dose) pill her uterus will allow, without bleeding. This may mean titrating downwards, trying a pill lower in the same ladder – if not already tried and found to cause BTB.

4.148 What if BTB does occur? Does she need a higher dose or different formulation?

Maybe! A higher dose pill (or a phasic or gestodene variety, see Qs 4.157–8) might be appropriate. *But first and foremost, important alternative causes of the bleeding must first be excluded* (see Table 4.12). I am aware of a young woman who was seen by a number of different doctors and nurses during 1991, complaining of BTB. They kept trying different brands without success until someone passed a speculum and, tragically, found an inoperable carcinoma of the cervix. She had had a reportedly negative cervical smear 1 year previously, but this was no excuse for the failure to examine. Note also carefully *all* the other possibilities in the Table; also Q 4.28 *re* tricycling.

Table 4.12 Checklist in cases of possible 'breakthrough bleeding' (BTB) in pill-takers

A *note of caution*: first eliminate other possible causes!

The following checklist is modified from the book by Sapire (see Further Reading):

Disease – EXAMINE the cervix. It is not unknown for bleeding from an invasive cancer to be wrongly attributed to BTB. Chlamydia can cause a blood stained discharge due to endometritis

Disorder of pregnancy causing bleeding (e.g. abortion, trophoblastic tumour)

Default – missed pill(s). Remember that the BTB may start 2 or 3 days later and be very persistent thereafter

Drugs – especially enzyme-inducers, see Qs 00-00

Diarrhoea with VOMITTING – diarrhoea alone has to be very severe to impair absorption significantly, see Q 4.00

Disturbance of absorption – likewise has to be very marked to be relevant, e.g. after *massive* gut resection. (Ileostomy cases studied have had no demonstrable absorption problems)

Diet – gut flora involved in recycling EE may be reduced in VEGETARIANS. Could sometimes be a factor in BTB, but not usually an important effect

Duration too short – minimal BTB which is tolerable may resolve after 2–3 months, see Q 4.00 *

finally, after the above have been excluded:

Dose — if she is taking a monophasic, try a phasic pill
    — increase the progestogen component
    — try a different progestogen
    — consider using a 50 μg pill such as Ovran (see Qs 4.00–00)

* Alternatively, the bleeding may sometimes be an end-organ effect, especially if in the second or third packet of a 'tricycle', see Q 4.00.

We are, finally in a position to consider how best to put the above facts and principles into practice. *The objective is that each woman receives the least long-term metabolic impact that her uterus will allow, i.e. the lowest dose of contraceptive steroids which is just, but only just, above her own bleeding threshold.*

4.149 What is the normal choice for the first pill prescription?

There is no proven 'best buy'. But the first choice of pill should in my view *normally* be made from those in Table 4.10, according to prescriber or *client* preference, and taking note of the comments in the 'Remarks' column. In general one does not choose the more complicated triphasics (see Qs 4.158–64) or 20-μg pills when future compliance is suspect. Pills known to have a relatively high rate of BTB are also best kept for trial later, when a new user is better able to cope (but all users must be advised about BTB should it occur). Microgynon/Ovranette from Table 4.11 is an additional option, but not a good choice for smokers or acne sufferers (see Q 4.220).

4.150 Which women may need consideration of a stronger formulation (50 μg) from the outset?

Those women who are known to have reduced bioavailability of the COC:

1 Women on long-term enzyme-inducing drugs (see Qs 4.31–3 and 4.188).

2 Rarely, women with established malabsorption problems (e.g. *massive* small bowel resection).

In addition:

3 *Some* women who have had a previous contraceptive failure with the COC and yet claiming perfect compliance or having missed no more than one tablet. But unlike 1 and 2, most of these should be given a standard formulation or the same (monophasic) as they previously had, only now tricycling the packets plus a shortened PFI after every third pack. (See Q 4.24.)

4.151 What pill should follow if BTB is unacceptable after 1–3 months' trial and there is no other explanation?

Provided that the other causes in the list in Table 4.12 have been carefully excluded, if BTB occurs and is unacceptable early on, or persists beyond about three cycles, the next strongest brand up the 'ladder' in Figure 4.9 may be tried. In general, gestodene-containing COCs have a good reputation for cycle control. Phasic pills may come into their own here, especially if the cycle control problem includes absent WTB. But the excessively progestagen dominant (less 'lipid friendly') brands Eugynon 30/Ovran 30 and Conova 30 are best avoided, unless indicated for special medical/therapeutic reasons.

If after trying lower dose options BTB can only be prevented by a 50 μg oestrogen pill, for that particular woman the latter need not be considered a 'strong' brand. I explain this to women as at Q 4.36. Obviously this 'titrating' process is not helped by the lack of provision by the manufacturers of a good range of doses, especially for the newer progestagens.

The answer to Q 4.151 is different for BTB late in a sequence of tricycling; if this applies see Q 4.29.

4.152 If cycle control is a big problem, and a 'third generation' progestagen is preferred, may one prescribe two pills, for example one 'Marvelon' plus one 'Mercilon 20' daily to construct that 50 μg desogestrel product which ought to be but isn't marketed?!

Yes, I would support this, but in selected cases with due caution as for other situations outside the strict terms of the Data Sheet, and with meticulous record keeping. See Q 4.34. I think it would be more easily justified as accepted practice in long-term users of enzyme-inducer drugs, who have been proved to have lower bioavailability of the COC. *Here*, if a rare thrombotic or other serious CVS event occurred it would be more difficult to establish that there had not been another cause for the bleeding problem – perhaps at the end-organ (see Q 4.154) – and hence that 'too much' oestrogen was not being given by the two pills a day regimen.

4.153 Later on, if there is good cycle control, among established asymptomatic COC-users, should one try moving down the ladder?

At the time of repeat prescription, the possibility of trying a lower-dose brand (if available) should always be considered. Otherwise one will never know whether they might not be equally suited to a lower and probably safer dose. If no lower dose exists, both prescriber and taker of the pill can have the satisfaction of knowing that metabolic risks and hence probable risk of side-effects have been minimized within the context of marketed products.

4.154 Low blood levels of the artificial hormones usually cause BTB – but is all BTB caused by low blood levels?

No. It is true that BTB is not a totally accurate marker of blood levels, and indeed variability in BTB or WTB with the same blood level could be caused by variation at the end-organ (the endometrium). This is indubitably true, and probably explains much of the light BTB common in the first one to two cycles and the late tricycle bleeding discussed at Q 4.29.

But women find BTB annoying in any event. Why give more drug than the minimum to prevent the annoying symptom? The dose administered should be only just above (and not enormously above) the bleeding threshold: whether mediated by low blood level or an unusually susceptible end organ. Hence titration downwards in those *without* BTB is still logical. But caution is essential in the reverse situation, as stressed already at Q 4.148 and Table 4.12 – remember particularly to check for chlamydia!

4.155 Should women with BTB be advised to take additional precautions? Can they rely on their COC?

It has been suggested that attempting to find the best choice of pill by titrating downwards at follow-up, in the way described above, will lead to breakthrough conceptions. Yet pill-takers who conceive rarely report having had BTB beforehand. That conceptions rarely occur unless pills are (also) missed is, I believe, for the following reasons:

1   First, it is a tribute to the fact that even the current low-dose pills are amazingly effective, with back-up contraceptive mechanisms (notably the progestagen 'block' to cervical mucus penetration by sperm) operating even if breakthrough ovulation should occur.

2 Second, it seems that (fortunately) BTB is an early warning – usually occurring when there is more circulating artificial steroid than the minimum to permit conception – in compliant women. (It may well be true, though, that BTB implies a reduced *margin for error*, so these women ought to be more careful than usual about not lengthening the PFI, Q 4.15–7.)

3 Thirdly, it is likely that the bleeding from the uterus itself temporarily enhances the anti-implantation contraceptive mechanism.

4 Fourthly, while present, BTB probably reduces coital frequency!

4.156 How would you summarize this policy?

All we want to do is give the lowest metabolic impact to the woman that her endometrium will allow. I would stress however that this prescribing system is based on the *hypothesis of Figure 4.11*, which is only now being rigorously tested. I would ask the reader to judge its plausibility and my view that it should be followed, pending the discovery of any better scheme.

4.157 What should be the second choice of pill if there are non-bleeding side-effects?

See below, Qs 4.228–9 and Tables 4.14 and 4.15

The pros and cons of phasic pills

4.158 What are phasic pills and what are their advantages?

Their main claimed advantage is that they tend to give a better bleeding pattern for a given (low) dose of hormones, using the given progestagen. For example, Logynon/Trinordiol gives an average daily dose of 92 μg of LNG (combined with 32.4 μg of EE). If this low dose of progestagen were used in a daily fixed-dose regimen, the incidence of BTB would be unacceptable.

Unexpectedly, the same has *not* been demonstrated for the gestodene-containing triphasics in Table 4.10, when compared with their actually slightly lower-dose monophasic equivalents! However all the gestodene combined pills are reported to give better cycle control than the levonorgestrel- or norethisterone-containing triphasics, particularly in early months of use.

All except one triphasic (Synphase) imitate the normal menstrual cycle to some extent, in particular by there being a higher proportion of the progestagen to the oestrogen in the second half of the pill-taking cycle. Histologically, this leads to the production of an endometrium which appears more like the normal secretory phase, with more gland formation and the presence of spiral aterioles. This improved histology probably lies behind the good WTB which occurs (some patients complain it is too good!).

4.159 What about the other postulated advantage, that the approximation to the normal cycle will itself lead to a reduction in long-term side-effects?

That is unlikely I think, though not impossible. On the contrary, some of the beneficial effects – which seem to relate to the very fact that the pill-cycle produces more stable hormone levels and is *not* the same as the normal cycle (see Q 4.51) – might also be reduced. As yet, we just do not know.

4.160 What are the disadvantages of phasic OCs?

These can be listed as follows:

1 An increase in the time required to explain the pill packet to the user.

2 An increase in the risk of pill-taking errors – though some companies have made the newer packaging much more 'user-friendly'.

3 A reduction in the margin for such errors (particularly in view of the low dose being taken in the very first phase right after the 'contraceptively dangerous' pill-free time – see Q 4.21).

4 Some women complain of symptoms which imitate the premenstrual syndrome, such as breast tenderness, in the last phase of pill-taking before the withdrawal bleed.

5 They are obviously not a good choice for women with (non-focal) migraines or anyone prone to headaches or mood changes or any symptom which tends to be precipitated by hormone fluctuations.

6 In the UK they are extra expensive to the Health Service, since the pharmacist or dispensing doctor is paid a separate dispensing fee for each of the three phases – and even for the *placebo* phases of Logynon ED and Trinovum ED! (like Femodene ED).

7 A small problem with postponing withdrawal bleeds (see Q 4.163), and for the same reason they are not suitable for tricycling (see Q 4.28).

8 Studies in Holland, Australia and New Zealand have all found that triphasics are definitely over-represented, among the COCs reportedly in use, by pill-takers presenting with unwanted 'breakthrough' conceptions. The reasons may include compliance problems due to complexity of the packaging and also relatively lower innate efficacy – see 3 above in this answer.

4.161 So for whom might phasic OCs be chosen?

1 The main indication is for cycle control with low dose, especially to get a good withdrawal bleed.
(*Note* however that in both the norethisterone and gestodene pill ladders the phasics are not actually quite the lowest dose products).

2 Upon request, if the woman likes the idea of 'imitating the menstrual cycle'; they usefully increase choice if side effects occur with monophasic products.

3 The gestodene triphasic brands (Tri-Minulet/Triadene) appear on the available data to have the edge on Trinordiol/Logynon for cycle control and to be more 'lipid friendly' (see Q 4.136). They could be appropriate for women with risk factors for circulatory disease, especially if BTB or absent withdrawal bleeding are problems.

4.162 What are your views specifically about BiNovum and Synphase?

1 *BiNovum* in my view is a brand which has almost no place now that TriNovum is available. TriNovum gives a lower mean daily dose (750 μg instead of 833 μg), gives at least as good cycle control, and has much better packaging.

2 *Synphase*. This may be useful for women experiencing BTB in the middle of the packet of a fixed-dose brand, especially Ovysmen/Brevinor. It is the only triphasic pill which has the highest progestagen to oestrogen ratio in the middle phase. However in comparison with Trinovum there is a negligible reduction in mean daily progestagen (714 μg rather than 750 μg), and it has rather unhelpful packaging.

4.163 How may a woman postpone the withdrawal bleed on a phasic pill?

There is no problem with Synphase. As with fixed-dose pills, see Q 4.238, two packets may simply be taken in a row without the usual 7-day break; but if this is tried with one of the other phasic brands, BTB is likely to occur early in the new packet because of the abrupt drop in progestagen from the higher level in the last phase of the previous packet.

There are two possible solutions, as in Figure 4.12.

Contraceptive efficacy will be maintained throughout either scheme.

1 First, tablets from the last phase of a 'spare' packet may be taken, thereby giving 7, 10 or 14 days' postponement according to the phasic brand in question.

2 Alternatively, the woman may follow immediately with a packet of the 'nearest' fixed dose brand up the same ladder in Figure 4.10 and Table 4.10 (i.e. the nearest equivalent to the final phase of her phasic pill). To be specific, this means postponing 'periods' with triphasics (see Table 4.13).

4.164 What is the future for triphasics?

They are currently very popular in the USA. But the list of problems at Q 4.160 makes them unlikely I think to be as successful here against the monophasic competition.

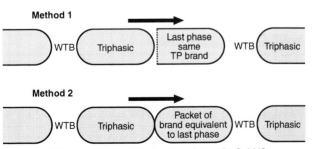

Figure 4.12 How to postpone periods with triphasic pills. Q 4.163.
Note: for Synphase just run on packets

Table 4.13 Postponing 'periods' with triphasics

Name of phasic*	Brand to follow* to delay WTB using method 2 of Figure 4.12
Logynon	Microgynon
Tri-Minulet	Minulet†
TriNovum	Neocon
Binovum	Neocon
Synphase	Synphase

*Or the identical equivalent by another manufacturer from Table 4.10 – the alternatives are Trinordiol, Ovranette, Triadene, Femodene and Norimin.
†There would be a small risk of a BTB episode here since Minulet has 25 µg less gestodene than phase 3 of Tri-Minulet

FOLLOW-UP ARRANGEMENTS: THE MONITORING OF THOSE SIDE-EFFECTS AND COMPLICATIONS PARTICULARLY RELEVANT TO COC SAFETY

4.165 What are the main aspects of pill monitoring, once the 'safest' pill brand has been identified for the individual as in Qs 4.133–56?

After careful selection and counselling as described above, the list of what can (and should) be done during long term monitoring is short – but important.

In summary, good practice would be to:

1 Advise in advance about the warning symptoms in Q 4.176 below.

2 Look for the onset of any new cardiovascular risk factors, especially if one is already present (e.g. age 35 in all smokers).

3 Look for the warning signs, primarily a rise in blood pressure (see Q 4.170), or the onset of or change in character or worsening of migraines (see Qs 4.124–8). The woman needs to be prospectively advised about the latter (i.e. more specifically than just the list at Q 4.176)

4 Arrange 3-yearly routine cervical cytology, with a *routine* bimanual no more frequently than that (see Q 4.167).

5 Teach breast awareness and self-examination (*without it becoming a nerve-racking ritual*) along with a good leaflet; and with periodic medical examination for reassurance, and referral for assessment or mammography as indicated.

6 Advise *re* special situations, notably immobilization, major surgery, or the treatment for varicose veins (see Qs 4.177 and 4.178).

4.166 How often should pill-takers be seen, and by whom?

In my opinion, everything depends on whether the pill-taker is one of the 'safer' women or not (see Qs 4.103–4). The prescriber should mentally classify the pill-taker into one of the two categories – a form of triage really – on which follow-up arrangements depend.

1 The ordinary 'safer' women are seen 3 months after the first pill prescription, or any change of brand, for BP check and symptom assessment, as well as answer any queries. Subsequent visits are usually 6-monthly, but the frequency in this low-risk group can be further reduced.

   It is good practice and an appropriate use of scarce resources for the checks for women to be regularly delegated to the practice nurse, so long as she is family planning-trained (ENB Course 901 or equivalent). There must be an agreed protocol for when she should call in the doctor. One example: even if she has only been taught the technique of smear taking and not full bimanual examination, she can and should be taught how to move the cervix so as to elicit cervical excitation tenderness.

2 The women with any of the relative contraindications in Qs 4.103–32 or with any important chronic illness should normally be seen by the doctor: with a low threshold for more frequent visits, perhaps 1 month after the first prescription, and if necessary more frequently than 6-monthly thereafter. It could also be appropriate for a nurse in whom you have confidence – fully family planning trained – to care for this category too. But the main point is that whoever, either she or you as the doctor, should recognize that pill-takers in this category 2 are 'very different animals!' Take just two examples: the migraineurs are much more likely (though still unlikely with good care) to get strokes; and the heavy smokers have an inbuilt 20 times greater risk of having a heart attack than the risk-factor-free pill-takers in category 1 (see Q 4.86).

4.167 Ideally, shouldn't all pill-takers have a full pelvic examination at least annually?

No, I consider this part of medical mythology. Please turn to Q 4.62. Though most of the disorders listed there can be picked up by a careful bimanual examination (BME), everything listed is also *less* likely to happen in pill-takers than in, for example, the partners of intermittent condom-users! Those are the ones at increased risk of ovarian cysts (benign or malignant), fibroids, endometriosis, ectopics, etc., if you can persuade them to come in, not the pill-takers! So BMEs need only be done routinely at the 3-yearly smear.

4.168 How frequently should the blood pressure (BP) be measured, and why is it so important?

BP should be measured pretreatment and thereafter at 3 months, at 6 months, and then at least annually in category 1 women (see Q 4.166). Studies have shown that nearly all COC-users have a measurable small increase in both systolic and diastolic BP. Such elevations by no more than 5 mmHg in women without other risk factors are of no concern; but all degrees of clinical hypertension should be detected:

1 *Moderate hypertension* – above 160/95 – because it can become irreversible. (Malignant hypertension has rarely been attributed to the COC.) But it is fully reversible if the pill is discontinued promptly. Secondly there is an increased risk of haemorrhagic strokes, including subarachnoid haemorrhage.

2 *Mild hypertension* – above 135/85 – this should be taken seriously especially if there are circulatory risk factors (see Q 4.170).

4.169 At what levels of BP should the pill be discontinued?

It is generally agreed that *repeated* readings at or above 160/95 would be too high both for starting and continuing with the COC.

4.170 When should a rather small rise in BP, perhaps not out of the normotensive range, nevertheless lead to a consideration of change of method?

Behind this question are the studies which show that hypertension acts as a marker for an increased risk of arterial disease. Studies by the life insurance companies, of large populations, have shown that raised BP is associated with a small but measurable reduction in life expectancy, even in women. While it is not certain that pill-induced mild hypertension has the same significance as the idiopathic variety, it would be prudent to assume that it does. Faced therefore with a 33-year-old, heavy-smoking woman with a BP repeatedly around 135/85 – knowing that before pill-taking it was, say, 110/70 – one would prefer she switched to another method of birth control right away rather than continuing to the upper limit of 35 years.

4.171 So can the BP be used as an ongoing test of liability to arterial disease?

This is what I am suggesting. In other words, for years pill-prescribers have longed for a simple clinical test – for example, a reagent which could be added to a woman's urine in the clinic and would turn it green if she could safely continue with the COC and red if she should discontinue. It is my view that we have that test already – not perfect, but usable in the same kind of way. A rise in BP is like a red or at least pink test, implying that the woman (especially if she already has a risk factor) has now entered a category at increased risk of arterial thrombosis.

4.172 Can patients on hypotensive treatment be legitimately given the COC?

The POP would be a better choice (see Q 5.48). But the COC may be acceptable in a young, non-smoking woman who will accept no other method of birth control, and then only after full consultation with the physician supervising control of the hypertension.

> Note: This presupposes that the woman's hypertension is not pill related. It would not be acceptable for a woman whose hypertension was induced by the COC (and readily reversible by simply stopping it in favour say of the POP), then to be given antihypertensive drugs in order to enable her to stay on it. There can be few occasions when treating the side-effects of one drug by other powerful drugs can be anything but bad medicine.

4.173 What types of migraine indicate that the combined pill should be stopped?

Please reread Qs 4.124–8. To recap, any change in the character of migraine to include any symptoms (Q 4.126) which are focal and explicable by transient cerebral ischaemia, or to become more severe and crescendo in nature: these mean the *oestrogen* of the combined pill should be stopped immediately and for ever. This is for fear that the transient ischaemia might become permanent by a thrombotic stroke. But the POP and injectables may be started right away.

4.174 What about the occurrence of the woman's first ever migraine attack while taking the COC? Should she stop the method?

Yes, at the time, this is also an indication to stop the COC. But if it had no serious sequelae on that first occasion and no attack thereafter includes focal symptoms, I consider that subsequent cautious COC use is acceptable. However she must be warned in simple terms about the important symptoms to watch out for in future (see Q 4.126).

4.175 What about 'ordinary' headaches occurring on the COC?

These are not a contraindication, more in the nature of a common, more or less tolerable, side-effect and one for which the woman may or may not ask help. If so, it is well worth ascertaining *whether the headaches tend to occur in the pill-free week*. If they do, the tricycle regimen, using the lowest acceptable fixed-dose formulation, leads, at worst, to the woman experiencing only five headaches a year instead of 13! (see Q 4.28).

4.176 What symptoms should lead pill-users to take urgent medical advice (potential major problems)?

Pill-users should be told to (a) transfer at once to another effective method of birth control and (b) come under medical care without delay, pending diagnosis and treatment, if any of the following should occur (this list ought to be a form of revision of the chapter so far!):

1 Severe pain in the calf of one leg (see Qs 4.83 and 4.218 *re* deep venous thrombosis).

2 Severe central pain in the chest or sharp pains on either side of the chest aggravated by breathing – could be myocardial infarction or pulmonary embolism (see Q 4.83).

3 Unexplained breathlessness with or without the coughing of blood-stained sputum – could be pulmonary embolism (see Q 4.83).

4 Severe pain in the abdomen (see Q 4.202).

5 Any unusually severe, prolonged headache, especially if it is the first ever attack or gets progressively worse (crescendo

migraine), or is associated with the symptoms at 6–9 below (see Qs 4.124–32).

6 A bad fainting attack or collapse, with or without focal epilepsy.

7 Weakness or very marked numbness suddenly affecting one side or one part of the body.

8 Sudden marked disturbance of vision, especially loss of a visual field or teichopsia (see Qs 4.126, 4.190).

9 Sudden disturbance of the ability to speak normally (nominal aphasia).

10 A severe and generalized skin rash (which could be erythema multiforme).

Most of the above are potentially thrombotic or embolic catastrophes in the making; but often there is a non-pill-related explanation.

Clinical signs which may not be complaints but still demand urgent action (including stopping the COC) are:

11 The onset of jaundice (see Qs 4.196 and 4.197).

12 High blood pressure (i.e. above 160/95, see Qs 4.168 and 4.169).

The pill should also normally be discontinued forthwith if immobilization is necessary after an accident or emergency major or leg surgery is required (see Qs 4.177–4.181 below).

Implications of surgery

4.177 Should a combined pill-user discontinue treatment before elective major surgery?

It all depends on the nature of the surgery. If it is major, or minor but associated with hypotension or immobilization:

1 The COC should be discontinued at least 4 weeks before the operation.

2 It should also not be recommenced until the first menstrual period which is at least 2 weeks after full mobilization. The reason for this rule is the well-established increased risk of deep venous thrombosis (DVT) postoperatively, and the potential for this to be increased by the prothrombotic changes caused by oestrogens.

> Note: For the reason that they are oestrogen-free, the above rule does *not* apply to the POP nor to progestagen-only injectables/implants/rings which may be continued without a break during major surgery. Indeed they may be chosen to cover the time on a waiting-list (see Q 4.180)

4.178 Should the COC be stopped for a minor operation such as laparoscopic sterilization?

This is definitely unnecessary since the risk of postoperative DVT is vanishingly small after such minor surgery. The same applies to dental extraction. 'Iatrogenic' pregnancies seem frequently to be caused this way. However, since thromboembolism occurred after 3 of 438 laparoscopic cholecystectomies in a 1993 report from Sydney (1 was fatal), avoid COC use in *complex* laparoscopies.

4.179 What about minor leg surgery, such as complex operative arthroscopy, or ligation of varicose veins? Or injection treatment for leg veins?

This is quite another matter. Oestrogen-containing therapy should be discontinued 4 weeks before either such surgery or sclerotherapy, and avoided for the duration of leg bandaging thereafter.

4.180 What contraception is suitable before and after surgery while the COC is contraindicated?

Progestagen-only methods are all appropriate. A good choice might be DMPA (see Q 4.177). The first injection may be given at any time in the woman's pill-taking cycle, after which she just finishes the current packet. If irregular bleeding is a problem, a new packet of her usual pill may be started as early as 2 weeks after full mobilization, without waiting for the expiry of the 12 week's duration of the injection.

4.181 What should be done if a patient who is a pill-taker is admitted as an emergency for major surgery or orthopaedic treatment with immobilization?

In these circumstances the risk of DVT is high, especially in the obese. The COC should be discontinued at once and careful consideration given to the use of subcutaneous heparin prophylaxis. This would be particularly important for gynaecological, orthopaedic and cancer surgery.

Do not forget to ask the young girl on traction, after falling from her boyfriend's motor bike, to stop taking her pills.

DEALING WITH OTHER SIDE-EFFECTS AND EVENTS DURING PILL-USE

4.182 What general points can be made about the so-called 'minor' side-effects?

1 First and foremost they frequently do not seem minor to the woman affected!

2 Many of them are common in the general population, hence it is difficult to be sure that the COC is to blame in an individual case.

3 The frequency of complaint depends on many factors, including anxiety about possible harm due to the therapy.

4 Many can be classified under two main headings:
   (a) those related to cycle control (see Qs 4.149–4.156);
   (b) those which are also common in pregnancy.

4.183 Which are the pregnancy-mimicking minor side-effects?

The order below is alphabetical. Most are dealt with in more detail below.

Common:

1 breast enlargement and bloatedness with fluid retention;

2 cramps and pains in the legs;

3 cystitis and other urinary infections;

4 depression and loss of libido;

5 gingivitis;

6 headaches;

7 nausea;

8 vaginal discharge (non-specific) and cervical 'erosion';

9 weight gain.

Less common:

1 breast pain (see Q 4.214, 4.229);

2 chloasma (see Q 4.222);

3 galactorrhoea (see Q 4.214);

4 superficial thrombophlebitis (see Q 4.122).

There are some more serious conditions which are similarly commoner in pregnancy. For example, some immune disorders (see

Q 4.226); chorea, cardiomyopathy, pemphigoid gestationis, hae-molytic uraemic syndrome and cholestatic jaundice of pregnancy; not to mention hypertension and venous and arterial thrombosis.

Subsequent questions consider the management of side-effects, considered by systems – excluding the circulatory system (already dealt with in some detail).

Central nervous system

4.184 Is depression commoner among pill-takers than controls, and how can it be managed?

In the RCGP study it was shown that for every 130 depressed pill-users there were 100 who were non-OC-using controls. This implies that only 30 of the 130 could really blame the COC, even in the much higher doses then given. But there are some who are free from depression when off treatment, with recurrence when rechallenged. In a proportion of patients altered tryptophan me-tabolism leads to lowered pyridoxine levels. In these pyridoxine 50 mg daily may be beneficial, taking up to 2 months to be effective. Others may require a change of progestagen or change of method, with or without antidepressant therapy.

Depression could also be secondary to other pill side-effects (e.g. headaches, or loss of libido). But the Oxford/FPA Study (1985) ruled out any link between the COC and 'serious' psychiatric illness – which includes severe depression needing hospital refer-ral.

4.185 How does the COC affect libido?

Loss of libido is reported particularly among those who are also depressed. Many extrinsic factors may explain this, including placebo reaction to the COC or frustrated desire for a child. However, there are certainly some cases where there is a real physiological effect of the hormones.

Contrariwise, in some women libido is actually increased because the method is so reliable, non-intercourse-related, and often reduces premenstrual tension. This makes woman-initiated sexual activity more probable late in the pill cycle than it is late in the normal cycle.

4.186 How should one manage the complaint of loss of libido?

1   First, discuss fully psychosexual aspects of the relationship, and the marital and family circumstances.

2 Second, check whether part of the problem is soreness or dryness – which could be caused locally by *thrush*, or a vulval skin eruption.

3 Use of a water-soluble lubricant may help.

4 Finally, consider changing to a more oestrogen-dominant pill (see Q 4.229 and Table 4.15).

4.187 How may the COC affect epilepsy?

The condition is not initiated by the COC. The attack rate is often reduced, though rarely it may be increased. Avoid *triphasic* COCs (see Q 4.160). Liver enzyme-inducer antiepileptic therapy is one of the few indications for a 50-μg oestrogen COC with *tricycling* (see Qs 4.33–6). Moreover, regardless of therapy, if fits are commonly initiated around the pill-free time tricycling a monophasic may reduce their frequency. Injectables are another good option (see Q 5.91(12)).

4.188 If epileptics and others on chronic enzyme-inducing treatments are on the pill, how should they be managed? (See Q 4.30 and following)

First, please read Qs 4.15–37 before this answer.

I used to advise *shortening* the PFIs. But pending the marketing of the active 24 + 4 placebo packs mentioned at Q 4.8, it simplifies compliance to eliminate most of them: by using the *tricycle regimen*. This also appears to improve epilepsy control (see Q 4.28), though no comparative trial has been published. After three consecutive packets the woman should still shorten the PFI, arbitrarily to just 4 days. Diary cards may be helpful.

If the woman complains of BTB, exclude another cause (see Q 4.148); then the next step is to try two tablets a day, e.g. of a 30- or 35-μg fixed-dose pill. If necessary the combined oestrogen content of the two pills per day can be increased to 100 μg (maximum), titrated against the BTB. In this way the usual policy of giving the minimum dose of both hormones to be just above the threshold for bleeding (see Qs 4.148–9) can be followed. The epileptic can be reassured that she is 'climbing a down escalator' (see Q 4.36).

Caution is necessary when enzyme inducers are withdrawn, since it takes some weeks for the liver's level of excretory function to revert to normal. See Q 4.37 for the details.

4.189 What about headaches and migraines?

These critically important subjects were considered earlier, under 'risk factors' (see Qs 4.124–32) and 'monitoring' (see Qs 4.173–4.175)

4.190 How can the pill affect the eyes?

If any acute visual disturbance occurs the woman should be told to stop the pill at once, pending further investigation.

1 At worst, acute loss of vision in one eye could be caused by retinal artery or vein thrombosis or haemorrhage.

2 Loss of a field of vision may signify transient cerebral ischaemia. This must be taken seriously, see Qs 4.124–8.

3 Blurring of vision may be a normal manifestation of diffuse 'common' migraine. If it occurs completely unassociated with headaches, fundoscopy should be performed. In a few cases dilated retinal veins have been found. Since this finding is linked with an increased risk of retinal vein thrombosis, oestrogen-containing pills should be recommended only on the authority of an ophthalmologist (whose opinion should be sought without delay).

4.191 What about the pill and contact lenses?

An increased likelihood of discomfort or even corneal damage among contact lens users taking the COC was reported with the old hard lenses (and stronger pills). It is believed to be explained by a slight degree of corneal oedema. With modern soft lenses and low-dose pills this problem is now uncommon. If it occurs, the woman should see her optician, and a brand containing the lowest possible dose of both steroids should be tried. Rarely, women have to make a straight choice between their contact lenses and this contraceptive method.

4.192 Does the pill cause or aggravate glaucoma?

There is no evidence of any effect even among those with a family history: though of course intraocular pressure rarely rises significantly during the peak childbearing years.

4.193 Does the COC cause nausea or vomiting?

Nausea may occur in the first cycle and occasionally recurs after the PFI with the first few pills of each packet. Vomiting is most unusual, but if within 3 hours it could interfere with absorption of a tablet and hence affect cycle control and efficacy (see Q 4.28).

Both symptoms are oestrogen related and are thus not so frequent with modern pills. They are commoner in very underweight women, and in them may be intolerable, starting with the very first tablet and with every COC tried. More usually perseverance is rewarded. Use tablets with 30 or only 20 μg of oestrogen – or oestrogen-free (i.e. the POP). Nausea may also be helped by taking the pill at night rather than in the morning.

Vomiting starting for the first time after several months of trouble-free pill-taking should not be attributed to the pill. Consider pregnancy for one thing.

4.194 How often is weight gain on the COC truly due to it, and how may it be minimized?

The fear of this is one of the things that most puts young women off the pill. Yet clearly not all weight gain is caused by the pill. Most studies of modern pills show weight changes roughly as follows: weight gain of more than 2 kg in 15–20%; loss of more than 2 kg in 15–20%; unchanged or within that range, the remainder . . . . There is a kind of cyclical weight gain which is oestrogen linked (see Q 4.229) and due to fluid retention. This tends to be shed with a diuresis in the pill-free week.

Sustained weight gain can be marked in some individual women due mainly to an increase in appetite. Major change may imply unusual metabolic disturbance by steroid hormones, as also with injectables (see Q 5.94).

Apart from appropriate dietary advice, lower-dose brands of different progestagens may be tried; see Q 4.180 – before transferring to a different method such as the POP.

4.195 How should jaundice in a COC-user be managed?

First, the pill should be stopped immediately, since it has additive effects on liver metabolism. If some form of infectious hepatitis is diagnosed the COC is normally not restarted until at least 3 months after the liver function tests have returned to normal (6 months following a severe attack).

Abnormal liver function tests caused by any other mechanism (e.g. cirrhosis) contraindicate the method, though the POP may be usable (see Q 5.52).

4.196 How often is jaundice caused by the pill?

Rarely. Cholestatic jaundice is commoner among COC-users and also in pregnancy. A past history in either context contraindicates the pill. Gilbert's disease is incidental and benign.

4.197 Does the COC cause gallstones?

The latest research shows that the increased risk of this condition among COC-users is significant only during the early years of pill-taking. This suggests that the risk applies primarily to predisposed women. Studies of bile biochemistry have shown that contraceptive steroids can accelerate cholelithiasis.

4.198 If a woman has had definitive treatment for gallstones may she use the COC?

If the treatment was medical, the COC would be contraindicated because of the risk of recurrence. If the woman has had definitive surgical treatment by cholecystectomy, many surgeons will permit cautious use of the COC if no other method is acceptable.

4.199 Is acute pancreatitis linked with the COC?

Yes, in part perhaps through the link with gall-bladder disease. Most of the sporadic cases had cofactors like obesity, alcohol abuse, hypertriglyceridaemia, or lipid problems, and there have been few reports since the advent of sub-50-μg pills. If a woman has an attack of this condition on the COC artificial oestrogen would be absolutely or (very strongly) relatively contraindicated thereafter but she could transfer to a progestogen-only method.

4.200 What are the presentation and management of COC-related benign liver tumours (see Q 4.82)?

They present with abdominal pain and an upper abdominal mass, and sometimes with a life-threatening haemoperitoneum. The treatment is surgical removal. Subsequently both the COC and progestagen-only methods should be avoided (see Q 5.51).

4.201 Is the COC, like cigarettes, linked with Crohn's disease?

This example of inflammatory bowel disease is discussed in Q 4.112. In case-control studies past pill-use was commoner only among women with colonic Crohn's of the non-granulomatous variety. The condition often resolved if the COCs were discontinued. It would be logical if the woman could give up cigarettes as well!

In other inflammatory bowel disorders as well the COC is relatively contraindicated and it would be important to take the advice of the specialist before continuing the COC.

4.202 What is the differential diagnosis of abdominal pain which could be related to COC use?

1 Thrombosis of major intra-abdominal vessels such as the hepatic veins or a mesenteric artery or vein;

2 gallstones (see Q 4.197);

3 pancreatitis (see Q 4.199);

4 liver adenoma (see Q 4.200);

5 Crohn's disease (see Q 4.201);

6 porphyria (Q 4.76).

Much more commonly the pain will have an unrelated aetiology!

Respiratory system

Note: If unexplained chest pain or dyspnoea occur consider pulmonary embolism (see Q 4.176).

4.203 Does the COC promote allergic rhinitis or asthma?

There is some tenuous evidence of a causal association between COC use and these conditions, particularly the former (see Q 4.225). But many with both complaints continue to use modern COCs with apparent impunity.

Urinary system

4.204 What is the link between COC use and urinary tract infections?

Several studies have shown that such infections are commoner in OC-users than in controls. Women on the pill may have more frequent intercourse, thus increasing their risk of so-called 'honeymoon cystitis'. But some studies have also shown an increased incidence of symptomless bacteriuria in COC-users, resolving when the pill is stopped. This suggests a causal link, so it may sometimes be worth transferring to another method (but the choice of an occlusive cap needs to be carefully made – see Q 3.51).

Hypertension in association with renal disease is managed routinely (see Qs 4.168–4.172).

Reproductive system – obstetrics

4.205 What are the risks to the fetus if the woman continues to take the COC during early pregnancy?

In animal research, sex steroids can certainly be teratogens. Stilboestrol is a non-steroidal oestrogen which can harm the human fetus, often with very delayed manifestations; and the complex literature about deliberate hormone use (eg the former hormone pregnancy tests) in early pregnancy includes some studies which suggest an increased incidence of rare congenital abnormalities.

The copious literature is largely reassuring about the COC. The rate of birth defects in the Oxford/FPA and RCGP studies following COC exposure in pregnancy was no higher than expected in any group of women having a planned baby. In a major Connecticut study of 1370 abnormal babies there was no increase in COC use during the pregnancies compared with the mothers of normal infants. Studies of national birth defect registers in Hungary and Finland also strongly suggest that pill use in pregnancy has no effect on visible malformations, though multiple births are commoner.

The rule that a pregnant woman should avoid all drugs, especially in the first trimester, remains the ideal. But the situation envisaged by the question is not uncommon – can the woman be given any kind of risk estimate? She can certainly not be promised a normal baby. Quite apart from the uncertainty about rare anomalies, at least 2% of all babies show an important abnormality. An old much-quoted estimate by the Population Council, based on treatments in the 1960s – that a possible attributable abnormality might occur in 7/10 000 COC-exposed pregnancies – has been updated. Bracken (1990) found a risk ratio from COC of 0.99 (i.e. no detectable change) for all important malformations, in a meta-analysis of 12 prospective studies. This agrees with the better case-control studies.

Note that the risk after failed postcoital hormone treatment, which is given before implantation, would be expected to be even less than this low estimate (see Q 7.15).

4.206 Is there any residual fetal risk for ex-pill-users?

Here the balance of the published work is heavily tilted towards complete absence of risk. In 1981 an expert scientific group of the WHO declared categorically that there was no evidence of any adverse effects on the fetus of pill use prior to conception. The only residual anxiety relates to the fact that alterations in mineral and vitamin levels have been observed in OC-users (see Q 4.90, Table 4.7). These may take a few weeks to revert to normal; and supplementation with vitamins (perhaps most importantly folic acid) at and after conception has been shown to reduce the risk of neural tube defects in women with a previously affected baby.

4.207 Should women stop the COC well ahead of conception?

Some authorities advise that they should discontinue the pill and use a mechanical method of contraception for two to three cycles. This has not been proved to help, though it should certainly do no harm. Ultrasound scanning has lessened the importance of this for dating of the pregnancy. Although most authorities do not consider them important, some couples do find it reassuring that there are no detectable changes from normal in vitamin and mineral metabolism by about 2 months post pill. The FPA now recommends waiting for one natural period before trying to get pregnant.

A woman who conceives sooner than any of these arbitrary times should, in the light of Q 4.206, be very strongly reassured. Avoiding drugs and cigarettes is far more important! Along with an adequate, balanced diet, the Chief Medical Officer recommends a daily dose of 0.4 mg folic acid as prophylaxis against neural tube defects, starting before conception.

For trophoblastic disease, see Q 4.69.

Reproductive system – gynaecology

4.208 How does the COC affect the symptoms associated with the menstrual cycle?

Beneficially in most respects (see the summary list at Q 4.49). *Premenstrual syndrome* was less common overall in the RCGP study. But any prescriber knows that individual pill-takers do complain of a similar symptom-complex towards the end of each packet, with fluid retention, breast tenderness and depression/irritability predominating. These symptoms seem to be commoner on phasic pills. However, overall they remain more frequent in (so-called) normal cycles than in pill-taking cycles.

Similarly, most women notice the menstrual flow to be both lighter and less painful, but a minority who normally have light menses actually report the reverse.

BTB, absent WTB and secondary amenorrhoea after COC use are considered elsewhere (see Qs 4.10, 4.54–4.60 and 4.143–4.156). Remember all the non-pill causes of BTB (Table 4.12)!

4.209 What is the effect of COCs on pelvic infection, functional ovarian cysts and fibroids?

See Qs 4.52, 4.53 and 4.99.

4.210 What effect does the combined pill have on endometriosis?

This condition is sometimes treated but more often maintained in suppression by a progestagen-dominant COC such as Eugynon 30 or Microgynon 30, best on a tricycle basis (see Q 4.28).

There is also a strong clinical impression that it is less common among users of combined OCs, and this has received confirmation from the RCGP and Oxford/FPA studies.

The most significant gynaecological benefit of the COC is of course protection against two cancers (see Qs 4.67–4.72).

4.211 Does the COC cause vaginal discharge?

Do not attribute this to the pill without first eliminating other causes.

1 *Cervical erosion* (now better known as ectopy). This was definitely commoner in the prospective studies based on COCs containing 50 μg or more of oestrogen. It still occurs, though less frequently, on modern pills and requires treatment only if the woman complains of a discharge.

2 On the other hand, some women on progestagen-dominant pills complain of vaginal dryness.

3 It is still generally believed that *thrush (candidiasis)* is more frequent in COC-users. Yet a paper with the title 'The pill does not cause 'thrush'' was published in the *British Journal of Obstetrics and Gynaecology* in 1985. The journal would never have allowed such a title if this study of over 1300 women attending three departments of genitourinary medicine in

England had been the slightest bit equivocal! Other recent studies are confirmatory.

This is perhaps because current low-oestrogen pills have less pregnancy-mimicking effect on the glycogen content of vaginal cells. In practice it should certainly not be assumed that modern pills are to blame in any case of recurrent thrush. Genitourinary medicine experts currently recommend for such cases the daily application of any standard imidazole cream to the anogenital skin, continuing for many weeks if not indefinitely.

4 *Trichomonas vaginitis.* COCs seem to provide some (as yet unexplained) protection against this, but none against the transmission of other STDs.

4.212 Does the COC affect other vaginal conditions?

1 There is a suggestion from research in the USA that the COC protects against the rare *toxic shock syndrome.*

2 No effect either way has been reported on the incidence of *anaerobic vaginosis.*

4.213 How should the complaint of vaginal discharge be managed?

1 It is important to establish the cause by pelvic examination, with speculum examination of the cervix, and relevant microbiology.

2 Whenever relevant there should always be a low threshold for referral to a department of genitourinary medicine, and contact tracing if any true STD is identified. If genital warts or trichomoniasis are present such referral is particularly important (whether or not the woman is a pill-taker), since both may act as markers for more serious STDs.

3 If there is a symptomatic cervical ectopy (erosion), and the smear/colposcopy is negative, this may be dealt with by cryocautery as an outpatient.

The breasts

4.214 What effect does the COC have on the breasts?

For benign breast disease see Q 4.82, and for breast cancer see Qs 4.73–4.80. Most women notice an increase in size of their breasts and some change in texture. These effects may be acceptable, but breast tenderness is less so. The latter may occur with any pill formulation but seems particularly associated with the last phase of phasic brands.

Galactorrhoea among pill-takers is rare and needs investigation (plasma prolactin). A pituitary adenoma or microadenoma should be definitely excluded before dismissing this as a minor side-effect.

4.215 Should the combined pill be used during lactation?

In my view the answer is a definite no, on several counts. First it is an 'overkill' since practically 100% contraception can be obtained by the combination of lactation with the POP (see Q 5.54). Secondly, the COC frequently reduces the volume and quality of milk. and thirdly a larger dose of hormone is being given to the breast-fed infant than would be the case with the POP.

Musculoskeletal system

4.216 If given to young, postpubertal girls, will the COC cause stunting of growth? Indeed, are any other adverse effects more likely in very young teenagers than in the older young woman?

Given in high dose to young female animals, oestrogen alone can lead to premature closure of the epiphyses. However there is no evidence that a daily dose of 30 μg or even 50 μg of EE, especially when taken with progestagen, has this effect in postpubertal girls. Menstruation normally starts when adult weight and height have mostly been achieved. Pill taking should always be delayed until menstruation is established.

Young teenagers need much counselling (see Qs 8.10–11), if the COC is to be prescribed at all. The risks they run are great, affecting so many aspects of emotional development, sexual and reproductive health. But they are the risks of early sexual activity. There are no risks specific to the COC (including the risk of breast cancer under age 35, see Q 4.73) which are known to be greater when it is started at 13 than at 23. So the strictly pharmacological considerations are not different from those for a woman in her early 20s.

4.217 Is the COC associated with carpal-tunnel syndrome, primary Raynaud's disease, chilblains and cramps in the legs?

All these associations have been described, and some are probably causal, especially the first two in the list. Raynaud's *phenomenon* may be a manifestation of a contraindicating condition (such as a collagen disease which might itself promote arterial disease), so the symptom must be investigated.

Otherwise if these problems are troublesome it is worth a trial of discontinuation of the COC; but it may also be continued if the patient so desires.

4.218 How should one assess the complaint of leg pains and cramps?

Careful assessment and examination are important. If bilateral the symptom is less likely to be significant but look for water retention, varicose veins, chilblains or associated Raynaud's phenomenon.

If unilateral, deep venous thrombosis must be excluded. If in doubt the pill should be stopped and the patient referred for further investigation. Her contraceptive future depends on an accurate diagnosis being made.

4.219 How may the COC affect arthritis and related disorders?

A reduction in rheumatoid arthritis risk has emerged in some studies but not others. A 1990 meta-analysis suggests COCs may slow progression of the disease. Tenosynovitis and a form of allergic polyarthritis may occur, but causation has not been proved. For SLE, see Q 4.113.

Cutaneous system

4.220 Which skin conditions may be improved by COCs – and which COCs?

Acne, seborrhoea and sometimes hirsutism may all be benefited by oestrogen-dominant COCs (and indeed may be exacerbated by the reverse) (see Q 4.228).

4.221 Should Dianette be considered as a combined pill or as a treatment for acne and hirsutism?

It should be considered primarily as the latter, though with a very useful secondary effect that it is an effective contraceptive. As shown in Table 4.15, it should normally be tried only after lack of adequate benefit has been obtained by trying the oestrogen-dominant COCs listed. This is partly because the long-term epidemiology of cyproterone acetate has not been so well studied, in large populations, as the progestagens of the COCs. Yet Dianette appears safe for long-term use in selected cases, especially (after full investigation) in the polycystic ovary syndrome (Q 4.58).

4.222 Which skin conditions are more common in COC-users?

1 *Chloasma/melasma*. This 'pregnancy mask' may develop in women on the COC after exposure to sunlight, just as in pregnancy. The condition may be very slow to fade after the pill is stopped. Mild degrees may be masked by careful use of cosmetics and tolerated if exposure to sun can be reduced. A progestagen-only contraceptive may help, but the condition can also recur with the POP. A non-hormonal method may have to be chosen.

2 *Photosensitivity*. This is more common in COC-takers. Very rarely it may be the first manifestation of one of the prophyrias. Once acquired, like chloasma it tends to be permanent even if the pill is discontinued.

3 *Pemphigoid (herpes) gestationis*. If this serious skin condition occurs it absolutely contraindicates the COC.

4 Telangiectasia, rosacea, neurodermatitis, spider naevi, erythema multiforme, erythema nodosum, eczema, and possibly other allergic skin disorders – all these have been described as possibly causally associated or exacerbated by COCs, in a minority of women. Melanoma is discussed at Q 4.103.

4.223 What action should be taken if such skin problems present in a COC-taker?

First, discontinue the COC. Severe conditions such as erythema multiforme or pemphigoid gestationis would normally mean future avoidance of this method. If the condition has an immune/allergic basis it is usually unclear whether the COC steroids are the actual allergens (see Q 4.227). According to the views of the woman herself, therefore, and any dermatologist involved, if the condition is mild she may be cautiously rechallenged with a low-dose COC perhaps containing a different progestagen, or with the POP. Recurrence would suggest another method.

4.224 Does the COC cause gingivitis? Any other oral problems?

Hypertrophic gingivitis is a rare but well-recognized complication of COC use. Lesser degrees are more common, as in pregnancy. Symptoms are minimized by good oral hygiene.

'Dry socket', a painful state after tooth extraction, is also said to be commoner in COC-users.

Allergies and inflammations

4.225 What effect does the COC have on immune mechanisms?

Several studies on immunoglobulins have suggested that artifical sex steroids can modify immune mechanisms. The effects are of a similar nature to, but less marked than, those associated with pregnancy. A study from France, however, in which antibodies to EE were reported in patients suffering from venous thrombosis, has not been confirmed.

The RCGP Study in particular among the prospective studies showed an increase in inflammations and some disorders which are believed to have an immune basis. However, as shown in Figure 4.13 these are partly balanced by a well-established protective effect against thyroid over- and under-activity, and possibly rheumatoid arthritis (see Q 4.219). Once again, as with both malignant and benign tumours (Figs. 4.6, 4.7), combination OCs seem to be capable of causing both benefical and adverse effects within the same medical field. Causative associations are not all proven by any means and the magnitude of the effects described in Figure 4.13 is mostly small; but we badly need more information.

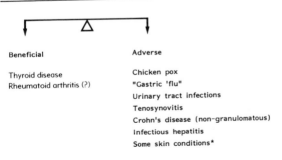

Some apparent associations of COC-use with immune disorders/inflammations

Beneficial

Thyroid disease
Rheumatoid arthritis (?)

Adverse

Chicken pox
"Gastric 'flu"
Urinary tract infections
Tenosynovitis
Crohn's disease (non-granulomatous)
Infectious hepatitis
Some skin conditions*

* See text

Figure 4.13 Immune disorders/inflammations and the pill. Q 4.225

4.226 Does use of the COC promote transmission of HIV infection? or make AIDS more or less likely after infection?

To cut a long story short, 'no' seems the current best answer to both questions – though this field of research is notoriously difficult. Effective contraception is obviously important for any woman known to be HIV positive, so the COC is a useful option to be able to use as well as the condom. This does not appear to worsen the prognosis.

Studies among prostitutes in Nairobi were the first to suggest an increase in the likelihood of seroconversion to HIV positive if the COC were used; but a causative link has not yet been established.

4.227 Do women sometimes become allergic to the COC hormones, or in COC-users is there an increased tendency to react to other allergens?

Data exist to suggest that either may occur. For example, in vitro studies of blood lymphocytes suggested hypersensitivity to mestranol in two cases (one of erythema multiforme, one of erythema nodosum). On the other hand I have had a case of erythema nodosum who was able to go back on the same brand of COC without suffering any recurrence.

4.228 Are there any guidelines for selecting the next pill if a patient complains of any minor side-effect and wishes to continue the method?

> **Note: Never forget there may be another, non-pill-related, explanation for any side-effect, and that a side-effect may be caused or highlighted because of anxiety or a psychosexual problem.** See the Preface. This applies particularly to this and the next question, and the linked Tables 4.14 and 4.15.

With modern COCs, an emotional or psychosexual explanation becomes more probable (though *not* invariable, see Q 4.193) if a woman keeps on returning with a wide assortment of side-effects after only taking a few tablets, and nothing ever seems to suit.

On first principles, first take a history and, as appropriate, then examine. After that, if the side-effect relates to BTB or absent WTB she should either be switched to a phasic pill or moved 'higher up the ladder' (see Q 4.151).

Table 4.14 Which second choice of pill? A: Relative oestrogen excess

Symptoms	Conditions
Nausea Dizziness 'Premenstrual tension' and irritability Cyclical weight gain (fluid) 'Bloating' Vaginal discharge (no infection) Some cases of breast fullness/pain	Benign breast disease Fibroids Endometriosis
Treat with progestagen-dominant COC, such as Loestrin 30, Microgynon 30, Eugynon 30 (but with caution regarding lipids, see Q 4.139)	

Table 4.15 Which second choice of pill? B: Relative progestagen excess

Symptoms	Conditions

Dryness of vagina
Some cases of:
  Sustained weight gain
  Depression
  Loss of libido
  Lassitude
  Breast tenderness
	Acne/seborrhoea
	Hirsutism

Treat with oestrogen-dominant COC, such as Marvelon, Gracial or Dianette (an acne treatment which is also contraceptive, containing 35 μg of EE combined with 2 mg cyproterone acetate); or possibly Norinyl-I (50 μg oestrogen).	

See Q 4.229.

For all other minor side-effects there are two empirical rules and two more specific ones. The empirical rules are:

1 Reduce the dose where possible (this will normally be the dose of the progestagen, as nearly all pill-takers should be on 30–35 μg of the oestrogen).

2 Alternatively, switch to another progestagen ladder (Fig. 4.10). For the more specific rules, see Q 4.229.

4.229 What are the more specific rules?

1 For side-effects or conditions which have become associated (through clinical experience, and sometimes by formal research) with a relative excess of the oestrogen, prescribe a more progestagen-dominant COC.

2 Conversely, for symptoms which have become associated with the progestagen, prescribe an oestrogen-dominant COC. This policy is summarized in Tables 4.14 and 4.15.

SPECIAL CONSIDERATIONS: WHEN TO COME OFF THE PILL?

4.230 Are there benefits to be gained from taking breaks from COC use? Is duration of use of any relevance?

From the point of view of *preservation of fertility*, the answer is a categorical no on both counts (see Qs 4.61–2). In relation to *circulatory disease* duration of use may have an effect, though not shown in recent good studies (see Qs 4.87–8), and probably mainly relevant to smokers.

However, even if the limited evidence on that score is believed, there is no real value to be expected from taking breaks; that is, *unless the breaks are so long as to have a real influence on total accumulated duration of use (Fig. 4.14).*

It is worth reminding any woman asking that during 10 years she has in fact taken 130 breaks. Moreover, there is increasing evidence that the body tends to restore metabolic changes towards normal during each PFI (see Q 4.26).

Metabolic risk markers show no apparent progression beyond 2 years' continuous use. So it could even be argued that repeated restarting of the COC might be more harmful than the relatively steady-state situation that is maintained during sustained use.

The main problem with breaks of a few months' at a time was well shown in a study in which one quarter of young women

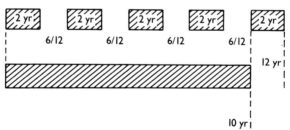

Figure 4.14 Breaks and accumulated duration of use of the COC. Q 4.230.
The blocks represent segments of pill-taking duration (in which the only breaks taken are the pill-free weeks). Note how a woman who takes 6-monthly breaks every 2 years still accumulates 10 years of total duration in 12 years.

had unwanted pregnancies, during a planned break of just 6 months.

4.231 What about duration of use and cancer risk? (Qs 4.00–00)

There are studies which show beneficial effects on cancer of the ovary and endometrium, and others showing possible harmful effects on cancer of the cervix and breast. In each of these opposite categories both the beneficial and the adverse effects described were greater with increasing duration of use!

Short breaks are again unlikely to be relevant, as the evidence points to total duration. Reducing the total duration of use when young does appear in several studies to be beneficial for breast cancer risk, so there is logic in not continuing the COC method when contraception is not required, e.g. between partners.

Since at present it is impossible to state with certainty whether the good effects of pill use outweigh the adverse effects on cancer overall (see Q 4.66), though they may do so, it is equally impossible to assess accurately the changes on both sides of the equation caused by increased duration of use. See below, Q 4.232 and Table 4.16. The pros and cons seem roughly in balance.

Table 4.16 Management by age, smoking and duration of COC use

A: Age and COC use Age (yr)					
	30	35	40	45	50
Smoker	Review	Change method	(COC contraindicated for contraception) (POP and HRT usable)		
Non-smoker —		Review	Review	Review	Non-hormonal method, or no method now if post menopause
B: Accumulated duration of use Duration (yr)					
	4–5	10	15	20	25+
Smoker	Review	Second review	?Change method	Change method	—
Non-smoker	—	Review	Review	Review	Review

Both smokers and non-smokers with a relevant family history of breast cancer or other risk factor should review duration of use carefully at about 4 years (see Qs 4.73, 4.103).

4.232 How much should *age per se* influence prescribing, with regard to both cardiovascular system (CVS) risk and cancer?

CVS risks and age

Here opinions have changed since the last edition of this book, triggered by the landmark decision of the US FDA's Fertility and Maternal Health Drugs Advisory Committee in October 1989. Their recommendation, subsequently endorsed by the FDA itself, was for:

> The removal of all age limits on the use of (combined) oral contraceptives by healthy non-smoking women – i.e. free of all risk factors.

Was this a cavalier decision, flying in the face of previously agreed practice? I think not, because:

1 Non-smoking pill-takers are actually much 'safer' than we used to think (Q 4.86).

2 Modern prescribing and monitoring are more structured and careful (Q 4.98–181).

3 The pills themselves are believed to be safer (see Q 4.133).

4 Above all, we now have a much better appreciation of the benefits to gynaecological health of the COC for women, most particularly older women (see Q 8.38).

In short, even if the CVS risks climb somewhat with age, the benefits increase at least as much and the risk/benefit ratio is therefore unchanged if not improved. *But only for healthy non-smokers!*

Note: The important issue of how to diagnose the menopause when it is masked by the COC or other hormones is discussed at Qs 5.61–4, 5.121, 8.44–6.

Cancer risks with age

These show a general increase. But the COC does not appear to increase breast cancer risk when used by the older woman (see Q 4.76), and protects against cancer of the ovary and endometrium whose incidence rises above age 40. Hence the new FDA-based policy permitting use of the COC by an older age group should lead if anything to an overall reduction in cancer risk. But see Q 8.38.

4.233 If a smoker really does give up cigarettes at age 35, may she continue to take the COC? And if so, until what age?

There are no good data about this important question, for both practical and ethical reasons. Ex-smokers are a rare breed and their CVS morbidity would need examining prospectively with and without continuing to take the pill. We can extrapolate to some extent from the British Regional Heart Study of 7735 *men*, which reported that in ex-smokers of up to 20 cigarettes a day no excess risk of ischaemic heart disease (IHD) was observed in those who had quit 6–10 years prior to the screening, compared with never-smokers. However heavy ex-smokers (>20 per day) still had a significantly higher risk after 11–20 years.

Other studies show a marked early decline in risk of IHD, due to loss of the acute metabolic effects of smoking; but they suggest in men that it takes 10 years to return to the levels seen in never-smokers. If this delay is due to early coronary atheroma generated by years of smoking, one must be concerned about the prothrombotic effects of ethinyloestradiol in any COC (Q 8.41).

In a 1990 report from the US in *women* ex-smokers, 'the increase in risk of a first myocardial infarction dissipated after 2–3 years'. This is more rapid than among the British men, but it does not establish safety if COCs had been taken and continued to be taken. The ex-smoker cannot be reassured like the risk-factor free woman about continuing with the pill until her menopause (Q 4.232), though in my view this is not absolutely contraindicated.

4.234 Please would you summarize how age and duration of use should influence long-term prescribing?

Please see Table 4.16. For overall cancer risk, duration of use is treated as neutral in the table because it affects the size of benefits as well as of risks (see Q 4.231). And as just seen (see Q 4.232), cancer risk with increasing age is probably reduced by COC use. With regard to CVS risk, duration is considered in the table as mainly relevant to women with risk factors.

SOME REVISION QUESTIONS

4.235 What are the medical myths about prescribing the pill?

The following list is not exhaustive, but includes some important examples currently believed by some health care professionals. *Pill myths* – Do not prescribe the COC if:

Myth	Actuality The COC is:	
Wish to optimize fertility	Beneficial	Q 4.62
Fibroids	Beneficial	Q 4.82
Current amenorrhoea, after investigation	Beneficial (sometimes)	Q 4.58
Past amenorrhoea, resolved	Neutral	Q 4.60
Recent menarche (if cycling)	Neutral	Q 4.216
History of gestational diabetes	Neutral (watch weight)	Q 4.116
Varicose veins (no past thrombosis)	Neutral	Q 4.122
Thrush	Neutral	Q 4.211
Recent trophoblastic disease (hCG now normal)	Neutral	Q 4.69
Sickle cell trait	Neutral	Q 4.108
Thalassaemia	Neutral	Q 4.105
Epilepsy (allowing for drug interactions)	Neutral (sometimes beneficial)	Q 4.187
Migraine (non-focal, tolerable, no change)	RC	Q 4.131
Cervical neoplasia (preinvasive)	RC	Q 4.72
Hyperprolactinaemia	RC	Q 4.58
Wish to minimize overall cancer risk	Unknown, but avoiding COC might even increase this risk.	Q 4.67

RC = relative contraindication

4.236 What are the pill myths relating to continuing use of the method?

Myth	Actuality	
1 There should be a break from pill use every few years	False	Q 4.230
2 Duration of pill use should never be more than 5 (or 10) years at a time	False	Q 4.230

3 The pill should be stopped in all women reaching 35 years of age	Smokers (or if risk factors)	Q 4.232
4 The COC should be stopped before all surgery	Only for major or leg surgery	Q 4.177
5 Prolonged absence of withdrawal bleeds (to preserve fertility)	Irrelevant	Q 4.10

There are also myths which many doctors share with pill-takers about 'missed pills' (see Qs 4.17, 4.242 and 7.18(e)).

4.237 In what important situations do doctors commonly forget to enquire whether the patient is on an oestrogen-containing pill?

1 Emergency admissions, involving surgery or confinement to bed

2 When elective arrangements are made for a major operation, or for surgery or sclerotherapy for varicose veins.

3 When any potentially interacting drugs are prescribed – especially rifampicin and griseofulvin.

4 When arranging any laboratory test, especially of the blood. Results of many tests may be modified by the COC (see Table 4.7).

SOME QUESTIONS ASKED BY USERS ABOUT THE COC

The majority of such questions will readily be answered by reference to the earlier questions in this chapter.

4.238 I am told thrombosis has to do with clots – I have clots with my periods so does this mean that I can't use the pill?

Far from it! Clots with the periods just means that they are heavy, and could well improve dramatically if you went on the pill – the COC would be better than the POP.

4.239 Can I postpone having a period?

Certainly. The bleeding you get between packets of pills is actually entirely caused by you when you take a 7-day break between packets. It is really a 'withdrawal bleed' rather than a proper period, and there is no reason why from time to time you should not run two packets on to each other so there is no break and therefore no bleeding. The rules are a little different, however, for so-called phasic pills (see Q 4.163). Also it is not recommended that you simply take pill packets endlessly without any breaks – unless there is a special reason and then we recommend the so-called tricycle regimen (see Q 4.28, Fig. 4.4).

4.240 Do I always have to see periods at weekends?

Certainly not. If it happens to have worked out that your periods are tending to come at weekends on the COC, all you need to do is to take some extra pills one month to move your withdrawal bleeding to a more convenient time. Discuss with your doctor which pills to take if it happens to be a phased type (see Q 4.163).

4.241 My 'period' is much lighter than normal, almost absent in fact and a different colour – does this matter?

No, anything from quite average sort of bleeding through to nothing at all can be normal for the response of an individual woman's womb to the stopping of the pill's hormones. Should you have no periods at all 2 months in a row, you should take prompt advice to eliminate the possibility of pregnancy and also to discuss whether you should start the next packet. This action should be taken even if you have only missed one withdrawal bleed when you missed pills – or if there is earlier vomiting, diarrhoea or treatment with an interacting drug (see Qs 4.28–4.31).

(Many other questions are asked about issues related to bleeding on the COC, whether normal, abnormal, or absent. These can be answered by reference to Qs 4.10, 4.29, 4.35, 4.46, 4.55–60, 4.149–63, 8.16 (18–26).

4.242 Is it safe to make love in the 7 days between pill packets?

Yes: but only if no pills have been missed (by forgetting, stomach upset or drug interaction) towards the end of the previous packet, and also only if you do in fact start another packet after the pill-free week (see Qs 4.21, 4.28–4.31 and 8.16(16)). *Beware*, particularly when you come off the pill for any reason, including because of being sterilized.

4.243 Which are the most 'dangerous' pills to be missed – presumably in the middle of the month?

Not so, the middle of the month is the least bad time to miss pills, though you should not make a habit of missing any . . . . The worst pills to be missed are any that result in lengthening of the pill-free time (see Qs 4.19–4.25). Never be late starting your next packet! something lots of people don't even consider as missing a pill.

4.244 Are there any problems in pill taking for flight crews?

It is easy for them, or other air-travellers, to become confused about regular pill-taking because of passing through different time zones. The effectiveness problem is greatest when flying due West, since the new bed-time pill might be late, many hours more than a day later than the preceding one. One solution is a watch which gives the time at their home base as well as local time. If in doubt on arrival at a new destination or if deciding to switch to morning rather than evening pill taking with a new pack, air-travellers should err on the side of taking a pill too early rather than late: leaving only 6.5 rather than 7.5 days between packets.

4.245 My skin has got worse on the pill, yet I was told it should get better – why is this?

It all depends on the severity of your acne and which pill you have been given. The recommended ones are at Q 4.229 (Table 4.15).

4.246 Can I use a sunbed if I am on the pill?

Yes.

4.247 Does using either the COC or the POP delay the menopause?

No. This occurs as a result of an inexorable process of egg loss which seems to be unaffected by anything. It even occurs at the same time as it otherwise would in women who as a result of surgery have been left with only one ovary.

4.248 Can I take antihistamines and the pill?

The ones given by your GP, or which you may purchase in the chemist, seem to cause no important change in the effectiveness of your pill. Other medicines may do, however (see Qs 4.30 and 4.31, Table 4.3), and the warning sign of an interaction can be bleeding during tablet-taking. Always tell any doctor that you take the pill.

4.249 Is it true that you are more likely to get drunk if you are on the pill?

Some research published in 1984 suggested this, since it showed that alcohol leaves the body more slowly in pill-users than in non-pill-users. Subsequently, other researchers in Australia found the opposite, that pill-takers recovered from the effects of alcohol *more* quickly than non-takers! But the take-home message about which there is no argument is that *all* women should be extra careful about alcohol. This is because their smaller livers make it have a bigger effect than in men, both short term and long term (meaning that the risk of liver damage is greater in women).

5 Oestrogen-free hormonal contraception

BACKGROUND AND MECHANISMS

5.1 What are progestagen-only pills (POPs)?

In the UK these pills contain a microdose of one of three progestagens, either from the norethisterone group (norethisterone and ethynodiol diacetate) or levonorgestrel. They are taken on a continuous daily basis.

The first brand of this type contained chlormadinone acetate but it was withdrawn 1 year after introduction in 1969 when toxicity tests using the Beagle bitch showed that this progestagen tended to cause breast nodules, which could become malignant. As with Depo-Provera (see Q 5.104), it is now realized that this breed of dog is a highly inappropriate animal model.

5.2 Which POPs are in current use?

See Table 5.1. POPs account for no more than 8% of the UK oral contraceptive market.

5.3 How much is known about the POP method?

The short answer is: still remarkably little. No large cohort studies are in progress, and case-control studies have not been attempted because of the low prevalence of use. Hence we are forced to draw on the few metabolic and clinical studies available; and otherwise to extrapolate from available data on the combined pill (adjusting in an admittedly arbitrary way for absence of artificial oestrogen and presence of a particularly small dose of the progestagen).

Table 5.1 Progestagen-only pills in the UK

Name	No. of tablets per packet	Progestagen	Dose (μg)
Microval/Norgeston	35	Levonorgestrel	30
Neogest	35	Levonorgestrel	37.5*
Micronor/Noriday	28	Norethisterone	350
Femulen	28	Ethynodiol diacetate	500

* Plus 37.5 μg of inactive isomer — so best not used (see Q 4.135)
A desogestrel POP is expected on the market in the late 1990s.

5.4 What is the mode of action of POPs?

This is summarized in Table 5.2. The main action has previously been thought to be the alteration in the cervical mucus. But there is also a considerable effect on ovulation, in most women and in most cycles – around 60% – and more in older women. Ovulation may be abolished completely leading to amenorrhoea; but even without this there are varying degrees of interference with the ovulatory process as described in Q 5.5.

It must therefore be understood at the outset that the hormonal environment of a previously cycling woman on the POP is the *resultant of the direct effect of the exogenous progestagen and an amount of ovarian activity which varies* – both between women and between cycles. This explains the very varied menstrual pattern which is observed, and is also relevant to other side-effects.

5.5 What effects can the POP have on ovarian function?

In individual women, or in the same woman in different menstrual cycles, the effects vary. Although the patterns have been described in four groups, this is for convenience. The situation is better described as a spectrum running from no interference with the ovarian cycle, though to complete quiescence of the ovaries and no follicular or luteal activity.

In a short-term study (1980), Swedish workers have described four main groups in this continuum (percentage of cycles in parentheses):

1 Cycles showing almost no change from normal, with apparently normal ovulation, minimal shortening of the luteal phase, and progesterone levels within normal limits (40%).

2 Normal follicular phase but marked shortening of the luteal phase, with lower progesterone levels for a shorter time (21%).

3 Follicular activity with higher peak oestrogen levels than usual; but no ovulation and no progesterone production. Ultrasound scans of the ovaries in these women show the formation of abnormal follicles or functional cysts, which may be single or multiple (23%).

4 Diminished follicular activity, low oestrogen levels, no corpus luteum formation and no endogenous progesterone production. Ultrasound scanning confirms quiescent ovaries (16%).

Table 5.2 Various progestagen delivery systems (all except COC are oestrogen-free)

	Oral		Injectable		Implant	Vaginal ring
	COC	POP	NET-EN	DMPA	Norplant	LNG ring (WHO)
Administration						
Frequency	Daily	Daily	2-monthly	3-monthly	5-yearly	3-monthly
Progestagen dose	Low	Ultra-low	High	High	Ultra-low	Ultra-low
Blood levels	Rapidly fluctuating		Initial peak then decline		Constant	Constant
First pass through liver	Yes	Yes	No	No	No	No
Major mechanisms						
Ovary: ↓ Ovulation*	+++	+	++	+++	++	+
Cervical mucus: ↓ sperm penetrability	Yes	Yes	Yes	Yes	Yes	Yes
Endometrium: ↓ receptivity to blastocyst	Yes	Yes	Yes	Yes	Yes	Yes
Use effectiveness	0.2–3	0.3–4	<2	0–1	0–1	3
Menstrual pattern	Regular	Often irregular	Irregular	Very irregular	Irregular	Irregular
Amenorrhoea during use	Rare	Occasional	Common	Very common	Common	Common
Reversibility						
Immediate termination possible?	Yes	Yes	No	No	Yes	Yes
By woman herself at any time?	Yes	Yes	No	No	No	Yes
Time to first likely conception from first omitted dose/removal	3 months	c. 1 month	c. 3 months	6 months	c. 1 month	c. 1 month

* By two mechanisms – no preovulatory follicles formed, plus no LH surges occur.

229

5.6 How do the changes described in the last question show themselves in the menstrual pattern and affect the risk of contraceptive failure?

1 A majority of the women experiencing cycles of the type in Group 1 above will have regular periods. They are not immune to breakthrough bleeding (BTB), however, probably because of direct effects of the artificial progestagen on the endometrium. Here ovulation is the norm, the pharmacological effects on the pituitary/ovarian axis are minimal; but this means that they are also the group with the highest risk of breakthrough pregnancy. They are relying chiefly on the mucus and perhaps sometimes the endometrial effects for contraception (Fig. 5.1).

2 Groups 2 and 3, which show varying degrees of cycle disturbance, short of complete abolition, merge with each other and are therefore together in the middle column of Figure 5.1. It is from among these women that extra-frequent or erratic, irregular bleeds will be reported: the endometrium no longer receives adequate endogenous progesterone, and many of those in Group 3 also have increased oestrogen stimulation from the increased follicular activity. The bleeding pattern is a *resultant* of this abnormal ovarian activity and the (rather rapid) fluctuations each 24 hours in the level of exogenous progestagen. It would appear that it is in cycles showing the patterns of Groups 2 and 3 that symptomatic or asymptomatic functional ovarian cysts may be formed. The risk of breakthrough pregnancy is considerably less than in Group 1, probably almost nil since such a cycle is anovular (though the woman could always have a Group 1-type cycle in another month).

3 In Group 4 at the extreme of the continuum, there is either complete amenorrhoea, or intermittent, very light bleeding. This is caused by irregular shedding of the endometrium receiving much less oestrogen than usual and only the saw-tooth pattern of daily exogenous progestagen administration. The risk of contraceptive failure here is nil. It is of course also the norm for POP-taking during lactation.

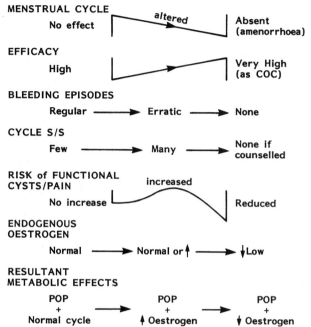

Figure 5.1 Spectrum of responses to the progestagen-only pill. Q 5.5, 5.6, 5.35 and 5.39.

Note the metabolic effects are minimal anyway in *all* the groups, across the 'spectrum'.

5.7 What then does amenorrhoea on the POP mean?

First, it may certainly be caused by pregnancy, and this must be excluded in the usual way. Once that explanation is ruled out, paradoxically the women experiencing prolonged episodes of amenorrhoea are the ones not ovulating and so actually at least risk of conception. It is from among the Group 1 POP-using women, who are experiencing regular periods and being regularly reassured thereby, that the majority of unplanned conceptions occur. See also Q 5.65 *re* possible risks of sustained amenorrhoea.

5.8 Are any particular POPs more likely to cause erratic periods or amenorrhoea?

As has to be said about so many aspects of POP use, the possibility of differences between the POPs has been inadequately studied. The Swedish studies quoted at Q 5.5 were not able to demonstrate any correlation between doses given or measured blood levels of the artificial progestagen and the types of ovarian reaction or the bleeding profile – even though the blood levels also showed wide patient-to-patient variation (see Q 5.9). So it appears that the main factor is the degree to which the end-organs, especially the ovary and the uterus, are susceptible to the effects of the POP in the blood.

5.9 In POP-takers is there the same variability in blood levels of the steroids as described for the COC (see Q 4.142)?

Yes. There is the same enormous variation between women who are apparently similar, taking the same POP and having their blood levels estimated at the same time after their last tablet was ingested. But variation in target-organ sensitivity appears more important (see Q 5.8) in causing bleeding side effects.

There is also (as for COC-users) the fact of variation, again about 10-fold, between the peak and trough blood levels each day within the same woman. This aspect is discussed at Qs 4.15 and 5.83 (Figs. 4.2, 5.3).

5.10 How does the enterohepatic cycle operate for the POP?

As in Figure 4.5 (see Q 4.14), after the artificial progestagen is absorbed liver metabolism creates metabolites which re-enter the lumen of the bowel, via the bile. But the action of the bowel flora does not result in reformation of active progestagen. Hence the achieved circulating levels of the POP are normally not dependent on hydrolysis by the intestinal flora and subsequent reabsorption of the progestagen; so antibiotics can have no effect on POP blood levels. However enzyme-inducing drugs may reduce the blood levels and affect efficacy, just as they do with the COC (see Q 5.28).

EFFECTIVENESS

5.11 What is the overall effectiveness of the POP?

As usual, reliability depends greatly on the motivation of the woman. An overall rate of 0.3–4/100 woman-years can be quoted, the higher rate occurring when patient compliance is poor, and particularly at very young ages, as discussed in Q 5.15. The lower rate applies particularly during *lactation* (Q 5.54).

5.12 What is the influence on the effectiveness of age, and of duration of use?

In the Oxford/Family Planning Association (FPA) study there was no evidence for the former view that the pregnancy rate increases with duration of use – if anything the figures are compatible with the reverse (as is found with practically all other methods).

However, there is a marked influence of age (see Table 5.3). The failure rate falls from 3.1/100 woman-years for the age of 25–29 to 0.3 for women above the age of 40. Possible explanations are as follows.

1 The usual influence of declining fertility with age, shown for example also for the IUD (see Q 6.11).

2 Related to 1, it is well known that the prevalence of abnormal menstrual cycles increases with increasing age, and this is likely to predispose to abnormalities of ovulation (Groups 2–4, as discussed at Q 5.5). Although not reported, it would be expected that the older women in the Oxford/FPA study had a greater incidence of irregular bleeding and amenorrhoea; whereas the younger women would tend to have ovarian cycles which were more 'resistant' to the effect of the exogenous progestagen, and hence more would be ovulating and at greater risk of conception. They would necessarily be relying solely on the other two main effects of the method (on the mucus and endometrium).

Table 5.3 Progestagen-only pill — user-failure rates/100 woman-years Oxford/ FPA Study (1985 report) — all women married and aged above 25, any duration of use.

All ages	Age (years)			
	25–29	30–34	35–39	40+
0.9	3.1	2.0	1.0	0.3

NB: These figures are different from those given in Table 0.1, because they are based on nearly twice as many woman-years of observation.

3 Older women tend to have less frequent intercourse.

4 It is possibly also true that the younger women were less consistent in their pill taking.

5.13 Do other factors affect the effectiveness of POPs? What about body weight?

The Oxford/FPA study was unable to show any statistically significant difference between the failure rate according to which particular POP brand was used, though appreciable variation was noted. Cigarette smoking did not appear to be of importance.

Body weight.   The Oxford/FPA study did show a trend to higher pregnancy rates with increasing weight. Though not statistically significant, this has to be taken seriously in view of the significance of similar analyses of data now available for other progestagen-only methods. With both the levonorgestrel-releasing vaginal ring (Qs 5.152) and Norplant (Qs 5.146–51) – specifically in trials of the higher-silica polymer 373 (an older subcutaneous implant which had a higher failure rate overall) – the pregnancy rate was positively correlated to increasing weight. The ring in particular is such a similar method that I feel the weight effect has to be considered real for the POP also, until a larger POP study settles the issue. *There is no proof that weight is not important.*

5.14 Why does the weight effect on efficacy show up with low-dose progestagen methods and not with the combined pill and injectables?

My explanation for this is that the COC and injectables are just too effective, in users of whatever weight, for this trend – which would after all be expected for any drug – to be detectable in studies of a realistic size. The doses given by the progestagen-only methods of Q 5.13 are nearer the minimum for efficacy, so something like weight can exert a detectable influence on the failure rate.

5.15 What are the implications of the findings with regard to efficacy?

1 *For the young.* Unfortunately the Oxford/FPA study does not include women under the age of 25. However, extrapolating from Table 5.3, the expected failure rate is likely to be quite high, say 4/100 woman-years, especially since compliance tends to be less good in the young. However some studies

which included many women in their twenties have shown acceptable failure rates of 1–2/100 woman-years. So with careful selection and education of users the POP is certainly on the list of options for the young.

2 *For older women.* The main implication of these findings, more positively, is the remarkable efficacy of the method in the older woman. Since that is precisely the group who may need to transfer from the COC (see Q 4.114, Table 4.8), it is useful to be able to state quite truthfully to a woman over 40: 'Your chances of conceiving if you are a regular taker of the POP are the same as for a 25-year old taking a modern combined pill.' (The Oxford/FPA study gives method-plus-user failure rates of around 0.3 in both instances.)

3 *For the overweight.* See Q 5.13. For the time being I feel we should warn women weighing above 70 kg (11 stone) of the possibility of a higher failure rate than as quoted in Q 5.11. If nothing else is suitable, the use of two POPs per day may be considered particularly in the under 30s, with careful counselling and record keeping for the reasons at Q 4.34.

5.16 For those users who are still ovulating, how long does the contraceptive effect on the cervical mucus last, following each dose?

As illustrated in Figure 5.2, following one tablet the effect is maximal about 4 hours later, but there is some return of sperm penetrability around 24 hours. Although regular POP taking abolishes this, making the mucus normally impenetrable throughout the 24 hours, at least in some women the mucus effect is likely to be at its lowest around the time that each new tablet is taken. Figure 5.2 actually derives from some work in the late 1960s using the POP megestrol acetate (0.5 mg). Similar data are available for levonorgestrel and there is no reason to believe that the general principles derived from Figure 5.2 would not hold good for all currently marketed POP brands.

Scanning electron microscope (SEM) studies have shown a characteristic tight mesh of microfibrils in mucus obtained from women using various microdose progestagens – when the progestagenic effect is maximal. However, in cycling women (Group 1 in Q 5.5), if the mucus is sampled at mid-cycle as little as 36 hours after the last tablet was taken the SEM appearances are already nearly back to the normal open mesh of oestrogenic mucus which

SPERM PENETRATION TEST

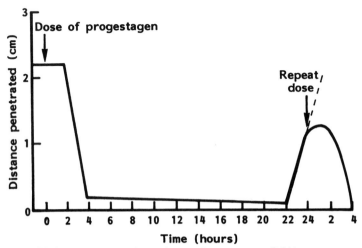

Figure 5.2 Sperm penetration of cervical mucus after progestagen. Q 5.16.
Note minimum reduction in sperm penetration between 4 hours and 22 hours after a
single dose of megestrol acetate (0.5 mg). Unlike the rest of the figure, the effect of a
repeat dose is presumed, not experimental.
(Redrawn from Cox HJE 1968 The pre-coital use of minidosage progestagens. Journal
of Reproduction and Fertility Supplement 5: 167–172, Figure 1)

sperm can readily penetrate. Such studies are prone to artefacts,
but others showing rapid loss of associated cellular and biochemical
changes in mucus after discontinuation of progestagens, confirm
Figure 5.2: that the contraceptive effect of the POP on mucus
disappears if a woman is as much as 12 hours late in taking her
tablet. Hence a much stricter rule must be observed (see Q 5.20).

5.17 What endometrial effects have been described in POP-users?

As with other tissues, observations differ according to the variable
amount of endogenous ovarian activity superimposed on the direct
effect of the progestagen (see Q 5.5 and Fig. 5.1).

That said, blockade of progesterone receptors occurs, and
characteristic changes have been described in the histology of the
endometrium on both light and electron microscopy. Uterine
glands diminish both in number and in diameter. These and

associated biochemical effects are believed to reduce the likelihood of successful implantation.

5.18 How important is the endometrial effect, how long does it take to develop and how readily is it lost?

The answers to all these questions are largely unknown. The mucus effect has been more fully studied, but the endometrial effect may well be a useful back-up during long-term POP use, particularly when ovulation is not abolished.

5.19 For maximum efficacy of the POP, how and when should it be taken?

As implied by Figure 5.2, and the answer to Q 5.16, the answer to 'how?' is: 'extremely regularly'. Indeed I always tell prospective POP-users that the POP is 'a package deal'. In other words 'here is your packet of pills, now get your partner to give you a present – an alarm watch!' Non-breastfeeders are encouraged to take their tablets at precisely the same time each day (plus or minus 1 *hour*). There is very much more leeway during full lactation (Q 5.6, 5.23, 5.24), since ovulation is then inhibited and the situation is like taking the COC.

It is often concluded from Figure 5.2 that the best regular pill-taking time is in the early evening, if the woman usually has intercourse when she goes to bed. However, that may not be an easy time for good compliance. And the hard data in Figure 5.2 relate to taking only the first tablet in cycling women: it is believed that the mucus effect is thereafter sustained for at least 27 hours with modern POPs.

Marginally, in that minority who have fertile ovulations at all on the POP, the worst time for regular pill taking is just before the commonest time for intercourse: since the woman would then be *regularly* relying on the tablet taken 24 hours earlier. But if she finds that is her easiest time to remember, no problem. It is often satisfactory to recommend pill taking at the time of a main meal (breakfast, lunch or supper) or absolutely *anytime in lactation*.

5.20 What rule do you recommend for missed POPs?

Bearing in mind the spectrum of effects of this method on different women and in different cycles (see Q 5.5), and the lack of data about the relative importance of the contraceptive effects in Table 5.2, it has not surprisingly proved difficult to reach agreement on the matter of 'rules'.

1   There is good agreement among the authorities on one point: since the mucus effect is so quickly lost, *extra precautions should begin if a woman is more than 3 hours late* in taking her POP (27 hours since the last tablet).

2   The difficult part of the advice is: for how long should loss of contraception be assumed? From 1985 to 1992 in the UK the FPA recommended in its instruction leaflets that *an additional contraceptive method should be used just for the next 48 hours. But in the 1993 leaflets 7 days is now specified* (see below).

5.21   Most manufacturers' data sheets have said for years that a late POP means 14 days' loss of protection. Does it take that long to restore the efficacy of the POP?

No – most authorities feel that this is far too long:

1   The pill-free-week problem is non-existent here (cf. Qs 4.15–24).

2   The hostile mucus effect seems to be maximal (and sustained) within no more than 48 hours.

3   Even a 2-day rule allows about 5 days for the recommenced POP to have its contraceptive effect on the endometrium. (Even if sperm managed to penetrate the mucus before the 2 days of extra contraception started, it would be at least 5 days before any blastocyst would start implanting.)

5.22   So why are you now recommending 7 days additional precautions, if one pill (or more) is missed for more than 3 hours?

1   The main reason is pragmatic. After much campaigning for them to come into line with scientific knowledge and clinical practice, the manufacturers of POPs are prepared finally to accept a reduction from 14 days for the duration of lost protection when a tablet is taken late. However their head offices which are all outside the UK will apparently not accept a reduction to less than 7 days.

2   Secondly, 7 days' extra precautions would, conveniently, be the same duration as in the rule for missed combined pills (see Q 4.16). The 48-hour rule did always seem illogical to women switching from the COC, when the prescriber said it was not quite as effective and kept stressing how much less margin for error her new pill would have!

3 Thirdly, given the fact that considerably more than half of POP-users actually obtain their main contraception by a block to ovulation (those, especially the older women, whose cycles are in the Groups 2, 3 and 4 of Q 5.5 above): 7 days would allow longer for any lost ovarian suppression to be restored. This may or may not be important in some women: there are no data.

In my opinion this new advice is preferable: it is not too demanding, it errs on the side of caution and it is more consistent with the COC. But the confusion caused by any such change is unfortunate, especially as the 2-day advice at Q 5.20 was not shown to cause avoidable pregnancies.

5.23 When should emergency postcoital contraception be considered in addition, if POP tablets are missed?

In my opinion, this decision should be based on *the mucus effect*. Thus this intervention should be offered up to 72 hours after any unprotected intercourse which occurred following the 3 hours delay which might lead to loss of the mucus effect, and before two pills had been taken to restore it (see Q.7.18(f)). Seven days of extra precautions should then follow, as in the basic new advice.

Note: In full lactation the advice at Qs 5.19–23 is too strict – see p 292.

5.24 How long does it take to establish efficacy when starting the POP?

The contraceptive effect on the mucus develops very rapidly (Fig. 5.2). We do not know the minimum time needed to establish the antiovulation or anti-implantation effects. However, with a first day start and hence taking 7–14 pills before it would occur, any POP-induced interference with fertile ovulation ought theoretically to be as great as it will be in later cycles. So no extra precautions are now advised with a first day start and this seems adequate.

5.25 What therefore are the recommended starting routines with the POP?

See Table 5.4 (p. 253), and important footnote.

5.26 What advice should be given to a woman who vomits a tablet and fails to replace it successfully within 3 hours?

She should take extra precautions as well as taking her tablets for the duration of the illness and for 7 days thereafter.

5.27 Should any action be taken if a POP-user requires antibiotic treatment?

Yes if the antibiotic is an enzyme-inducer! This means rifampicin or griseofulvin. Otherwise no action is required since, as explained at Q 5.10, ordinary broad-spectrum antibiotics can have no effects on the blood level of the active exogenous progestagen.

5.28 Should the POP be avoided for women using enzyme-inducing drugs?

Enzyme-inducers do lower progestagen as well as oestrogen blood levels, and the failure rate of the POP would therefore be expected to increase. (The drugs concerned are in Table 4.3, Q 4.31.) Extra precautions should be advised during and for at least 7 days after any short-term treatment (longer after rifampicin, see Q4.37) Long term, a better hormonal option might be an injectable along with a shortened gap between injections (see Q 5.89). If the POP is preferred Professor Orme of Liverpool suggests that the dose be increased to two, three or even up to four POP tablets per day – depending on factors like young age or obesity. Even then the woman should be warned that the efficacy of such a regimen is not well established. And as usual, since this is not supported by the Data Sheets, very careful records are essential.

5.29 Can the small dose of progestagen in the POP influence other drugs?

Since the effect of the COC on other drugs is for most practical purposes negligible (see Q 4.41), the effect of the lower dose in the POP can certainly be disregarded.

ADVANTAGES AND BENEFICIAL SIDE- EFFECTS

5.30 What are the advantages of the POP?

1 *Acceptable efficacy*, in the range of 0.3–5/100 woman-years. Higher efficacy applies in the older women, for whom combined oral contraceptives (COCs) might be contraindicated.

2 *No epidemiological evidence, so far, of increased risk* of either circulatory or malignant disease. Again this not certain because of inadequate study; plus any (good or bad) effects

may very well vary between women because of the variable impact of the POP on the hypothalamo-pituitary-ovarian axis.

3 *Avoidance of all side-effects in which artificial oestrogens are implicated.*

4 *Minimization of any side-effects in which progestagens are implicated.*

5 *Minimal alteration in all metabolic variables* which have been measured (see Qs 5.39–5.46).

6 *Good general tolerance* – especially suitable for women who complain of side-effects with other hormonal methods, or in whom the latter are contraindicated.

7 *Most minor symptoms of the COC are not a problem,* such as weight gain, nausea, headaches and loss of libido.

8 *Return of women's fertility on discontinuation more rapid* than after the COC.

9 The tiny dose means *minimal effect on lactation*, and levels of the artificial steroids within breast milk seem to be negligible.

10 *No harmful effect from overdose*, even when taken by a child.

5.31 Do the beneficial effects listed at Q 4.49 also apply to the POP?

1 Some do – most of the *contraceptive benefits*, for example.

2 Some women report improvement in *symptoms of the menstrual cycle*, notably premenstrual symptoms, mastalgia and dysmenorrhoea. Others report the reverse (see Qs 5.32 and 5.67).

3 Protection against *pelvic infection* is extremely probable, though not yet actually proven for the POP (see Qs 4.52 and 5.91).

4 For the remaining items listed in Q 4.49 there is so far no evidence to suggest that the beneficial effect applies to the POP. Indeed in the case of two of them (extrauterine pregnancies and functional ovarian cysts) the method may even increase the risk.

MAIN PROBLEMS AND DISADVANTAGES

5.32 What are the main problems of the POP?

1 The need for *obsessional regularity in pill taking* (see Q 5.19) and attention to the daily timing thereof. Not suitable for the disorganized.

2 *Alteration of the menstrual pattern* is the main problem, except in breastfeeders. The reasons are explained at Q 5.5. According to that Swedish study one can predict to some extent the type of change that the POP will produce. Women normally having long follicular/short luteal phases were more likely to be in Group 4 on the POP (tending to have episodes of amenorrhoea). Those with regular or short cycles – who had relatively short follicular but long luteal phases – were more likely to enter Group 1 and have somewhat more regular bleeding. In general, the duration and volume of flow may change, and there may be intermenstrual episodes. The latter may necessitate a curettage in some older women – (see Q 5.52(7)). Alternatively the woman may develop amenorrhoea.

All in all cycle irregularity is the commonest reason for abandoning the method. Yet a woman can be told that irregularity means the method is probably more effective in her particular case (see Q 5.6). Another disadvantage therefore is that:

3 Precisely in those women with the most acceptable, regular cycles, the risk of pregnancy is greatest.

4 A small number of women develop symptomatic *functional ovarian cysts* (see Q 5.34), causing pain which may sometimes be severe enough to imitate an ectopic pregnancy.

5 *Pregnancies in POP–users are more likely to be ectopic* than are pregnancies occurring in the general population. As for the IUD (see Qs 6.29 and 6.32), it is not thought that the POP actually increases the risk of ectopics in a population of POP-users; indeed the reverse is probably true.

5.33 What is the risk of ectopic pregnancy? Why do ectopics occur in POP-users?

When compared with sexually active non-pregnant controls studies have shown a *reduced* risk of ectopic pregnancy in POP-users. This is to be expected because the method often interferes with ovulation, and with fertilization. Moreover the effect of the POP on cervical mucus should reduce the risk of tubal damage from pelvic infection.

However in some studies the likelihood of any breakthrough pregnancy which actually happens being ectopic is increased. Possible explanations include the following:

1 A selection effect, exactly as described for the IUD (please see Q 6.30), if there is pre-existing tubal damage and fertilization

occurs. The numerator of ectopics is reduced, but if the denominator of POP 'breakthrough' pregnancies is reduced even more, the *relative* frequency of ectopics among the conceptions will increase.

2 Progestagens do modify tubal function. Overall contractility and the rate of ovum transport are decreased, the latter probably from a reduction in the number of ciliated cells.

Of the two, the first explanation is thought by far the more important. See Q 6.30–2. Ectopics can only happen if normal ovulation occurs, followed by fertilization – i.e. the risk relates only to a subgroup of Group 1 in Q 5.5.

5.34 How frequent are functional ovarian cysts among POP-users?

In a Margaret Pyke Centre (MPC) study, functional ovarian cysts (FOCs) as diagnosed by ultrasound occurred in as many as half the POP-users (12/21), as compared to four out of the 21 controls. Most of these were asymptomatic but seven women – all of them POP-users – complained of some pain; one required admission for rest and analgesia. It is also clinical experience that some POP-users are diagnosed as cases of ectopic pregnancy (menstrual irregularity plus one-sided pain and a tender mass) but laparoscopy shows only a functional cyst, or evidence that one has recently ruptured.

5.35 What is the cause of FOCs?

The precise causation of FOCs remains undefined. It is clearly due to an abnormality of ovulation which is succeeded by accumulation of fluid within the follicle or corpus luteum. On the basis of the groups defined at Q 5.5 one would expect the frequency to be no different from a control population in Group 1, and actually reduced in the group with quiescent ovaries, Group 4. The increased frequency would be expected to manifest itself in Groups 2 and 3, especially 3 (see Q 5.53 for the clinical implications).

5.36 Does the POP affect neoplasia?

Little is known, for the reasons discussed at Qs 4.65 and 5.3. The UK National Case Contral Study (NCCS) (see Q 4.73) found a significant apparent protective association with breast cancer. This needs confirmation.

If there is any real influence of the POP on carcinogenesis it will be subjected to two important considerations:

1 Any effects may be (slightly) beneficial on some cancers, adverse on others (as for the COC, see Q 4.66), and related in each case to duration of use.

2 The effects may be expected to depend in part on the amount of interaction with the woman's menstrual cycle, i.e. her 'Group' in Q 5.5.

For the present one can truthfully state to any woman: 'there is no evidence to suggest that any POP increases the risk of cancer'.

5.37 What effect does the POP have on trophoblastic disease?

See Q 4.69 for a discussion of the reasons why the COC, and also for the time being the POP, should normally not be used until hCG levels are undetectable.

5.38 What is the influence of the POP on benign tumours, such as benign breast disease and fibroids?

There is no evidence that any of the tumours mentioned at Q 4.82 are influenced, either way. The story is again likely to be most complex.

If we take benign breast disease (BBD) or fibroids as examples, the data suggest that progestagens reduce the incidence of both these conditions. So Groups 1, 2 and especially Group 4 (amenorrhoeic) women (see Q 5.5) would be expected to see a benefit. One could hypothesize, however, that the complete opposite would be true of women who are in Group 3, with increased follicular activity and therefore more oestrogenic stimulus to their BBD or fibroids. As so often with the POP, there are no hard data to confirm or refute this hypothesis.

5.39 What are the effects of the POP on metabolism?

Unfortunately, although this has been slightly better studied than the epidemiology, there are few good studies of modern POPs. Moreover, the studies can be faulted on at least one of the following counts:

1 Inadequate attention to confounding variables – meaning that the changes seen might be due to characteristics of the woman for whom a POP was chosen, rather than the POP itself.

2 Lack of attention to the different metabolic responses to be expected, according to whether the users respond to the POP as in the Groups 1,2, 3 or 4 of Q 5.5. Figure 5.1 shows that the

resultant metabolic effects might well vary: from (in Group 1) those of the normal menstrual cycle with normal ovarian oestrogen plus a small effect from the POP, to the situation (Group 4) where the progestagen is unopposed because of abnormally low endogenous oestrogen production. Despite these limitations, the overall findings of the metabolic studies are most reassuring, as discussed in the next questions.

5.40 What are the effects of the POP on coagulation and fibrinolysis?

1 Numerous studies have shown that the POP, unlike COCs, has no important measurable effect on blood clotting, platelet aggregation or fibrinolytic activity.

2 One interesting study looked at prostacyclin and thromboxane levels. Among COC-users prostacyclin levels were decreased (favouring platelet aggregation). There was no change in the POP group, and in the latter, particularly among women using levonorgestrel alone, the thromboxane concentrations were depressed. Since thromboxane enhances platelet aggregation, this could even indicate a decreased risk of thrombosis in POP-users.

5.41 Presumably, the POP may therefore be used by women with a definite past history of thromboembolism, even if COC related?

Yes, definitely (see Q 5.49). But most Data Sheets for POPs still do not say this. The norethisterone products are particularly interesting. 'Primolut N' is norethisterone 5 mg and often used for gynaecological indications such as menorrhagia, in doses up to 15 mg daily. There is no mention of past thrombosis as a contraindication. Yet it is there in the Data Sheets of both Micronor and Noriday – each containing (see Table 5.1) $1/45$ of the daily dose of norethisterone in the Primolut regimens!

5.42 What are the effects on blood lipids, especially high-density lipoprotein-cholesterol (HDL-C)?

The POPs currently available seem to have little effect on all the main aspects of lipid metabolism; but in one or two studies the important subfraction HDL_2-C was slightly depressed with POPs containing either levonorgestrel or norethisterone. *This might be expected to happen less in those POP–users who have more endogenous oestrogen from their own ovaries (Groups 1–3 of Q 5.5)*, and therefore there must be some concern about hypo-oestrogenism in those who are amenorrhoeic, Group 4. What we strongly desire is the marketing of the more 'lipid-friendly' progestagens (see Q 4.136) as POPs: these would be preferable, especially for those women with Cardiovascular risk factors for whom the POP is often chosen (Q 5.49).

5.43 What are the effects on carbohydrate metabolism?

Once again a consensus view is that the effects are minimal. However, some studies have shown that long-term users have a slight deterioration in glucose tolerance and a tendency to hyper-insulinism. It has been suggested that this effect is greater in users of the levonorgestrel POPs than those from the norethisterone group, but this finding has not been confirmed. Some studies cannot exclude the possibility that adverse metabolic findings are the result of selection of the POP by users who are more likely to have them anyway – see the Indications in Q 5.49.

5.44 May the POP be used by frank diabetics?

Certainly – after the diaphragm or sheath the POP is the method of choice. Workers in Edinburgh have found that with 350 µg norethisterone POPs no increase in insulin dosage appeared necessary and there was no change in the incidence and severity of retinopathy. They consider the POP to be an ideal choice from the metabolic point of view. In addition only one pregnancy occurred among 50 women during the period of observation (1050 woman-months) and the woman concerned omitted a number of pills.

Generally diabetics have exceptionally good compliance since they take their pill with each evening dose of insulin.

5.45 Would you use current POPs in a diabetic with evidence of tissue damage, especially arteriopathy?

Usually not – for the reasons alluded to at Qs 5.42, 5.43 and 5.51, though they are not absolutely contraindicated. Here would be another indication for 'lipid-friendly' POPs, e.g. containing gesto-dene or desogestrel.

5.46 Have any other metabolic effects been described?

1 When progestagens are administered alone they have little if any effect on hepatic secretion of plasma proteins – cf. the COC, Q 4.68.

2 Thyroid and pituitary-adrenal function also appear to be unaffected.

3 Progestagens beneficially affect the biochemistry and physiology of cervical mucus (see Q 5.16), thereby probably protecting the user against pelvic infection.

4 They also appear to improve aspects of erythrocyte metabolism in sickle cell anaemia (see Q 5.93).

5.47 So, does the POP affect the risk of circulatory disease?

We lack adequate data. In the Oxford/FPA study there were just two cases of venous thromboembolism and two of stroke in 3303 woman-years of study. Considering the women were in the older age group and in general more likely to have other risk factors for circulatory disease, this seems a highly acceptable incidence. It is also unlikely to have any significant link with the method.

Although we can be sure that the absence of artificial oestrogen does not increase the risk of thrombosis, we cannot be so sure about the effect on arterial disease. However, the marketed POPs have in general no more than a minimal effect on HDL-C (see Q 5.41) and appear not to affect blood pressure (see Q 5.48 below).

5.48 Does the POP affect blood pressure?

Apparently not: studies have shown *neither* the slight rise in systolic and diastolic pressure which occurs in almost all individuals given oestrogen-containing preparations, *nor* any increase in the incidence of clinical hypertension. *COC-induced hypertension reverts to normal on the POP*. The same appears to apply to DMPA and other oestrogen-free methods in this chapter. *Progestagens appear adversely to affect blood pressure only if oestrogens are also administered.*

In a POP-user another cause (notably essential hypertension) should be sought if hypertension is diagnosed.

SELECTION OF USERS AND OF FORMULATIONS

5.49 For whom is the POP method particularly indicated?

As a working rule: *Contraindications to or side-effects with the COC, and a hormonal method is preferred? Try the POP.* Or, more specifically:

1 *Women above 35 who smoke cigarettes* (healthy non-smokers, usually, might just as well continue to take an appropriate COC, see Q 4.232). At present use of the POP can be continued until the menopause. However, there is a small question mark about minimal atherogenesis due to the unopposed artificial progestagen, especially during prolonged amenorrhoea (see Qs 5.39, 5.42 and 5.43).

2 *Oestrogen-linked contraindications or side-effects on the COC.* Some of those listed on the left of Table 4.14 may improve. The POP should not be chosen preferentially for conditions such as endometriosis, since it does not reliably suppress endogenous oestrogen. But the main point is that this category also includes:

3 *History of or any predisposition to thromboembolism, including known prothrombotic coagulation factor changes*: since adverse effects on clotting mechanisms have not been demonstrated (see Q 5.40). It follows, accordingly:

4 *Chronic systemic diseases* in which oestrogen is the hormone which might exacerbate the condition (e.g. systemic lupus erythematosis (SLE)) or where there is an extra thrombosis risk (e.g. some severe cases of *Crohn's*, (Q 4.112) and, again *SLE* (Q 4.113). *Sickle cell disease* is another example . But, see Q 5.93, DMPA may be an even better option.

5 Patients with *diabetes* or *obesity*. Diabetics do particularly well on the POP, especially with regard to compliance (see Q 5.44). *There are efficacy considerations for the obese (see Q 5.13–5).*

6 Patients with *hypertension*, either related to the COC *or* other varieties if well controlled by treatment.

7 Patients with *migraine* (including, with appropriate caution and advice, young women with migraines which are severe, focal, or have begun for the first time on the COC). See Qs 4.124–8.

8 During *lactation* (see Qs 5.54 and 5.55). This is a well-established indication, in which the method has the highest efficacy.

9 At the *woman's choice*. This might apply to a young reliable pill-taker who prefers a hormonal method, yet wishes to use the least possible amount of exogenous hormone.

5.50 What are the contraindications to the POP?

A long list of conditions contraindicating use of POPs may be found in the manufacturers' data sheets, but most are there for medicolegal reasons, with no epidemiological basis.

In general and with the exceptions suggested below, *the absolute contraindications to the COC are only relative contraindications* (of varying importance). Moreover (see Q 4.102) any list of contraindications must be to some extent a matter of personal judgement, and, with the POP, also informed guesswork – bearing in mind the dearth of data.

5.51 What then are the absolute contraindications to the POP, in your view?

So far as possible these are listed in the same order as for the COC (see Q 4.101).

1 *Past severe arterial disease, or current exceptionally high risk of the same.* Pending further information I would not prescribe the POP long term to a woman known to have current ischaemic heart disease including angina or to have already suffered a thrombotic stroke; nor to women with marked and multiple risk factors (e.g. a 45-year-old heavy smoking hypertensive diabetic!) – or if so one would discontinue the method if they became amenorrhoeic (see Qs 5.42 and 5.65)

   Severe hereditary lipid abnormalities with a poor prognosis come into this category because of 'exceptionally high risk'. However the POP may be prescribed with extra counselling and supervision in the presence of milder abnormalities with a good prognosis (see Q 5.52). All this caution could probably cease if only there were a 'lipid-friendly' POP! (see Q 4.136).

2 Any *serious side–effect occurring on the COC and not clearly due only to oestrogen* – or associated with past progestagen-only use. Liver adenoma and severe past steroid-associated cholestatic jaundice would come here since it is not clear with which of the two hormones in the COC they are primarily linked. Also in this category:

3 *Recent trophoblastic disease* (see Q 4.69).
   As for all medical methods, we must add:

4 *Undiagnosed abnormal genital tract bleeding* since the POP will confuse diagnosis.

5 Actual or possible *pregnancy*.

6 The woman's own continuing uncertainty about POP safety, even after full counselling.

Contraindication (almost absolute, or 'strong relative') which is specific to the POP among pills:

7 Previous *ectopic pregnancy* (see Q 5.33), especially in a nulliparous woman. Her one precious remaining tube deserves maximum protection (e.g. by the COC), plus ectopics are life-endangering. However for an informed multiparous woman aged 35 this history might well be only a relative contraindication. Hence I have placed it in this intermediate category.

5.52 What are only relative contraindications to the POP, in your view? (i.e. it may certainly be used, but with caution and sometimes special monitoring).

Here there is much obvious overlap with Q 5.49.

1 *Risk factors for arterial disease.* This category includes established hypertension once it has been diagnosed and controlled and also focal migraine (see Qs 4.124–30). The presence of more than one risk factor can be tolerated more readily than with the COC – but with the presently available POPs there are limits (see Q 5.51, section (1)). Prothrombotic coagulation factor abnormalities are actually included above as 'indications', since they should not be worsened at all by the POP. Likewise, there is not the oestrogen-related concern about thrombotic stroke in migraine, including focal migraine – though it may be affected (see Q 4.129).

Lipid abnormalities might be slightly worsened by the POP, especially in Group 4 (see Q 5.5) amenorrhoeic women: however I still consider that if they have a good prognosis they are only a reason for caution. Hence mild elevation of cholesterol to above 7.5 mmol/l, which is an absolute contraindication to the COC, would only relatively contraindicate the POP.

2 *Sex–steroid–dependent cancer.* Seek the advice of the oncologist looking after your patient, particularly for breast cancer. As mentioned at Q 5.36, POP use was less commonly reported in women with breast cancer under age 36 than among controls. There is also no evidence that the POP affects the prognosis after breast cancer is diagnosed. Caution should still be exercised and the final decision should be the woman's own after counselling.

3 *Current liver disorders* with persistent biochemical change.

4 *Relevant interacting drugs.* These are rather strong relative contraindications since the progestagen dose of the POP is already so low; but the dose can be increased in selected cases (see Q 5.28). Caution is also necessary in *severe* malabsorption states (though available studies actually show surprisingly good absorption of the artificial sex steroids, see Q 4.43–4).

5 *Chronic systemic diseases* (see Q 5.49 for important examples). The same comments as at Q 4.105 for the COC apply. The POP has the slight disadvantage of lesser efficacy, balanced by the likelihood that if hormones were one day shown to aggravate the particular systemic disease, the tiny dose in the POP ought to have less effect than the COC.

Relative contraindications specific to the POP among pills:

6 *Functional ovarian cysts* (FOCs). These are definitely associated with the POP (see Qs 5.34 and 5.53). A past history of hospitalization for severe pain resulting in this diagnosis would be a strong relative contraindication, whether occurring before or during use of the POP. However, some women may prefer to continue using the method, since most episodes of FOC formation will be practically asymptomatic.

7 *Unacceptability of irregular menstrual bleeding,* and arguably at the climacteric because such bleeding might cause a diagnostic problem (relating to endometrial carcinoma).

8 Where *complete protection against pregnancy is vital,* especially if the woman is likely to be at all erratic as a pill-taker. In my view the method is therefore *minimally* contraindicated for *teenagers* in general: chiefly because of its innately higher failure rate at this age (see Q 5.12) which may be increased by compliance problems. But the POP or one of the other progestagen-only methods would certainly be preferable to most IUDs if STD infection is a concern (Qs 4.52 and 5.46).

5.53 What are the clinical implications of an increased rate of FOCs?

1 In the past, before this problem was identified, a proportion of POP-users with FOCs must have been experiencing mild unilateral pain which they managed to control with simple analgesics. When reported, the prescriber has doubtless ex-

plained it as ovulation pain. (But ultrasound studies suggest that most FOCs are asymptomatic – see Q 5.34.)

2 It is likely that hormone production by functional cysts may explain some of the menstrual irregularity. For example, in half of the Group 3 women in the Swedish study (see Q 5.5) a high oestradiol followed by an abrupt fall was associated with a withdrawal bleed 72 hours later. This could well have been due to disappearance of a cyst.

3 The main risks of FOCs are those of unnecessary surgery, especially laparoscopy, and also some necessary surgery for acute events such as ovarian torsion. This is why the past history of *symptomatic* FOCs, either before use of the POP or while taking it, should now be considered a fairly strong relative contraindication.

In my experience, however, some women so much prefer this method to the alternatives that they are prepared to take the risk of recurrences. They should be advised to take prompt medical advice as indicated. In spite of the problem of distinguishing this syndrome from ectopic pregnancy, every effort should be made to avoid unnecessary laparoscopies or other surgery. This is where pelvic ultrasound and the ultrasensitive pregnancy tests which are becoming available for routine use can often be of the greatest value.

5.54 What are the effects of the POP on lactation?

The COC can reduce the volume and alter the constitution of milk. Some of the artificial steroids are transferred to the infant. By contrast the POP appears a suitable choice for lactating women. Indeed progestagens when administered alone, by any of the means discussed in this chapter, appear to reduce neither the volume of milk nor the duration of lactation, and some reports suggest that both may be increased. Careful studies on both norethisterone- and levonorgestrel-containing POPs show that the amount transferred to the milk is minute and most unlikely to present any hazard. Studies of the blood of suckling infants have been unable to demonstrate any progestagen, since the concentration is below the limits of the sensitivity of present assays.

Last, but not least, the contraceptive combination of lactation plus the POP is nearly 100% effective. See postscript, p. 292.

5.55 What are the implications for prescribing the POP during lactation?

1 First and foremost, the above findings need discussion. The prospective user may be interested to learn that, according to Scandinavian studies of 30-μg levonorgestrel POPs, after 2 years of lactation with regular POP taking the infant will have received at most the equivalent of one tablet! If this is not sufficiently reassuring, of course, another method should be adopted.

2 Another advantage is that the main symptom with the POP – irregular bleeding – is unlikely during lactational amenorrhoea, except when it is first commenced postpartum (see Q 5.56).

5.56 When should the POP be commenced after delivery?

1 Since, unlike the COC, the POP does not affect lactation nor the risk of venous thrombosis, it is medically safe to start it in the immediate postpartum period. However:

2 Studies have shown a greater likelihood of spotting and bleeding problems with starting early in the puerperium. So unless there are special reasons to start earlier, the fourth week (i.e. from around day 21, later if adequate alternative contraception) is usually chosen (Table 5.4), as with the COC.

5.57 How should weaning be managed in POP users?

Some women simply continue using the POP long term. However if greater efficacy is desired, when only a few feeds are being given

Table 5.4 Starting routines with the POP

	Start when?	Extra precautions?
Menstruating	1st or 2nd day of period	No
Postpartum		
(a) No lactation*	Day 21 (see Q 8.21)†	No
(b) Lactation*	About 4 weeks after delivery	No
Induced abortion/miscarriage	Same day or next day	No
Post COC	Instant switch	No

* Bleeding irregularities minimized by starting at or after the 4th week.
† See Q 8.21 re starting artificial hormones later on during postpartum amenorrhoea.
  Provided there is certainty that there is no chance of an early pregnancy, can start POP (or COC) any time plus 7 days, extra precautions.

in each 24 hours the COC can simply be started on the first day of any chosen menstrual bleed. The dose in the breast milk is not believed to have any relevance to the health of the baby, but the COC may hasten the end of lactation.

5.58 Which POP should be chosen?

After consideration of the contraindications (see Qs 5.51 and 5.52), there are few guidelines. Neogest is best avoided since it gives a useless dose of non-contraceptive dextro-norgestrel (see Q 4.135). Microval and Norgeston are possibly preferable to the other POPs during lactation since such a negligible amount reaches the breast milk (see Q 5.78).

No study has shown statistically different rates of effectiveness between the levonorgestrel POPs (Microval, Norgeston, Neogest) and the norethisterone group (Micronor, Noriday and Femulen). A 'best buy' can also not be stated for menstrual disturbance or any other minor side-effects. The initial choice of POP for cycling women is therefore arbitrary.

INITIAL MANAGEMENT AND FOLLOW-UP ARRANGEMENTS

5.59 What are the main aspects to convey during counselling?

The truth of the phrase 'forewarned is forearmed' is never so clear as in counselling about the unpredictable bleeding pattern of the POP (as indeed for all the oestrogen-free methods in this chapter). Its good efficacy, second only to the combined pill and injectables, especially in older women, should also be stressed – provided always that the rules for successful pill taking are followed (see Qs 5.19–5.28). As for other methods, a supplementary leaflet (e.g. that produced by the FPA) should always be supplied.

5.60 How should POP use be monitored?

POP monitoring should be much as for the COC (see Qs 4.165–6), but almost all users can be put into the 'safer' category 1.

1 A baseline blood pressure and weight are valuable.

2 Routine regular breast and cervical smear examinations are good screening practice, though not here believed to have any special relevance to the contraceptive method.

3 The woman should be seen 3 months after starting the POP and normally 6 monthly thereafter – but the interval may be extended, and all checks performed by the family-planning trained nurse, with recourse to a doctor only if problems arise, such as pelvic pain.

4 Otherwise routine examinations should be kept to a minimum. Blood pressure may be recorded annually, once 6-monthly checks have been entirely normal, and weight only needs to be measured against the baseline reading if the woman records an important change.

5.61 For how long may POP use be continued?

At present the answer is 'indefinitely' (until the menopause), in the absence of contraindications, multiple-risk factors, or the occurrence of important complications; but see Q 5.49 (1).

5.62 How can the menopause be diagnosed in older POP-users?

If a POP-user above the age of 45 develops prolonged amenorrhoea, yet was previously observing bleeding episodes, it can be difficult to distinguish between amenorrhoea secondary to the POP and the onset of the menopause.

1 Symptoms, especially hot flushes, can be a useful guide.

2 There is also evidence that a high level of follicle stimulating hormone (FSH) can be meaningful at the menopause despite continued POP-taking. Low levels, on the other hand, suggest that the woman is in Group 4 of Q 5.5, still potentially fertile, and should continue to use this or some alternative contraceptive method.

5.63 How do you act if the FSH is high in an older POP-user? Is there a practical protocol?

If the FSH is at menopause levels, my practice is to suggest that the woman discontinues the POP and transfers to a simple barrier method. The FSH is then repeated at 1 month, on two occasions if there is any doubt. If the woman is still amenorrhoeic, has vasomotor symptoms, and menopausal FSH results are again obtained, she may be advised that her chances of conception are low enough to discontinue alternative contraception – whether or not she now transfers to taking hormone replacement therapy (HRT). No guarantee of total infertility can be given, however, and she is warned to return for advice should she develop any subsequent (non-HRT-related) bleeding. And women who want more complete reassurance should continue a simple method of birth control until 1 year after the last spontaneous bleed.

5.64 What if FSH measurements are not available?

The advice should then be as usual for the diagnosis of the menopause: namely to discontinue hormonal contraception and use an alternative for at least 1 year of complete amenorrhoea, or for 2 years in women under 50 (but see Q 8.34).

5.65 Should I be concerned about hypo-oestrogenism in any POP-user who develops prolonged amenorrhoea, even when not related to the menopause?

This is a difficult one: there are no good data. *But* if you look again at Q 4.58, there has to be the possibility that women in Group 4 at Q 5.5, with quiescent ovaries and low plasma oestradiols, will be at increased risk eventually both of osteoporosis and of arterial disease associated with low HDL-C levels (see Q 5.42). Both those conditions will be exacerbated by heavy cigarette smoking, which has known adverse effects on plasma oestrogens and (separately) on the risk of arterial disease.

Arbitrarily, pending more data, I am currently suggesting that after 5 years' POP amenorrhoea, smokers (particularly) should have plasma oestradiols and a bone scan if this can be arranged. If the oestradiols are less than 100 pmol/l or the scan shows significant osteoporosis, either another contraceptive method should be chosen or there could be consideration of 'add-back' natural oestrogen by any chosen route. If the tests are not available, for women without oestrogen deficiency symptoms, present data are far too scanty to ban the option of continuing with POP (Q 5.100–1).

MANAGEMENT OF SIDE-EFFECTS OR COMPLICATIONS

5.66 What should be the second choice of POP if bleeding problems develop and cannot be tolerated?

1 First: examine the patient – for a coincidental gynaecological cause. (See Table 4.12 and Q 4.148!)

2 An understanding of the spectrum of individual reactions to the POP is of some help (see Qs 5.5 and 5.6). It would appear that the bleeding problems are concentrated in Groups 2 and 3. Group 1 cycles are generally the most acceptable. With good counselling, women in Group 4 can also accept their long episodes of amenorrhoea (but see Q 5.65). Careful assessment of the bleeding pattern therefore aids decision-making.

3 If it appears that a reduction in dose might transfer a woman from Group 2/3 to Group 1, one could for example switch from Femulen to Micronor/Noriday.

4 The reverse could be tried if reaching Group 4 seemed likely to be achieved thereby, i.e. a trial of Femulen, the strongest POP available. But this could be counterproductive, making the bleeding irregularity worse, if amenorrhoea did not result.

5 Switching between the levonorgestrel and norethisterone group POPs may be useful, but has to be empirical since their precise equivalence has not been worked out.

5.67 What minor side-effects have been described in POP-takers?

The short answer is that POP-users report almost any of the minor side-effects reported by COC-takers, but in general less frequently. In the Oxford/FPA study, headaches, psychological disturbance and hypertension were particularly associated with COCs as a cause of discontinuation of the method. However, menstrual disturbance and, interestingly, breast discomfort, were reported more commonly among POP-users. Mildly androgenic effects such as acne also occur.

5.68 Which second choice of POP should follow if non-bleeding minor side-effects develop?

The decision to change to a different POP has again to be empirical. For example, if headaches occur on a levonorgestrel POP, it may be worth transferring to one of the norethisterone group.

With support and reassurance, however, the subjective symptoms often disappear after a few months of continuing to take the same POP.

5.69 What action should be taken if a POP-user complains of low abdominal pain?

As usual, causes unrelated to contraception should first be excluded. But two particular possibilities must be borne in mind, especially as both also cause menstrual irregularity and perhaps a unilateral mass:

1 Ectopic pregnancy.

2 Pain due to the formation/torsion or rupture of a functional ovarian cyst. Referral for ultrasound and possible laparoscopy may be required. See Q 5.53.

5.70 Which symptoms should lead a POP-user to take urgent medical advice? Should she transfer to another method at once?

Abdominal pain is probably the only acute symptom with that implication among users of this method (see Qs 5.33 and 5.34). Neither for this, nor for any of the other symptoms in the COC list at Q 4.176 (which are mostly irrelevant as they relate to oestrogen), should the woman discontinue the POP instantly without first arranging another method. Continuing to take the POP for a few more days can do no significant harm – whereas an unplanned pregnancy might.

5.71 What should be done if a POP-user is immobilized after an accident or requires emergency major surgery?

There is no reason for a woman using any oestrogen-free preparation to discontinue the method in either of these clinical contexts.

5.72 What are the risks if a woman should become pregnant while taking the POP?

1 The main risk would be ectopic pregnancy (see Q 5.33).

2 The available findings concerning teratogenesis are extremely reassuring. No cases of congenital abnormality have been reported, though there have been no good large studies. In the Oxford/FPA study there were 30 accidental pregnancies in continuing POP-users. Of these seven were terminated, 15 ended in normal live births without any malformations, one was ectopic and a surprisingly high number (seven) ended in a spontaneous miscarriage. (This last observation has not been reported in other studies, so the researchers feel it can reasonably be ascribed to chance.)

See also Q 4.205 – the usual 'armchair thinking' about the POP would lead one to expect an even lower rate of fetal abnormalities in breakthrough POP pregnancies than with the COC – and the latter rate is already known to be remarkably low.

There is certainly no need to advise switching from the POP to another method for any arbitrary time before a planned conception (very debatably necessary even for the COC, see Q 4.207).

5.73 Are there any risks or benefits for ex-takers of the POP?

There are no data to support or refute any such ex-use effects. If they exist at all they are likely to be clinically insignificant.

QUESTIONS ASKED BY USERS ABOUT THE POP

The general public does not ask many questions about the POP, since few know of its existence as a separate method. Much confusion between these 'mini-pills' and low-dose combined pills has to be cleared up. The majority of questions by individual users are the same as those already answered, above. However, the following short list may be instructive.

5.74 Does the POP ever cause an abortion?

No. Although not its usual method of action, one possible way the POP operates on some occasions is by stopping implantation: the process by which a dividing fertilized egg becomes embedded in a lining of the womb. Stopping this is not now felt by most people to be causing an abortion, for the reasons explained at Qs 7.2 and 7.3. But the POP rarely if ever works this way, anyway.

Reading the question a different way, taking a large number of POPs (or combined pills for that matter) is most unlikely to stop a fully established implanted pregnancy.

5.75 If the POP is not so effective as the combined pill, why are some women recommended to use it?

Taken regularly, this method is only a little less effective than the combined pill, especially in women above the age of 35. Indeed above the age of 40 it is effective as the COC would be for a 25 year old. Otherwise the POP is chosen chiefly because of some medical reasons for not using the COC, which is certainly the normal first choice.

5.76 My period is overdue on the POP – what does this mean?

First, we must exclude the possibility that the method has let you down. Once that has been done, the most likely explanation is that the pill is preventing egg release. So paradoxically you will be more effectively protected from pregnancy than a girlfriend who is seeing regular periods on this pill (see Q 5.7).

5.77 I know that COC users do not see proper periods – is that also true of the bleeds I get on the POP?

On the POP, some episodes of bleeding are caused like normal periods. In these the special structure in your ovary known as a corpus luteum stops producing the two hormones which stimulate growth of the uterine lining, and this leads to it coming away, and hence a period. However, many POP-users have other bleeding or spotting episodes as well. These are either shorter or longer than a normal period and can be lighter or heavier. They are caused by irregular shedding of the womb lining, in turn caused by combined effects from the artificial hormone of the POP and the oestrogen and progesterone produced by your ovary (see Qs 5.4–5.6 and Fig. 5.1).

5.78 I am breastfeeding my baby and have been given the POP – won't this harm my baby?

Although a very tiny amount of the hormone does get into the breast milk, it has not been possible to show any changes in its quantity or in its quality. The amount taken by the baby is very small; for example with Microval or Norgeston your baby will take only the equivalent of one tablet if you continue to breastfeed for 2 years! In short, there are no reasons for believing that your baby will be harmed (see Qs 5.54 and 5.55).

However, there is no absolute proof that the POP would be completely harmless, and if you are unhappy it would be important to discuss another method with your family doctor or a local clinic.

BACKGROUND AND MECHANISMS

5.79   What are injectables?

The two available in the UK are progestagenic steroids given on a regular basis by deep intramuscular injection for contraception. Experience with them dates back to the early 1960s. DMPA (see below) has been used by over 15 million women world-wide, and it is licensed for contraceptive use in more than 90 countries.

5.80   What injectables are available in the UK?

1   Depot medroxyprogesterone acetate (DMPA). This is available in aqueous microcrystalline suspension and is normally given in a dose of 150 mg every 12 weeks. Other regimens have also been tried and proved effective.

2   Norethisterone oenanthate (NET EN, Noristerat, Norigest). This is available in a vehicle of benzyl benzoate and castor oil, the dose being 200 mg every 8 weeks. Other regimens are not now recommended.

Note: DMPA is an example of a pregnane progestagen, which appears to have more benign metabolic effects than either oestrane progestagens such as norethisterone or gonanes such as levonorgestrel – all derived from 19-nortestosterone.

5.81   What is the status and availability of injectables worldwide and in the UK?

DMPA has been repeatedly endorsed by the WHO and the International Planned Parenthood Federation (IPPF). It is currently available for long-term use in more than 90 countries, including the UK, Sweden, Germany, Denmark, the Netherlands and New Zealand. It has been repeatedly recommended for similar licensing by the obstetrical and gynaecological subcommittee of the USA

Food and Drug Administration (FDA), and finally received approval at the end of 1992. It is currently used by about 10 million women worldwide.

In the UK the Minister of Health finally agreed in 1984 to the earlier recommendation by the Committee on the Safety of Medicines (CSM) that the method could be used long-term for contraception by selected women after full counselling. It is currently used by a very small minority, less than 1% of women practising birth control in the UK. However, this is mostly because the option is offered so infrequently: most of those who do use it are very satisfied customers!

NET EN. This is less widely used, chiefly in Germany and a number of developing countries. It is now available in the UK, a product licence for antifertility use having been granted. Although it is only officially for short-term use at present, longer-term use is acceptable in selected patients after counselling.

5.82 What is the mode of action of injectables?

The primary action of the (relatively high) progestagen dose given by both injectables is to prevent ovulation. As with other hormonal methods, this is supplemented chiefly by contraceptive actions at the endometrial and mucus level. (See Q 5.4 and Table 5.2.)

5.83 Do injectables provide a steady dose?

No – see Figure 5.3. Although the levels fluctuate far less than any oral method (COC or POP), there is a much higher level initially, declining exponentially thereafter. This is one of the advantages of newer injectables, and also rings and implants (see below); in that all the latter release the hormone at a relatively constant or so-called zero-order rate.

5.84 What is known about individual variation in blood levels?

This exists, as for the oral methods. However, the variation is rather less marked since variable absorption from the gut and variable 'first-pass' metabolism (see Qs 4.30 and 4.31) are not involved. Blood levels seem to decline more rapidly in thin women (see Q 5.87). NET EN has a shorter duration of action than DMPA.

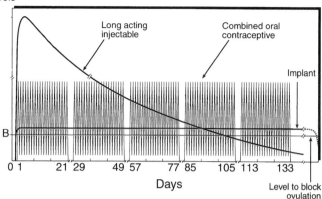

Figure 5.3 Blood levels of progestagen hormone in users of three delivery systems. Q 5.83.

This is a schematic representation for DMPA. After an injection there is a very high level – B indicates the level to block ovulation – then a decline as time passes. Oral contraceptives (the POP would be similar, without a 7-day break) show wide fluctuations – a sawtooth pattern. Implants lead to remarkably constant blood levels. (Adapted from Population Reports K2 May 1983 Population information program. John Hopkins University, Baltimore, Figure I)

5.85 What effects do injectables have on ovarian function?

Since ovulation is generally inhibited, the 'spectrum effect' described at Q 5.5 for the POP is much less marked with these agents. However follicular activity occurs, especially towards the end of the injection period and more in some women than others. This has not been as well studied as with the POP, but it means similarly that observed menstrual and other side-effects must be the *resultant* of effects of the exogenous and endogenous steroid hormones on the end-organs. More importantly, follicular oestradiol keeps serum concentrations in the range normally found in the early to middle follicular phase (90–290 pmol/l). This prevents clinical hypo-oestrogenism (whether as symptoms or signs) in the vast majority of users, but there is some concern at present about those with prolonged amenorrhoea and abnormally low oestradiol levels (see Qs 5.97, 5.100).

5.86 What is the overall effectiveness of injectables?

Among available reversible contraceptives the use-effectiveness of these methods is greater than the COC – since the factor of the user's memory is almost eliminated. The range of efficacy quoted for DMPA is 0–1/100 woman-years, and for NET EN 0.4–2/100 woman-years.

5.87 What factors influence the effectiveness of injectables?

As usual, the rate of failure is marginally higher in younger, more fertile women; and also paradoxically in women who are under-weight, especially in developing countries.

With NET EN it is essential not to massage the injection site (see Q 5.118) since this shortens the duration of action; this increased the pregnancy rate in early studies.

5.88 What are the recommended starting routines for injectables?

1 In menstruating women the first injection should be given before day 5 of the cycle. With either drug the contraceptive effect is said to be immediate. Yet, because of the analogy with the COC (Table 4.4), I advise extra precautions for 7 days if the first dose is later than day 2. Non-pregnant women on the POP or COC, can be given any time.

2 Postpartum (whether or not the woman is breastfeeding). It is now clear that the first injection should preferably be postponed until 5–6 weeks after the delivery. Earlier administration increases the likelihood of heavy and prolonged bleeding. However this is not inevitable and clinical judgement can be used if there is doubt whether the woman will return at the right time for her first dose. She must then be forewarned about the increased bleeding risk. Lactation is not inhibited.

3 Postmiscarriage or termination of pregnancy (first trimester). The injection is normally given within 7 days of the procedure and no extra precautions are required. After a late (second trimester) abortion some further delay may be recommended to reduce the risk of heavy and prolonged bleeding, similar to that just mentioned in item 2 above.

5.89 Do interactions with other drugs pose any problem with injectables?

1 There is certainly no problem with non-enzyme-inducing antibiotics, since the drug does not have to be absorbed from the gut.

2 Drugs inducing liver enzymes (see Q 4.33) pose a theoretical problem, particularly in the time just before the next injection is given (Fig. 5.3). It is recommended that the interval between injections is shortened to 10 weeks for DMPA; or even to 8 weeks in the more high risk situations, e.g. when the potent enzyme-inducer rifampicin is used.

Actually, in the developing world DMPA is used successfully for contraception during rifampicin treatment for tuberculosis and there are very few reports of breakthrough pregnancy occurring (even without this sensible policy of shortening of the injection interval).

5.90 Might injectables affect the action of other drugs?

In clinical practice this possibility can seemingly be disregarded.

ADVANTAGES AND BENEFITS

5.91 What are the beneficial effects of injectables?

These can be listed as follows:

Contraceptive benefits

1 *High effectiveness* – definitely greater than the COC (see Q 5.86). Freedom from 'fear of forgetting' – a problem with all pill methods.

2 Highly *convenient*, non-intercourse-related.

3 *Reversible* (though with some delay).

Non-contraceptive benefits

Most of those at Q 4.49 are believed to apply.

4 In many women there is a reduction in the disorders of the menstrual cycle:
  (a) *less heavy bleeding*, often culminating in amenorrhoea (which can be a health benefit in reducing the risk of

gynaecological disorders as listed at Q 4.50, but may have its own unproven problems as well Q 5.100);

(b) *less anaemia* – indeed the haemoglobin has been noted to rise regardless of the bleeding pattern, suggesting a direct haemopoietic effect;

(c) *less dysmenorrhoea;*

(d) *less symptoms of premenstrual tension* (not invariably);

(e) *no ovulation pain.*

Note: These improvements are variable, and dependent on the bleeding pattern experienced by individual women.

---

5 *Less pelvic inflammatory disease* (PID) – as for all progestagen-containing contraceptives (see Q 4.52). Confirmed by a WHO study (1985).

6 *Less extrauterine pregnancies* since ovulation is inhibited.

7 Possibly *less functional ovarian cysts* overall, for the same reason (see Q 4.53) – but this has not been well studied.

8 A possible reduction in the rate of *endometriosis*, which indeed can be treated by these agents.

9 Overdose extremely unlikely and would not be fatal.

10 *Beneficial social effects,* especially because the method is under a woman's control.

11 *Protection* against *endometrial cancer* (see Q 5.105).

It is not known how many of the other benefits described for the COC (Q 4.49) apply also to injectables, namely a reduction in risk of benign breast disease, fibroids, thyroid disease, toxic shock syndrome, *Trichomonas vaginitis* and ovarian cancer. But on theoretical grounds most are likely benefits, only waiting to be firmly established.

Benefits not (necessarily) shared with the COC

12 Beneficial effects on frank *sickle cell disease* (see Q 5.93).

13 *Aggression, mood swings and epileptic attacks*: especially in mentally handicapped patients, DMPA is reported as very beneficial if the timing of these problems is regularly premenstrual or menstrual. 'Tricycling' of the COC may be a way of obtaining a similar benefit (see Q 4.28).

14 *Lactation* is not suppressed, may even be enhanced due to increased production of prolactin – but POP appears even better, see Q 5.114.

15 Complete *freedom from side-effects due to oestrogen.*

5.92 In view of the above advantages, why has there been so much adverse publicity about injectables?

Mainly because of:

1 Unfounded excessive anxiety about *cancer* (the balance of the evidence is favourable! Q 5.105);

2 The possibility of *abuse* (by providers, 'pushing' the method on women or, worse, giving it without their knowledge or consent). This is a potential problem with any injection but one that is not best solved by banning a good product.

3 If side-effects occur, the impossibility of removing the injection once it has been given.

Yet overall safety is clearly greater than the COC. Indeed there have been no deaths proven to be caused by either injectable. Wherever it has been made available as a realistic choice, the fact that continuation rates are better than for most other methods refutes the view that patients are frequently forced to have it against their will.

5.93 What is the effect of DMPA on homozygous sickle cell disease?

A careful trial in the West Indies demonstrated a highly significant improvement in the haematological picture, and a reduction in the number of painful crises, in patients treated with 3-monthly injections of DMPA. It is suggested that this may be the method of choice both in SS and SC disease.

There are theoretical reasons for believing that all progestagen-containing contraceptives would be similarly beneficial, including the POP (see Q 5.46), NET EN, Norplant (see Q 5.147) and even perhaps the COC – though with the last the artificial oestrogen content has its own disadvantages (see Q 4.108).

MAIN PROBLEMS AND DISADVANTAGES

5.94 What are the main disadvantages of injectables?

1 First and foremost, the fact that *the injection cannot be removed once given*. This means that the method is irreversible for at

least 2–3 months (depending on the injectable used), and early side-effects would therefore have to be tolerated for a long time.

2 *Disturbance of menstruation* is so marked and variable, both between patients and within the same woman over time, that it has been called 'menstrual chaos'. With reassuring counselling *amenorrhoea* is usually very acceptable (see Q 5.117); however:

3 Possible, as yet unconfirmed, *loss of bone density* in users with long-term amenorrhoea (see Q 5.100). Other manifestations of *hypo–oestrogenism* including apparently adverse lipid effects are also possible (see Qs 5.85, 5.97, 5.111 and 5.112).

4 *Delay in the return, but no loss, of fertility* (see Q 5.113).

5 *Weight gain*. Most women gain weight, up to 2 kg (4.5 lb) in the first year, and a few do so very rapidly after the very first dose. This possibility must be discussed with users in advance. Women who are already overweight seem less likely to gain much weight than do thin women. The increase is thought to be due to increased appetite plus possibly an anabolic effect. It is not associated with fluid retention and diuretics are useless.

6 Possible *adverse effects on the fetus* (see Q 5.129).

7 *Galactorrhoea* may occur, with a raised prolactin (usually within the normal range).

8 *Mildly androgenic effects* such as acne are surprisingly uncommon.

9 *Enuresis* may recur in women who were enuretic at adolescence. This is believed to be caused by a relaxing effect of the progestagens on smooth muscle.

10 *Subjective effects*. These are many and varied – as with all hormonal methods. It is difficult to know how many are truly attributable to the method and how many to placebo reactions. The following have been reported:
   (a) lassitude;
   (b) depression (see Q 5.124)
   (c) loss of libido, vaginal dryness (relatively rare, but see Qs 5.100 and 5.101);
   (d) bloatedness;
   (e) dizziness;
   (f) breast symptoms (increase in size and tenderness);

(g) leg cramps;

(h) headaches.

5.95 What are the effects of injectables on metabolism?

Although many studies have been reported (particularly on DMPA) they tend to be poorly controlled especially for cigarette smoking, and may not allow adequately for the time since the last injection was given, individual variation, the presence or absence of ovarian activity, and so on. Endogenous oestrogen has a vital part to play in most women, more than with the COC, particularly in the last half of the time of effectiveness of each injection. However, neither ovulation nor functional cyst formation are common, and overall there is less individual variation between women in the amount of ovarian activity than with the POP (see Q 5.5).

5.96 What are the effects on blood coagulation and fibrinolysis?

To summarize much research, there is no effect of any significance on either of these, and DMPA and NET EN may certainly be used where there is a past history of venous thromboembolism.

5.97 What are the effects on blood lipids, especially HDL-C?

Available data about blood lipids are scanty and difficult to interpret. Most researchers have reassuringly found no effect or even a decrease in triglycerides or total cholesterol with both injectables. A few studies show a decrease (10–15%) in HDL-C levels with DMPA. In a prospective study of NET EN, HDL-C declined more markedly, by about 25% after the first injection, but did not change further with up to 4 years of use. These results may at least partly be related to the lower endogenous oestradiol production in users of injectables, and their relation to amenorrhoea and the overall clinical significance are not clear (see Q 5.102, and, *re* contraindications, Qs 5.110 and 5.112).

5.98 What are the effects on carbohydrate metabolism?

Some reports find an increase in insulin levels with both these injectables, but most report no change. The development of overt diabetes in women using DMPA for contraception has not been reported, and WHO does not consider this a contraindication to the method.

5.99 Are there any other metabolic effects?

Injectables do not appear adversely to affect liver function. Injectables can be used safely by women with a history of jaundice or current liver disease, including hepatitis B infection. Only minimal effects have been shown on plasma protein and vitamin metabolism.

5.100 What is the present information about a possible osteoporosis risk with injectables, especially DMPA? Is hypo-oestrogenism a problem?

Evidence is still too scanty for DMPA, and absent for NET EN. A New Zealand article published in the British Medical Journal in 1991 is stimulating further studies. In brief, that was a cross-sectional study of 30 current users of DMPA with a minimum 5 years' previous use and all with continuous amenorrhoea, compared with 30 premenopausal volunteers and 30 postmenopausal controls. The bone density values in the DMPA users were lower by about 7% compared with the premenopausal women. This is too small a reduction for any fracture risk and moreover the values were higher than in the postmenopausal women whose mean duration of relative oestrogen deficiency was similar (about 10 years).

There are many problems with this study. The laboratory and technical work may be good but they are let down by the basic design (there could be no knowledge of the bone status of the DMPA-users *prior to* starting the method) and the attempted matching process may well not have led to true comparability between the studied groups (risk of confounding). Four times as many DMPA users were smokers (40%) as the premenopausal controls, though the DMPA-related difference persisted when the (only) 21 women who were concordant for smoking habits were compared.

Quite separate studies of long-term DMPA users do show plasma oestradiols which can be less than 100 pmol/l, as after the menopause, and this is commoner in amenorrhoea and with cigarette smoking. With both the natural and premature menopause as a model – and both do lead to increased risk of osteoporosis and of arterial disease – pending further information I think we should be cautious (see Q 5.101).

5.101 How should long-term users of injectables be managed if they do become amenorrhoeic?

Pending more data, I suggest that, as for the same situation arising with the POP (see Q 5.65) and presumably NET EN, if available a plasma oestradiol is arranged for any DMPA-user – especially if she is a smoker – who has had continuous amenorrhoea for more than 5 years. A full lipid screen and bone scan would also be of some interest, but are not essential and likely to be even less available.

If levels of oestradiol are above 100 pmol/l and the bone scan is normal, and if the woman is happy with the injectable, it may continue to be used (long term), plus the usual follow-up. If the oestradiols are less than 100 pmol/l or the scan shows any significant loss in bone density: either another contraceptive method should be chosen or there could be consideration of 'add-back' natural oestrogen by any chosen route. (The percutaneous route is recommened, as usual, if there is a past history of thrombosis.) Older amenorrhoeic DMPA-users would almost always benefit from HRT, and I think it is wise to discontinue injectables by 45 anyway (Q 5.120). For younger women without oestrogen deficiency symptoms, if the tests are not available, data are too scanty to ban the option of continuing with the injectable.

> Note: All these proposals are tentative, for the time being and until we have better data.

5.102 What is the effect of injectables on circulatory disease and on hypertension?

Despite the reduction in HDL-C mentioned above (see Q 5.97), which is probably more important as just discussed in DMPA-users with amenorrhoea, there are no data suggesting that injectables increase the rate of development of atherosclerosis or increase the incidence of myocardial infarction or strokes. More epidemiological research is required.

5.103 What effects do injectables have on blood pressure?

Here is some good news: most studies show no significant change in either systolic or diastolic blood pressure in women using either injectable. Some reports even suggest a slight decrease in BP.

5.104 Do injectables affect neoplasia in animals?

Given enormous doses of DMPA, Beagle bitches (which are by nature prone to breast nodules) can develop malignant tumours of the breast. Two out of 12 rhesus monkeys given 50 times the human contraceptive dose in a 10-year trial developed endometrial carcinoma. No cases were observed in monkeys treated with the human dose or 10 times the human dose.

The animal models (Beagle bitches or rhesus monkeys) are believed by most authorities to be manifesting species-specific reactions which are not applicable to the human, or the doses used have been irrelevantly high.

5.105 What are the latest data about DMPA and cancer in the human?

Recent (1991) publications by WHO from good hospital-based case-control studies in developing countries provide the best data to date. The findings can be summarized:

1 *Endometrial cancer* – a protective effect, in fact a fivefold reduction in risk. There was also an ex-use protective effect detectable for at least 8 years after cessation of DMPA use. It seems the reduction in risk is as great for DMPA as for the COC.

2 *Epithelial ovarian cancer* – protective effect like with the COC (perhaps surprisingly) not demonstrated: but certainly no increase in risk either.

3 *Primary liver cancer* – no increased risk, and this was in countries (Thailand and Kenya) where hepatitis B is endemic.

4 *Cervical cancer* – no increased risk. This is the finding of a larger and better WHO study than that reported in 1984, which showed a small association with DMPA use. It confirms the suspicion at the time that the association was due to confounding by factors such as sexual activity and smoking.

5 *Breast cancer* – no overall association, but see Q 5.106.

Overall these results are very favourable to this much maligned method!

5.106 Does DMPA increase the risk of breast cancer?

Good news, again! (mostly, anyway). In the large WHO hospital-based case-control study from five centres, reported in *The Lancet* in October 1991, there was no link with breast cancer in the total population (869 cases, 11 890 controls), nor any increased risk with increased duration of use.

The only statistically increased risk was for use in the first 4 years after initial exposure, mainly in women under 35. Although this seems superficially similar to the positive findings among young long-term users in the 1989 New Zealand DMPA study, and those in the UK NCCS for young COC-users, unlike them the WHO study found *no duration-of-use effect*. There was no increase in risk among women who started DMPA more than 5 years previously.

DMPA may perhaps be bringing forward the appearance of cancers which would have become manifest later. On the other hand it is very plausible that the association in the WHO study is entirely caused by *detection bias*; recent users (who would necessarily be young) or their physicians being more likely to discover breast lumps in the first four years of DMPA use.

5.107 May DMPA be used in cases of trophoblastic disease?

In the UK it is recommended that DMPA, like all contraceptive steroids, should be avoided until hCG is undetectable (see Q 4.69). Thereafter there is no objection to this method, which can be a very suitable means of preventing pregnancy for the 2 years of designated follow-up.

5.108 Is there any evidence that injectables affect the development or growth of benign tumours?

It is difficult to assess the significance of two cases of benign liver tumours reported in the USA. Benign breast disease can sometimes deteriorate, according to clinical anecdotes. There are otherwise no reports of adverse effects on benign tumours, and it appears that the growth of uterine fibroids is usually inhibited.

SELECTION OF USERS AND OF FORMULATIONS

5.109 For whom are injectables particularly indicated?

1 First and foremost, if a *systemic, non-intercourse-related method* is chosen by the woman and other options (particularly those containing oestrogen) are contraindicated, or disliked.
   This includes the categories:
   (a) postvenous thromboembolism or known prothrombotic abnormality of coagulation. A good example of the latter is severe *SLE* (see Q 4.113);

(b) to cover relevant elective surgery (Q 4.180);

(c) *forgetful pill-takers.*

2 Women in whom *long-term progestagens are indicated,* e.g. some with perimenopausal problems, and those with endometriosis.

3 As an *alternative to the IUD* where the risk of PID is held to be high (e.g. the young woman whose partner may have multiple partners).

4 *Sickle cell disease* (see Q 5.93).

5 At the woman's choice.

5.110 What are the absolute contraindications to injectables?

These are identical to the first six relating to the POP (see Q 5.51), with the need for a little more caution (as also in Q 5.112 with respect to relative contraindications) because:

- The dose is larger.

- There is the aforementioned reversibility problem after any given injection is given.

- Amenorrhoea is more frequent (see Q 5.100)

1 *Past severe arterial disease, or current exceptionally high risk of the same.* Pending further information I would not prescribe an injectable long term to a woman known to have current ischaemic heart disease including angina or to have already suffered a thrombotic stroke; nor to women with marked and multiple risk factors (e.g. a 45-year-old heavy smoking hypertensive diabetic!) – or if so one would discontinue the method if they became amenorrhoeic (see Qs 5.97 and 5.100–1).

   Severe hereditary lipid abnormalities with a poor prognosis come into this category because of 'exceptionally high risk'. However, the injectable might be prescribed with extra counselling and supervision in the presence of milder abnormalities with a good prognosis (see Q 5.109). All this caution could probably cease if only there were a fully 'lipid-friendly' injectable on the market (see Q 4.136).

2 Any *serious side-effect occurring on the COC and not clearly due only to oestrogen* – or associated with past progestagen-only use. Liver adenoma and severe past steroid-associated cholestatic jaundice would come here since it is not clear with which of the two hormones in the COC they are primarily linked. Also in this category:

3 *Recent trophoblastic disease* (see Q 4.69).

As for all medical methods, we must add:

4 *Undiagnosed abnormal genital tract bleeding* since the injectable will confuse diagnosis.

5 Actual or possible *pregnancy*.

6 The woman's own continuing uncertainty about the safety of DMPA or NET EN, even after full counselling.

5.111 Why is past ectopic pregnancy not any kind of contraindication to injectables, whereas it is to the POP (and the vaginal ring)?

Because, like the COC, injectables almost always block ovulation and hence virtually eliminate the risk of an ectopic. The woman with damaged tubes of course remains still at risk of getting her ectopic later, when off the anovulant treatment.

5.112 What are the relative contraindications to injectables?

See Q 4.102 – here is my list:

1 *Risk factors for arterial disease*. This category includes established hypertension once it has been diagnosed and controlled and also focal migraine (see Qs 4.124–30). The presence of more than one risk factor can be tolerated more readily than with the COC – but there are limits, see Q 5.109(1). Prothrombotic coagulation factor abnormalities are actually included above as 'indications', since they should not be worsened at all by an injectable. Likewise, there is not the oestrogen-related concern about thrombotic stroke in migraine, including focal migraine – though it may be affected (see Q 4.129).

   Lipid abnormalities might perhaps be worsened by the injectables, especially in amenorrhoeic women: The POP, having less metabolic effects, would normally be a better choice (see Q 5.52, 5.65).

2 *Sex steroid–dependent cancer*. The POP is lower dose and more readily reversible (see Q 5.52). But seek the advice of the oncologist looking after your patient. There is no evidence that injectables worsen the prognosis after breast cancer is diagnosed, but there is no proof of the opposite either.

3 *Active liver disease* – caution required. Yet there are reports that patients with chronic active hepatitis may even improve on this treatment.

4 *Other chronic systemic diseases.* The same comments as at Q 4.105 for the COC apply. The great effectiveness as a contraceptive often helps to outweigh the continuing uncertainty as to what effect (either way) an injectable might have on the disease. With that proviso and given the reversibility problem, DMPA may be a good choice for the conditions listed as absolute (see Q 4.101) or relative (see Q 4.103) contraindications to the COC – including severe SLE or Crohn's disease.

5 *Unacceptability of menstrual irregularities*, especially cultural taboos associated with bleeding – or amenorrhoea.

6 *Obesity* – but see Q 5.117(3).

7 Past *severe endogenous depression* (above-average support needed).

8 Any woman who is *planning a pregnancy in the near future.* In fact this contraindication would become absolute if she wished to conceive within 6 months of the proposed injection.

9 *In the years leading up to the menopause* There are five concerns:
   (a) the effect on HDL-C (see Q 5.97), particularly if the woman were a smoker;
   (b) the possibility of hypo-oestrogenism increasing bone density loss as the ovaries begin to fail some time before the actual menopause (see Q 5.100).
These objections (a) and (b) might, in selected cases, be overcome by 'add-back' oestrogen replacement (see Q 5.101)
   (c) irregular bleeding may lead to the need for D&C;
   (d) the menopause may be masked (see Q 5.121);
   (e) the method is perhaps too strong, a 'contraceptive overkill' (see Q 8.33, 8.50).

5.113 What effects do injectables have on future fertility?

Return of fertility is slow, especially with DMPA. It is normal for conception to be delayed until about 8 months after the last injection (i.e. about 5 months after the last dose has 'officially' ceased to be active, see Table 5.2). The degree of delay – in ovulation, menstruation and conception – is unrelated to the duration of use or to the dose.

A study of parous women in Thailand showed that almost 95% of DMPA-users had conceived by 28 months after their last injection, a cumulative rate which was indistinguishable from that following discontinuation of the IUD or an oral contraceptive. Another finding is that underweight women regain their fertility faster.

Most importantly, as well as there being no evidence of a permanent infertility effect, secondary amenorrhoea of this variety is extremely treatable by standard ovulation induction methods.

Referral is advised, where specialist facilities are available, if amenorrhoea persists beyond about 9 months from the last injection.

5.114 What are the effects of injectables on lactation?

1 Both injectables appear to increase the volume of breast milk.

2 Most studies suggest no important change in its composition.

3 The amount of hormone transmitted to the infant in breast milk is very small, less than 0.5% of the maternal dose. The amount of exposure to hormone is markedly less with NET EN.

Although no long-term effects on infant growth and development have been reported, the amount of exposure to an artificial hormone is obviously greater than with the POP. In view of this minimal uncertainty, in my view it would be preferable *in this country* for most lactating women to use the POP, transferring to the injectable as one option when the child is weaned. (The combination of POP plus full lactation is sufficient, almost 100% effective contraception.)

If DMPA or NET EN are used in lactation, as for non-breastfeeders, the injection should ideally be given 5–6 weeks after delivery, this delay being helpful to minimize bleeding problems.

5.115 Which injectable should be chosen?

1 The natural first choice is DMPA, since its effects are better known, and it is marginally more effective. The injection is less uncomfortable and only needs to be given four times a year.

2 Possible reasons for selecting NET EN include:
   (a) reduced likelihood of complete amenorrhoea;
   (b) shorter time until spontaneous reversal of the effect if unacceptable side-effects were to develop after the first injection;
   (c) more rapid return of fertility after the last injection;
   (d) less risk of marked weight gain;
   (e) if DMPA proves unsatisfactory, as an empirical second choice.

5.116 What should be done at the first visit prior to giving an injectable?

1 A good *medical history* should be taken with special reference to the absolute and relative contraindications (see Qs 5.110 and 5.112).

2 Record the *weight*. This is more important than with other hormonal methods.

3 Record the *blood pressure*. This is desirable as a baseline, but on present evidence appears not to be especially relevant to the method.

4 Examine the *breasts* and teach breast self-examination/awareness with a good leaflet, not leading to a nerve-racking ritual.

5 Carry out a *pelvic examination and cervical smear* – again mainly as good preventive medicine. It is relevant to the method after childbirth to exclude the possibility of retained products; and sometimes to exclude a clinical pre-existing pregnancy.

5.117 What is the minimum information which should be conveyed at counselling?

Failure to counsel adequately has been the main cause of adverse publicity in this country. The following should be discussed.

1 *Amenorrhoea.* As Dr Wilson of Glasgow has declared, reassurance that a 'monthly clean-out' of the 'bad blood' is not necessary for good health may make all the difference between happy acceptance and chronic anxiety and dissatisfaction.

2 The opposite possibility of *frequent irregular bleeding*. Reassure the woman that medical advice is available if this should occur.

3 *Weight gain.* Not inevitable, as it is mainly caused by increased appetite.

4 *Delay in fertility return.* Women should be told on average it may take 9 months from the time of the last injection to conceive.

5 Theoretical *long-term risks*. The cancer balance seems on present evidence to be rather favourable to the method (see Q 5.105). The issues of arterial disease and osteoporosis, especially if there

were to be prolonged amenorrhoea are, still not fully resolved (see Qs 5.100–1). How much is told must depend on the doctor's judgement of the patient's understanding and background, but an opportunity for questions must be given and they must be frankly answered.

The information leaflet agreed between the manufacturing company and the UK Minister of Health should be given to each woman. She should be given time to read it before making up her mind, and any further questions then answered. The FPA also supplies a useful leaflet.

5.118 How are the injectables given?

By deep intramuscular injection, in this country usually into the upper outer quadrant of the buttock or outer thigh. The DMPA ampoule should be very thoroughly shaken to remove any sediment. NET EN should preferably be warmed to body temperature. The site of either injection should not be massaged.

5.119 What are the requirements for successful monitoring and follow-up?

1 Careful planning of the date for the next dose when each is given. Try to avoid the complexities of Qs 5.127 and 5.128 by explaining that if a planned date proves inconvenient, it is far better to ask for the next dose a week or two early than to be late . . . .

2 Equally important is ready access between injections to medical advice by telephone or in person, to deal with any anxieties arising.

3 Blood pressure is normally checked at least annually and weight at each visit in the first year; but thereafter, if stable, mainly at the patient's request.

4 Breast and cervical screening is performed according to local policies.

5.120 For how long, and to what age, may use of injectables be continued?

There are no known reasons for arbitrarily restricting the duration of use in younger women with adequate endogenous ovarian activity. The implications and management of prolonged amenorrhoea are discussed at Qs 5.100–1. The documented small reduction in HDL-C suggests that transferring to another method might be preferable at around age 45, or earlier for those with multiple CVS risk factors.

5.121 How can the menopause be diagnosed?

With difficulty – the scheme at Q 5.63 is not appropriate for injectables. The method has to be discontinued and alternative contraception practised: ideally for 12 months after the last spontaneous bleed, which may mean up to 24 months after the last injection in view of the unpredictability of the prolonged action (see Q 5.113). Vasomotor symptoms and FSH measurement(s) may help to shorten this time.

Injectables are actually by way of being a 'contraceptive overkill' around the climacteric (see Q 8.33, 8.50). Transfer to another method before age 45 is therefore normally preferable (see Q 5.120), with the added advantage of simplifying diagnosis of the menopause.

MANAGEMENT OF SIDE EFFECTS AND PRACTICAL PROBLEMS

5.122 How should non-acceptable, prolonged bleeding be managed?

1 The patient should be examined to exclude a gynaecological cause, especially retained products of conception or carcinoma. If the uterus is firm and non-tender, with a closed cervical os, it is unlikely that the bleeding has any cause other than as a side-effect of the injectable.

2 Possible treatments:
   (a) Give the next dose; but no earlier than 4 weeks since the last.
   (b) Give oestrogen (if not contraindicated). The preferred regimen is conjugated oestrogens (Premarin 1.25 mg daily for 21 days, repeated as necessary). However, simply giving one or more packets of any convenient 30 μg COC works well if not contraindicated. The extra progestagen matters not at all, so this is often convenient.
   (c) Haemostatics such as tranexamic acid and ethamsylate have been tried. They rarely work well, and there have been a few worrying case reports of serious thrombotic

events with the first. I think that that risk would outweigh the benefits for this indication.

(d) Curettage is a last resort.

(e) Iron treatment is rarely indicated to correct anaemia, since the actual amount lost over many days is usually not great.

It may be possible to help a woman through initial difficulties, particularly by 2(a) or 2(b) above. But irregular bleeding remains the commonest reason for discontinuing the method. The problem is most pronounced postpartum, often helped by delaying the first dose to 4–6 weeks.

5.123 How should amenorrhoea be managed?

1 First and foremost, pregnancy should be eliminated as the cause.

2 Secondly, the woman should be counselled as at Q 5.117(1). The establishment of prolonged amenorrhoea can often be the best solution for women with bleeding problems.

3 A short course of natural oestrogen to cause a withdrawal 'period' can sometimes be helpful as an adjunct to reassurance.

4 If the amenorrhoea exceeds 5 year's duration, see Q 5.101 above. The main concern *re* hypo-oestrogenism/osteoporosis primarily relates to smokers.

5.124 What about other minor side-effects?

Management can only be empirical, for example, switching to the other injectable or another method. Weight gain is the commonest complaint: dieting is possible but difficult. Diuretics are useless. Pyridoxine treatment may be tried if depression is reported (see Q 4.184), but there have been no good studies.

5.125 What symptoms should lead an injectable-user to take urgent medical advice?

Specifically related to the method, there are none – apart from the very rare occurrence of massive uterine 'flooding' (see Q 5.122).

5.126 Are prolonged immobilization or major surgery contraindications to injectables?

There is no need to discontinue either DMPA or NET EN before any kind of surgery. Indeed it may be a very satisfactory option instead of the combined pill for women at high risk of pregnancy while on the waiting list for major surgery. See Q 4.180 for the practical management.

5.127 How should one handle the problem of overdue injections? How can one maintain contraception without avoidably risking fetal exposure to the drug?

This is very difficult. Even if the woman is not amenorrhoeic, any bleeds give no information about when she may ovulate.

There is at least 1 week of leeway with each injection – the likelihood of conception during the 13th week with DMPA and the 9th week with NET EN is acceptably low. Beyond that, the risks of a very early pregnancy being 'on the way' begin to increase. One of the following courses of action might be followed, depending on the precise circumstances, and assuming intercourse has been continuing:

1 If the next dose is late by 3 days beyond 13 weeks with DMPA, prescribe the Yuzpe hormonal postcoital contraceptive (see Q 7.5) plus an immediate injection of the DMPA.

2 If the next dose is late by 5 days or, according to the legal case quoted at Q 7.11, 7 days beyond the 13 weeks, one could proceed in good faith to insert an intrauterine device (see Q 7.27) plus an immediate injection (unless the woman chose to switch to the IUD alone in future).

Counselling must include discussion of the (low) risk of harm to a fetus (see Q 5.117), and be fully recorded. Follow-up should be 100%, with exclusion of pregnancy about 3 weeks later.

5.128 What if the injection is more than a week beyond the 1 week 'leeway'?

This means beyond 14 weeks with DMPA. In a currently sexually active user one would have to follow the policy described at Q 8.21.

In brief, insist that she agrees to avoid all risk of conception – by abstinence, combinations of methods, whatever – for the next 10 or preferably 14 days. She then returns with an early morning urine. If this gives a negative result by one of the ultrasensitive slide pregnancy tests now available for primary care use (e.g. 'Clearview'), ideally sensitive to 50 IU/l of hCG, this can be interpreted as no conception up to 14 days previously, since when she had additionally agreed to be 'safe'. After discussion as at Q 5.127(2) above (recorded), one might then proceed with the next injection.

For extra security the couple should use the condom for a further 7 days and, again, there *must* be a follow-up visit to exclude pregnancy after 3–4 weeks.

5.129 What are the risks if a fetus is exposed to injectables?

1 There is no evidence of an increase in ectopic or miscarriage rates.

2 There is some concern that offspring of women exposed to DMPA during pregnancy, especially in the 4 weeks after an injection, are at increased risk of low birth weight and subsequent infant mortality. But it has been suggested this could be due to *confounding*, e.g. by social class.

3 Masculinization of the female fetus, particularly transient enlargement of the clitoris, and a possible increase in the incidence of hypospadias in males exposed to medroxyprogesterone acetate and similar hormones, have been reported. But no serious fetal malformation risks have been established with the very low doses used for contraception in DMPA and NET EN. Meaningful conclusions about what must be very low potential teratogenic risks are unlikely ever to be reached, because proceeding to term after exposure to injectables is such a rare event.

Every effort must of course continue to be made to prevent fetal exposure (see Q 5.127–8).

5.130 Are there any known risks or benefits for ex-users of injectables?

There are no established teratogenic effects on pregnancies among recent ex-users of injectables.

The only known problem is prolonged amenorrhoea and delayed return of fertility (see Q 5.113). There is a definite ex-use protective effect against carcinoma of the endometrium. Watch this space!

QUESTIONS ASKED BY USERS

General

Most questions asked are about DMPA, or Depo-Provera as it is best known by the general public.

5.131 What is in practice the most effective reversible contraceptive currently available?

Depo-Provera, with NET EN a close second.

5.132 Do injectables cause cancer in women?

This currently seems very unlikely and one cancer (of the lining of the womb) is less frequent (see Qs. 5.104–5.107).

5.133 But is it safe? How does the safety (freedom from health risk) of Depo-Provera compare with 'the pill'?

Overall, since it contains no oestrogen, its safety is believed to be greater than that of the combined pill. No deaths have been clearly blamed upon it (see Q 5.92).

5.134 Why are some people so opposed to Depo-Provera?

Mainly because of its potential for abuse, and the fact that if side-effects occur – and there are fewer overall than with the pill – the drug's action cannot be reversed once given. You have to wait for the last injection to wear off (see Q 5.94).

5.135 Is it a 'last resort' method?

The UK licence does require it to be used only after discussion of the more readily available alternatives and after full counselling with the special leaflet. But it can be an excellent second choice that is not 'second best' in any way.

5.136 Can I be too young to be given Depo-Provera?

Some doctors are reluctant to give it to very young teenagers, who are just beginning their normal menstrual cycle. There is no proof that it will ever cause fertility or other problems even then, and injectables would normally be preferable to insertion of an IUD, if that was the alternative choice (see Q 5.109).

5.137 Can I be too old to be given Depo-Provera?

Above the age of 45 injectables are stronger contraceptives than are really required, and there is an increasing risk of disease of the arteries. So other methods are usually preferable, especially in smokers not seeing 'periods' (see Qs 5.97 and 5.121).

5.138 Can the injection be given by my family doctor as well as through a clinic?

Yes – though some GPs may feel a bit uncertain about using the method. (Perhaps they should read this book!)

5.139 Where (on the body) is the injection given?

Usually into the upper outer region of the buttock, on either side; but it can sometimes be given into the shoulder or thigh muscles.

Questions asked by current users

5.140 Why can the injection not be given right after my baby?

If given too soon it tends to cause a lot of bleeding problems in the weeks after childbirth. These are less if it is given at about 5–6 weeks; but since it does not have any thrombosis problems it can sometimes be given much earlier, if you are prepared to accept the bleeding risk.

5.141 How long does the injection last?

Officially for 12 weeks, and each injection should be on time. This is for maximum safety against pregnancy. However, some women (and we do not know who they are in advance) go on being affected for much longer (see Q 5.142).

5.142 How far ahead should I discontinue injections if planning another baby?

You should plan about a year ahead, since it is quite usual (and nothing to worry about) for conception to be delayed that long.

5.143 Excess bleeding – will it harm me in any way if I can live with it?

The short answer is 'no'. You ought to be examined to eliminate any cause not related to the Depo-Provera. A blood test may be done to check that you are not anaemic, followed by iron treatment as required. Some treatments may be tried to stop the bleeding (see Q 5.122). Otherwise if you can live with an unpredictable bleeding pattern it will do you no harm. If you choose to have intercourse during bleeding that too is medically harmless.

The (near) future: non-oral routes for hormone administration

5.144 Why, first, should there be any interest in once a month injectables?

One problem with DMPA and NET EN is the initially too high levels which subsequently fall off rather unpredictably (Fig. 5.3).

An approach actually making use of this decline in levels is under study in association with WHO: once a month injectables containing small doses of either NET-EN plus oestradiol valerate (HRP 102) or DMPA plus oestradiol cypionate (HRP 112). This approach seems to give much more predictable bleeding patterns, the first bleed occurring about 2 weeks after the first injection, and then monthly, lasting for about 5 days, and without loss of efficacy.

5.145 What other developments can be expected?

The main advantage of non-oral routes on theoretical grounds is that they avoid giving the liver such a heavy initial *peak* metabolic load, via the hepatic portal vein. It is after all the liver which is intimately involved in the metabolism of clotting factors, lipid metabolism, the renin-angiotensin mechanisms involved in blood pressure control, among other important metabolic variables. The liver also suffers certain specific if rare pill-related disorders, such as hepatomas (benign and malignant) and cholestasis.

The current injectables are trail-blazers, foreshadowing the future, but leaving plenty of room for improvement. There are four main anticipated benefits of rings and implants:

1 no tablets to be remembered; ⎫ these advantages shared
                                  ⎬ by injectables
2 bypassing the liver;   ⎭

3 very long action with one treatment, yet quickly reversible;

4 constant blood levels, and less between-women variation.

I predict that the systemic steroid contraceptives of the future will always use a non-oral route.

SUBDERMAL IMPLANTS

5.146 What are contraceptive implants?

At present, those being tested contain a progestagen in a slow-release carrier, usually made of Silastic, a polymer of dimethylsiloxane. This delivers almost constant blood levels of the hormone (Fig. 5.3). One version called Norplant is already available in Scandinavia and the USA and expected to reach other countries in the near future, including the UK by 1994.

5.147 What is Norplant? How is it used?

Developed by the Population Council, this consists of six implants, each the size of a matchstick, implanted subdermally via a dedicated 11-gauge trocar under local anaesthesia. Trained clinicians can insert them in around 10 minutes, and remove them upon request in about twice that time. The implants release, after the first few weeks, about 40–50 µg levonorgestrel (LNG) per day, dropping to 30–35 µg per day after the first year through to 5 year of use.

The recommended site for insertion is the flexor surface of the forearm or upper arm, since implants at other sites tend to migrate under the skin, posing problems for removal.

Other features are summarized in Table 5.2.

5.148 What are the advantages of Norplant?

It has the same or better efficacy in comparison with DMPA, but a smaller biological effect than either DMPA or NET EN: more comparable to the POP. Hence it is believed to have the advantages already listed at Qs 5.30 and 5.31, plus some additional ones:

1 Absence of daily pill-taking routine, hence freedom from 'fear of forgetting'. This leads to high acceptability, excellent continuation rates, and the *failure rate* of the polymer 372 marketed version is about *0.2/100 woman–years* and appears to be unaffected by increasing body weight (cf. Q 5.13).

2 Long action with one treatment (at least 5 years).

3 Absence of the initial peak dose given orally to the liver.

4 Blood levels are steady rather than fluctuating (as the POP) or initially too high (as injectables). This reduces metabolic and most clinical side-effects.

5 No changes have been seen in blood pressure and metabolic changes are small, similar to those in users of LNG-containing POPs (see Q 5.39).

6 The implants are removable, reversing the method. The half-life of the LNG after implants are removed is about 2 days! In one study conception occurred within 1 year in 86% of women.

5.149 What are the disadvantages and problems of Norplant?

Ovulation occurs in only 10% of cycles in the first year, but once the release rate declines to 30 µg/day ovulation occurs more frequently (30–75% of cycles). This necessarily implies the same spectrum of ovarian effects in different women as was described at Q 5.5 for the POP. Yet the efficacy remains higher.

Similar problems result as with the POP:

1 Irregular and prolonged bleeding is the chief cause of requests for removal (involving 10% of women at 1 year).

2 Functional ovarian cysts are reported, but these are as usual mostly asymptomatic or can be managed conservatively. The Population Council estimates the need for surgical intervention at 0.03/100 woman-years of use.

3 The ectopic pregnancy rate was low, about 0.08/100 woman-years in the Phase III studies. Since ovulation is blocked more often pregnancies are probably even less likely to be ectopic than with the POP (though still more common among the pregnancies which do occur, because of the selection effect described at Q 5.40); and below the rate estimated for non-users of contraception.

4 Minor side-effects such as acne are also described, just as for the POP (see Q 5.67).

Specific problems:

5 There is inevitably some discomfort at insertion and removal.

6 Infection of the site, migration of an implant and difficult removal are infrequent complications.

7 Some women object to the cosmetic appearance of the implants.

5.150 When it becomes available, who might consider using Norplant?

Like injectables, the method combines most of the best attributes of the POP with no reliance on the user's memory. Hence the clinical indications are best summarized by a combination of the two lists at Qs 5.49 and 5.109, and in my view include lactation.

Contraindications are also as listed at Q 5.51, though item 7 (past ectopic) is, like a tendency to functional ovarian cysts, only a relative contraindication.

The developers believe that this method is so safe and effective that it can be considered as 'reversible sterilization', and as such it is likely to become very popular. It is a suitable minor procedure for general practice; training in insertion and removal is available (the MPC is involved).

5.151 What further improvements can be expected?

Implants that slowly biodegrade are under study (e.g. Capronor). The ideal hormone carrier would degrade in body tissue to a natural innocuous substance such as lactic acid and therefore would not have to be removed; however, it should also remain removable if desired.

Implants are also now under study which deliver the metabolically preferred progestagens (see Q 4.136) combined with oestrogens. Other contraceptive compounds will also be offered by this route, such as gonadotrophin releasing hormone analogues or antagonists.

CONTRACEPTIVE VAGINAL RINGS

5.152 What are vaginal rings?

Like implants, current versions use a Silastic carrier, which is in the shape of a ring between 5 and 6 cm in diameter and 4–10 mm thick. There are two main designs. In core-rings all the hormone is in a central core. In the shell design the inner core is hormone free, but encircled by a narrow hormone-filled band. Both types are then covered by Silastic tubing, giving controlled (zero-order) release to the vaginal mucosa.

Development of vaginal rings has followed two approaches (see Qs 5.153 and 5.157).

5.153 What is the LNG-ring? How is it used?

This design has many affinities with the POP. Since 1980, research coordinated by WHO has focused on versions releasing 20 μg LNG/day for 90 days. Like Norplant, they deliver almost constant blood levels.

These rings are not removed, except for replacement, though if so desired they can be removed before intercourse. They move freely within the vagina.

5.154 What are the advantages of LNG vaginal rings?

The blood levels achieved are equally steady but about half those when Norplant is in use. This somewhat increases the pregnancy rate (Table 5.2) to about 3/100 woman-years or the same as the POP, but further reduces the metabolic impact. Overall the advantages are as described for Norplant at Q 5.148, without the need for minor surgical procedures for insertion and removal. The method is under the woman's control.

5.155 What are the disadvantages of LNG-rings?

Again, most of these follow from its similarity to the POP. So the answer to Q 5.149 about Norplant applies on the whole to this method, including what is there said about functional cysts and ectopic pregnancies. Differences are:

1 A lower rate of bleeding irregularities is reported.

2 Minor non-bleeding side-effects – these are expected to be even less frequent than with Norplant, though there are insufficient data.

Specific problems:

3 In a study at the MPC during 1991–2 asymptomatic erythematous patches were discovered, apparently associated with the areas of contact of the rings with the vaginal fornices. At the time of writing it is not clear whether these are caused by physical pressure or a chemical effect, but they have (hopefully temporarily) put back marketing plans in the UK. The long-term effects on the vagina and cervix will need careful monitoring.

4 Vaginal discharge, irritation (not always associated with the patches mentioned at 3), odour and inadvertent expulsion have been specific complaints.

How acceptable these or future vaginal rings will prove to be is uncertain. Rings combine some of the inconvenience of a vaginal method with some of the systemic problems of hormones (but less of each than most alternatives).

5.156 Who might particularly consider using a progestagen-releasing vaginal ring?

The answer is probably the same kind of woman who would consider using Norplant (see Q 5.150). When compared with the latter, clearly this method avoids a minor operation for insertion and removal, and it is a method over which she has control. But she should be comfortable about having a foreign object in her vagina for a long period of time.

5.157 What is clinically the most promising type of ring?

The combined type. The combined pill is after all a very successful model from which to start. Workers in Brazil and Israel in the early 1980s showed that a standard pill (LNG 250 µg plus EE 50 µg), as formulated for oral use, was effective when taken vaginally.

Symptoms such as nausea were less frequent, though it is possible that this was due to achieving lower blood levels of oestrogen. See Q 7.21 for a possible application of this to emergency contraception.

Vaginal pills have never become popular, probably because daily compliance is still necessary. But a combined ring which releases 3-keto-desogestrel and EE has been studied at the MPC and elsewhere and shows much promise. It gives excellent cycle control with very few contraceptive failures . It can be retained for 3 weeks and removed for a withdrawal bleed during the fourth, thus closely imitating the combined pill (Mercilon by vagina!). Alternatively it can be used continuously perhaps for three calendar months at a time (analogous to tricycling, see Q 4.28).

5.158 What is the natural progesterone ring?

This is another WHO ring designed especially for *lactating women*. It releases over 3 months 5–10 mg/day of progesterone, thereby minimizing concerns about the composition of breast milk. With this method I would foresee the need for great care to transfer to a more effective method during weaning: if unwanted conceptions are to be avoided when the progesterone is no longer supplemented by the contraceptive effect of full lactation.

Other developments

Implants and rings, or other non-oral methods described below, using the third-generation progestogens gestodene and 3-keto-desogestrel are likely to be even more 'lipid friendly' than Norplant. Different lengths of a single 3-keto-desogestrel-releasing rod are being tested to determine the best release rates and duration of action.

5.159 Will the transdermal route be used for contraception?

Already we have transdermal oestrogen and combined oestrogen/progestogen patches for HRT. There is no *a priori* reason why this route should not also be used for combined or progestogen-only contraception, and not just for older women. However because larger doses must be used to achieve adequate cycle control, with present technology the patches would need to be rather large, posing cosmetic and perhaps comfort problems.

5.160 What are other theoretical routes?

For completeness, one should mention the rectal, transnasal and sublingual routes, all of which are in current use for other drugs. There are no known plans at present for routine contraception thereby.

Postscript: missed progestagen-only pills and lactation

All the strict instructions proposed at Qs 5.19–5.23 are designed for women who are not breastfeeding! *During lactation* ovulation is inhibited while there is sustained amenorrhoea, particularly during the first 6 months postpartum (see Fig. 1.3). Missing a POP is therefore like missing a COC in mid-packet (Q 4.19).

The 'leeway' must therefore go up, to at least 12 hours. But because breastfeeding varies in its intensity, it is probably wise to keep to the general policy of advising 7 days' added precautions. Some individuals, after discussion, may be told they may disregard it, and it would be most exceptional to find it necessary to offer emergency contraception, if they missed any tablets, to fully breastfeeding POP-users with amenorrhoea.

Intrauterine devices

BACKGROUND AND MECHANISMS

6.1   How would you define an intrauterine device?

This is any solid object which is wholly retained within the uterine cavity for the purpose of preventing pregnancy. Such devices are usually inserted via the cervical canal and may have marker thread(s) attached which are visible at the external os. There are currently three main types: inert, copper bearing and hormone releasing.

6.2   Should they be abbreviated IUD or IUCD?

Underlying this question is the possibility of confusion of 'intrauterine device' with 'intrauterine death' of a fetus. Hence many gynaecologists prefer IUCD, for IntraUterine Contraceptive Device. But this leads to problems in translation and moreover IUD is now well established in the world literature. An amusing compromise adopted by an expert committee of the World Health Organization (WHO) in the 1970s was the following: to use IUD (without full stops) for intrauterine device, and I.U.D. for intrauterine death! This agreed notation will be used here.

6.3   What is the history of IUDs?

An oft-quoted but poorly substantiated story describes the first IUD as a stone or stones placed in the uterus of camels in North Africa, to prevent pregnancies during long caravan journeys. One version of the story, however, suggests that the stones were actually put in the vagina, making the method more akin to a chastity belt than an IUD! Over 2500 years ago Hippocrates is credited with using a hollow lead tube to insert pessaries or other objects into human uteri. (The translations differ as to whether this was for contraception or other purposes.) Casanova recommended a gold ball; and as recently as 1950 one woman apparently used her wedding ring as a do-it-yourself IUD!

Cervicouterine stem pessaries were used from the late nineteenth century. They were made from material as exotic as ivory, glass, ebony and diamond-studded platinum, and were used for many purposes – including contraception. Some were shaped like collar-studs or had V-shaped flexible wings inserted into the lower uterine cavity. When the devices fractured, as they sometimes did, leaving just the intrauterine part in position, it was learnt that the latter (rather than the surface cap covering the external os) was the contraceptive. The first completely intrauterine device was a ring made of silkworm gut, described by Dr Richter of Braslaw. Later, silver wire was wound around the silkworm by Grafenberg and it is of interest that later versions were made of German silver, an alloy which contains *copper*. Now made of coiled stainless steel, the design is still one of the most widely used in the world (because it is so popular in China).

Many of the early devices were used as abortifacients as well as contraceptives, and the resultant haemorrhage and pelvic infection led to widespread condemnation by the medical profession. This retarded acceptance of the method, which was only really achieved in 1962 at the first International Conference on IUDs in New York City. The Lippes Loop was presented to this conference by its inventor, and became the standard inert device (see Fig. 6.1) against which many newer devices were compared: many now being bioactive, bearing copper or releasing hormones. The 'lay' terms 'loop'/'coil' are out-of-date and best not used.

6.4　How prevalent is use of the IUD?

In 1988 it was estimated that about 85 million IUDs were in use worldwide, 59 million of them in one country – China. In Britain, according to a recent survey (1991), IUDs are fitted in about 5% of women in the childbearing years.

6.5　What are the effects of IUD insertion on the genital tract?

Many cellular and biochemical changes have been described, but it is now clear that any IUD in situ long term acts chiefly by interfering with gametes and fertilization (Q 5.7).

1　All types of IUD lead to a marked increase in the number of leucocytes, both in the endometrium and in the uterine and tubal fluid. All the different types of white cell involved in a typical foreign body reaction are represented.

2　Inert and copper devices lead to elevated levels of many prostaglandins.

3　Copper enhances the foreign body reaction and leads to a range of biochemical changes in the endometrium, affecting enzyme systems and hormone receptors.

4　Copper ions are also toxic to sperm and blastocyst.

5　Progestagen-releasing IUDs alter endometrial histology with a decidual reaction and glandular atrophy, and block oestrogen

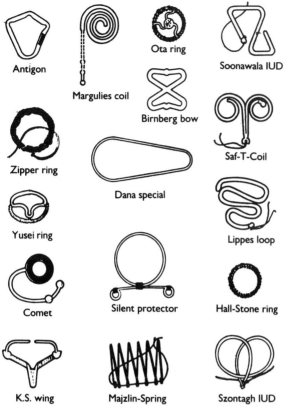

Antigon

Margulies coil

Ota ring

Birnberg bow

Soonawala IUD

Zipper ring

Dana special

Saf-T-Coil

Yusei ring

Lippes loop

Comet

Silent protector

Hall-Stone ring

K.S. wing

Majzlin-Spring

Szontagh IUD

Figure 6.1 Past inert IUDs – see Figures 6.8, 6.10 and 6.11 for bioactive IUDs. Q 6.3.

and progesterone receptors. They also markedly reduce the sperm penetrability of mucus to sperm.

6.6 Are there any known systemic effects of IUDs (outside the genital tract)?

An increase in some circulating immunoglobulins has been reported, but neither this nor the minute amount of copper entering the systemic circulation in copper IUD users is thought to be of clinical significance (except in Wilson's disease, see Q 6.80). Absorption of hormones or any other chemicals which are carried by bioactive devices must always be presumed; but systemic effects of the progestagen-releasing IUDs are small (and depend on the release rate).

Inert and copper IUDs have no effect on the pituitary or ovary. However uterine shedding starts 2–3 days before circulating levels of oestrogen and progesterone have reached the levels usual at the start of the menses in non-IUD-users.

6.7 So what is the main mode of action of IUDs?

The main effect is now believed to be by the blocking of fertilization. The inflammatory cells of the fluid in the whole genital tract (including the tubes) appear with all IUDs to impede sperm transport and fertilization. Actual phagocytosis of the sperm has been reported. In various studies of long-term IUD users viable sperm have rarely been found in the uterine cavity, the tubes or in aspirates of the pouch of Douglas, in clear contrast with the findings in sexually active controls.

Blastocysts have however been flushed from the cavities of other users, showing that the implantation-blocking effect is a back-up contraceptive mechanism. Also the remarkable effectiveness of IUDs when inserted postcoitally, up to 5 days after ovulation, indicates that they can still be remarkably efficacious when the action cannot be by blocking fertilization. To work by this mechanism IUDs seem only to require to be present in the uterus for the last 9 days of each cycle. This implies the need for caution whenever IUDs are removed (see Qs 6.13 and 6.14).

The progesterone or progestagen-releasing IUDs (see Qs 6.132–5) markedly impair the sperm penetrability of cervical-uterine fluid, as well as sometimes stopping fertile ovulation: so that the above anti-implantation effect is likely to be a redundant back-up mechanism.

6.8 So IUDs appear to act differently when they are in situ long term?

Certainly. The postfertilization effect is probably rare with all IUDs. But if a potential user has ethical problems about that possibility she should perhaps only use progestagen-releasing devices, when available.

6.9 Why are inert devices now no longer inserted in the UK?

Their market was taken by the copper IUDs. As the surface area of inert devices is reduced, so the bleeding and pain side-effects are minimized but the failure rate increases. By virtue of its additional contraceptive actions (see Q 6.5), copper enables smaller devices to be used without loss of efficacy. The major advantage of inert devices (long-term use through to the menopause) is disappearing with the steady increase in permissible duration of use of copper IUDs (see Q 6.129).

EFFECTIVENESS

6.10 What is the overall failure rate?

For all current devices this is low, in the range of 0.3–2.0/100 woman-years including pregnancies which are due to unrecognized expulsions (estimated at about one-third of the total in the first year).

Two IUD designs stand out as the most effective currently available. These are the levonorgestrel-releasing *LNG–20 μg IUD* discussed later (see Q 6.132), and the *Copper T 380A 'Slimline'* (and various clones bearing copper collars on the side arms). Based on no less than 16 000 woman-years of use in multicentre WHO and Population Council studies the latter can now be said to be at least as effective as the COC! (see Table 0.2). *Each year in the first 5 the failure rate is 0.3/100 woman–years, falling to 0.1 in years 6–8.*

The time has come to move away from using so often the present UK market-leader, the Nova T design. See Qs 6.90 and 6.91.

6.11 What factors influence failure rates (and other problems) of IUDs?

1 In fact, by far the most important is competence of the doctor or other professional inserting the device. Comparative studies invariably show that the difference between doctors, for all the problems – summarized at Q 6.22 – is greater than the difference between devices.

2 The second most important factor in comparative studies is the age and hence relative fertility of the population. Above 35, the first-year failure rate (of 0.1–0.5/100 woman-years with any device) is so good that IUDs become the method of choice for many older women (see Qs 6.20 and 6.23).

3 Duration of use (see Q 6.125).

6.12 Are the various aspects of device design almost irrelevant then?

No. Attention to the shape and size of a device and of its introducer, and the insertion technique, can all influence efficacy. The ideal design would maximize delivery of any bioactive agent such as copper to the most important (high fundal) zone, and minimize:

1 the likelihood of malposition (especially too low in the cavity);

2 the likelihood of expulsion;

3 the liability to and seriousness of uterine perforation (see Qs 6.42 and 6.44).

Also:

4 the severity and duration of bleeding and pain (see Q 6.71).

5 the liability to exacerbate pelvic infection (see Q 6.53);

The first three problems are all, whatever else, relevant to efficacy.

6.13 How can insufficient caution when removing an IUD cause iatrogenic pregnancy?

The answer follows from Q 6.7 above. If one of the major actions of IUDs is to block implantation, removal at any time before the last 9 days of the cycle can enable the blastocyst to arrive at a non-IUD-bearing uterus. Pregnancy could therefore result even if a women were being sterilized at the time of removal, and this has in fact been reported. A more serious risk would be a clip-induced ectopic, due to trapping the blastocyst in the tube. These events are rare because of the other contraceptive effects of in situ IUDs (see Q 6.5), but they are entirely preventable (see Q 8.16).

6.14 How can such pregnancies be avoided?

Either by removal during a period, or more usually by following a '7-day rule', that is advice in advance to abstain or use a barrier method for 7 days before any IUD is removed. Seven days is believed to allow sufficient time, namely that between ejaculation and the latest likely implantation, for the IUD to have its antinidatory effects in that cycle. The 7-day rule is particularly important prior to sterilization, for fear of that iatrogenic tubal ectopic. It is also wise before any attempted replacement of an IUD.

Occasionally an IUD has to be removed midcycle although it has been recently relied upon (e.g. see Q 6.61). Postcoital hormone treatment should be considered in such cases (see Ch. 7).

6.15 How can excessive caution about the time of insertion of IUDs cause iatrogenic pregnancies?

By slavish adherence to the *myth* that it is best to insert only during or just after the menses! If women are told to wait until after their next period, not a few return pregnant. Several US-based studies have shown that IUDs can be inserted with relative safety *on the day they are requested*, if the woman's history indicates she is unlikely to have an implanted pregnancy.

Especially relevant was a US study which showed a statistically significant doubling of the rate of *expulsion* if copper-T IUDs were inserted on days 1–5 of the cycle as compared with days 11–17. Since the patients were unaware of the expulsion (usually partial) in nearly 40% of the cases, extra pregnancies could actually be caused by only inserting IUDs during the menses.

Finally, of course, deliberate postcoital IUD insertion up to day 19 of a 28-day cycle (adjusted for cycle length) is very effective (see Q 6.7).

6.16 What is the likely explanation for a high expulsion rate when IUDs are inserted very early in the cycle?

The main increase in expulsion rate occurs when IUDs are inserted during the menstrual flow, and is probably linked with extra myometrial activity at that time due to prostaglandins. The intraluminal pressure can rise above 100 mmHg and the fundal cavity is also narrower at this time than it is midcycle.

6.17 So when are IUDs best inserted?

The answer is – not during heavy days of the menses but at any time from their ending phase through until about midcycle. At the Margaret Pyke Centre (MPC) we target days 4–14 of a normal cycle. Beyond that if intercourse has been continuing, postcoital insertion in good faith is still permissible up to 5 days after the calculated ovulation day (see Q 7.11), but with caution and counselling, good records and follow-up.

6.18 Should adjunctive contraceptive measures be recommended to IUD-users following insertion?

Many women select this method precisely because they desire a non-intercourse-related method. However, there are three arguments for a very positive attitude to this approach, ideally using a male or female condom, or if not a spermicide or the contraceptive sponge (see Q 3.55), particularly during intercourse at times when the user herself perceives an extra risk. These are:

1 To provide some protection against both sexually transmitted and non-specific pelvic infection (see Qs 6.48 and 6.49), since there is good evidence that 'spermicides are also germicides'. Nonoxynol-9 is insufficient protection against HIV though, hence condoms are preferable.

2 Especially in early months, to provide some protection in the event of unrecognized expulsion, which is common and may be unnoticed in the menstrual flow.

3 To reduce the relatively higher risk of method failure in the young (see Q 6.11). This is less important if the Copper-T 380S is used (see Q 6.10).

ADVANTAGES AND BENEFITS

6.19 What are the advantages of IUDs?

These can be listed:

1 the method is highly effective;

2 it has no known, unwanted *systemic* effects;

3 it is nearly always reversible (see Q 6.130);

4 it is independent of intercourse;

5 it does not require any day-to-day actions, such as taking a pill;

6 motivation is chiefly required around the time of insertion and never subsequently if side-effects are acceptable – it then being truly a 'default' method;

7 it is relatively cheap and easy to distribute;

8 it does not influence milk volume or composition; and finally

9 with sympathetic providers the method is under a woman's control and (a point of occasional relevance) if the threads are removed, can be undetectable by her partner.

What a wonderful list of advantages! Why then do we not at least *offer* this choice far more, *as a routine to all parous young women in stable relationships?*

6.20 For whom are IUDs indicated?

The answer is: *upon request* for contraception, unless the absolute contraindications apply (see Qs 6.79 and 6.80) or if the relative contraindications are unacceptable to the woman herself after discussion in the light of alternatives. More specifically, in view of the threats to fertility (see Q 6.23(d)), and the fact that these are not only more serious when there is no family but also more probable in the young, current IUDs are not first-choice methods for most women until they have had children. (I say 'most women': only women themselves can make a realistic assessment of their state of monogamy or otherwise.)

After childbearing IUDs are an excellent 'holding manoeuvre' until the time that the couple are certain that their family is complete (and the man perhaps volunteers for his vasectomy!). Alternatively the method may be so acceptable that it remains in use until final removal 1 year following the menopause.

6.21 Is it possible that newer IUDs may broaden the indications?

Certainly. The LNG20-IUD (see Qs 6.132 and 6.133) in particular, may 'rewrite the textbooks' in relation to use by young nulliparae at high risk of pelvic infection. Progestagen-releasing devices may also be of special value as definitive treatment for women with menorrhagia, or with climacteric symptoms (see Q 6.135).

MAIN PROBLEMS AND DISADVANTAGES

6.22 In summary, what are the major problems and disadvantages of intrauterine contraception?

These can be listed briefly as follows:

1 *Intrauterine pregnancy* – increased risk of miscarriage, hence of infection.

2 *Extrauterine pregnancy* (but no increase in overall population risk, see Q 6.30).

3 *Expulsion* with risks of pregnancy (see item 1).

4 *Perforation* with risks of pregnancy, also risk of IUD penetration of bowel/bladder and adhesion formation – and the risks of surgery;

5 *Malposition* of the device which may cause items 1,7 and 8 in this list, as wall as 'lost threads'.

6 *Pelvic infection/salpingitis.*

7 *Pain.*

8 *Abnormal bleeding* – this may be increased in amount, duration, and/or frequency.

> **Note:** All available data are reassuring concerning *carcinogenesis*, whether of endometrium/or cervix. Rare problems are considered at Qs 6.82, 6.111 and 6.116.

6.23 Can the problems in Q 6.22 be interconnected? Please give examples.

(a) *Insertion* – is capable (either directly or indirectly) of causing any one of the eight problems.

(b) *Pain* – may be a symptom of 1–6. Hence these should first be excluded before terming it a side-effect (i.e. something that the woman may or may not be able to 'live with'). Beware the stoical woman or the one who tries too hard to avoid troubling the doctor!

(c) *Bleeding* – might mean numbers 1, 2, 3, 5 (definitely) and 6 (sometimes). So this too is not necessarily just a side effect.

(d) *Fertility* – (again indirectly or directly) can be impaired by any of 1–6 (see Qs 6.25, 6.33, and 6.48).

(e) *'Lost threads'* – may signify any of 1, 3, 4 and 5 (see Q 6.32).

(f) *Malposition* of the device may cause numbers 1, 3, 7 and 8 in this list, as well as 'lost threads';

(g) *Age* – increases the risk of 2 (ectopics) and of 8 (heavy bleeding), anyway, whether or not an IUD be present. But it definitely *reduces* the risk of 1, 3 and 6 (see Qs 6.11, 6.37 and 6.48).

(h) *Duration of use* – may increase the risk of 2 (mainly, it is thought, through increasing age). But it *reduces* almost all the other problems! i.e. 1,3,6,7 and 8 (see Qs 6.124–6.129).

It is instructive to consider further examples, such as: which of the eight IUD problems in Q 6.22 would pose special problems in nulliparae?

Intrauterine pregnancy (IUD in situ)

6.24 Does intrauterine pregnancy pose problems for IUD-users? In the first place, is there an increased risk of teratogenesis?

There is absolutely no evidence for an increased risk of any of the commoner fetal abnormalities, whether the device be present at the time of conception or during organogenesis – at least for the inert and copper-containing types. Proof of this is (as usual) impossible, especially as 2% of all babies have an abnormality, and most particularly for the rarer disorders. There are as yet no adequate data concerning any possible effects of progesterone – or a progestagen-containing device – on a continuing pregnancy.

6.25 Should the device be removed, and if so, surely this will increase the risk of miscarriage?

Paradoxically the 'obvious' course of action – which is to leave the device alone, so as to avoid disturbing the pregnancy – has been shown to lead to a high rate of miscarriage (above 50%). Moreover, more often than expected this occurs in the second trimester with dangerous complications, particularly haemorrhage and sepsis. Septic second-trimester abortions were 26 times more frequent in one study. There is also evidence that the risks of antepartum haemorrhage, of preterm delivery and of stillbirth are increased if the IUD remains present.

Such problems are not restricted to the Dalkon Shield, although first reported for that device. Tatum (inventor of the first T-device) produced good evidence that removal of a copper device in the early part of pregnancy reduced the spontaneous abortion rate from 54% to 20%.

6.26 How should removal of the device be managed?

First, the woman should be counselled and warned that she is at increased risk of miscarriage whatever is done, but that the risk can be reduced considerably by gentle removal of the device. This should then be performed, at the earliest possible stage in pregnancy, whenever the threads of the device are still accessible. If the threads are (already) missing, consider the possibility of perforation, and in all cases categorize/supervise the pregnancy as 'high risk' (see Q 6.25). See also Q 6.28 re-ensuring that the location of the IUD is established after delivery.

In rare cases of heavy bleeding or leakage of liquor the woman may need immediate admission. Usually she may continue as an outpatient, with appropriate advice about the subsequent occurrence of any pain, or more bleeding than the slight show to be expected at IUD removal.

6.27 What if the outcome after counselling is to be a legal abortion?

Clearly the removal of the device is then best performed at the time of termination. In my view there should be routine chlamydia testing and antibiotic cover for such procedures. This is indicated even more strongly:

1 if the woman is first seen with an IUD-associated incomplete abortion (take swabs first), or

2 if medical induction of the termination be planned, with mifepristone and/or prostaglandins (PGs).

This is because of anecdotes of very severe infections, implying that the presence of the foreign body increases the sepsis risk. In 2, I advise that the IUD is removed at the time of the first administration of the treatment, whether mifepristone or PG pessary, and not left to come away with the products of conception.

6.28 What if the original IUD is never found following spontaneous or induced abortion? Or at full term?

It is unbelievable how often the original presence of an IUD gets forgotten, especially after delivery. Women may then finish up with two IUD devices, or even one in their uterus and one still at large, free in the abdomen . . . . This is indefensible.

One can readily exclude either an embedded or perforated device with plain abdominal X-rays supplemented by ultrasound scanning if available (see Q 6.36).

Extrauterine pregnancy

6.29 What is the risk of extrauterine pregnancy when an IUD-user becomes pregnant, and is the rate really increased?

No! to the second question. First and foremost, since the last edition of this book it is now clearly established that: *copper IUDs do not increase the overall risk of ectopics in a population, as compared with suitable non–IUD-using controls.*

The rate of ectopics is fundamentally dependent on the rate of pelvic infection (see Qs 6.49–50) in that community. Because in situ copper IUDs drastically reduce fertilization rates (see Q 6.7), even women with damaged tubes, who will be at definite risk of an ectopic when they come to try for a pregnancy, may well escape this while using an IUD.

The risk among current users of the Progestasert (progesterone-containing) IUD appears to have been truly higher; but the more potent LNG IUD seems to block fertilization so well that in the Population Council study (1991) no ectopics at all occurred during a massive 3371 woman-years of use!

6.30 But surely ectopics are commoner among IUD conceptions?

Precisely so, but this does not invalidate the above answer. As a working rule, the ratio increases roughly tenfold. Thus approximately 1 in 10–20 IUD-associated pregnancies will be extrauterine if the background rate is 1 in 100–200 pregnancies among non-IUD users. My assessment of the literature is as follows:

1 In the first place, IUDs do not prevent extrauterine pregnancy quite as well as they prevent intrauterine pregnancy. Hence there will be such a great reduction in the *denominator* of uterine pregnancies as to lead to an increased *rate*, even though the *numerator* of ectopic pregnancies is also reduced (but not by so much).

It may help to use real numbers:

	Annual conceptions (no.)	Ectopics (no.)	Ratio
Ordinarily, in a society, let the ectopic rate be 1 in 100 pregnancies. Assuming no infertility, if 1000 women use no contraception:	1000	10	1 : 100
If the same 1000 women use a copper IUD with a 1st-year failure rate of 1/100 woman-years:	10	1	1 : 10
Difference:	990	9	

Thus although 1 in 10 of the IUD conceptions is ectopic, this is actually a valuable reduction of 9 in the expected number in the population. The ratio is higher because of the massive reduction of 990 in the number of conceptions. And very probably, even the one woman who has an ectopic while using the IUD was due to get one (along with the other nine women) in the future, anyway, when trying to conceive.

A similar explanation holds for the apparently increased *rate* of ectopics among conceptions with the POP, which nevertheless also protects against ectopics as compared with non-contracepting controls (probably better than the IUD does though less well than the COC).

2 There is a second mechanism, which could also be operating. If IUD-related or exacerbated inflammation occurred in the tubes of IUD-users, this could lead to interference with the movement of any fertilized ovum. This would allow some true IUD-related ectopics to occur.

As we have just seen there is no real need to invoke this second explanation to explain the observed rates. Yet my view is that this second mechanism may explain some ectopics, the IUD thus being a co-factor for a *few* tube-damaging infections (see Q 6.53–4), especially as chlamydia can be notoriously silent. But such ectopics may well not happen until after the IUD is removed. And even then the lifestyle of the woman or her partner is really more responsible than the IUD.

6.31 Is there an increased risk of ectopics with duration of use?

Some studies show this, others, especially of the new *banded* IUDs, do not. It is presently thought that the apparent association is mainly because longer-term users are also older – and the proportion of pregnancies which are ectopic rises with age in the general population.

6.32 What are the implications for management?

The main point is that, even if only by the above *selection* mechanism (more ectopics being allowed to happen *relative* to the intrauterine pregnancies), once an IUD-user is pregnant she could well have an ectopic. So the clinical slogan is:

> Every IUD-user with menstrual irregularity and pelvic discomfort has an ectopic pregnancy till proved otherwise.

In practice every IUD-user in whom pregnancy is suspected, with or without a positive pregnancy test, should have a pelvic examination to detect adnexal tenderness; and each IUD-user should be warned prospectively, backed by a leaflet, that any marked pelvic pain should always receive prompt medical attention, particularly if her period is late.

Beware also of the IUD-user who has just been sterilized. She could have a clip-induced ectopic if she was not advised appropriately (Q 6.13, 6.14) not to rely on the IUD for 7 days presurgery.

6.33 Is past tubal pregnancy a contraindication to IUD use?

In my view this is a relative contraindication in parous women and absolutely contraindicates the copper IUD method for nulliparae (see Q 6.80). Although *the method does not increase the overall risk of ectopics in a population*, it does as we have seen sometimes selectively fail to prevent them. The woman concerned should surely use a method which will provide maximal protection to her one remaining tube. Another poor choice would therefore be the progestagen-only pill (see Q 5.33). Good choices would be the combined pill or an injectable/implant, or the LNG-IUD when available (see Q 6.132), or even a very conscientiously used barrier method.

'Lost threads'

6.34 What is the differential diagnosis of 'lost threads' with IUDs?

The first possibility is that the threads are in fact present but not being palpated by the user. This may be due to her inexperience, or the threads may have retreated to just within the external os. If the threads are truly absent then the differential diagnosis is as shown in Table 6.1.

6.35 What are the 'do's and don'ts' of the management of 'lost threads'?

The first message from Table 6.1 is another IUD 'slogan', namely that:

> IUD-users with lost threads either are already pregnant, or at increased risk of becoming pregnant.

This is hardly surprising: the device is just as *absent* from the uterine cavity after perforation as after expulsion, and if the IUD is only malpositioned this might still leave part of the cavity unprotected.

1 All such women therefore need to be advised to use an alternative contraceptive method until the protective presence of an IUD has been established.

Table 6.1 Differential diagnosis of 'lost threads' with IUDs

Main diagnoses A: Not pregnant	Clinical clues	B: Pregnant	Clinical clues
(1) Device in uterus. Threads cut too short, or caught up around device during original insertion or avulsed at a previous removal attempt; or device itself malpositioned	(a) Periods likely to be those characteristic of IUD in situ (b) Uterus normal size	(4) Device in situ + pregnancy	(a) Amenorrhoea (b) Pregnancy test likely to be positive, with clinically enlarged uterus (sufficient to pull up thread)
(2) Unrecognized expulsion	(a) Recent periods as woman's normal pattern (b) Uterus normal size	(5) Unrecognized expulsion + pregnancy	(a) Amenorrhoea, following one or more apparently normal periods (i.e. unmodified by IUD) (b) Signs of pregnancy variably present (may be too early on first presentation)
(3) Perforation of uterus	As (2) plus (rarely) mass or actual IUD palpated on bimanual examination	(6) Perforation of uterus + pregnancy	As (5) plus (rarely) mass or actual IUD identified on bimanual examination

2 Consider also the possible need for postcoital contraception, especially if recent expulsion is diagnosed (see Q 7.18).

3 In general, X-rays and any form of intrauterine manipulation should be arranged in the follicular phase of the menstrual cycle, for fear of disturbing a pregnancy.

4 Above all, women with this problem need full explanations and supportive counselling throughout the management, which is described below (see Q 6.36).

6.36 What is the recommended protocol for the management of 'lost threads'?

I recommend the following very practical scheme (Fig. 6.2). Diagnosis and treatment are simultaneous in most cases, with minimum use of hospital facilities:

1 *Exclude implanted pregnancy.* Take a careful menstrual history, do a bimanual examination and if indicated perform the most sensitive pregnancy test available. If the woman is pregnant, the management is primarily that of the pregnancy itself. *Note: However*, if an IUD is not recovered in the products of conception, or at full term in the placenta, an X-ray should be taken before assuming expulsion (as opposed to perforation or malposition).

In the absence of pregnancy, proceed as follows: *during the follicular phase of the cycle*, but preferably *not* during heavy days of the menstrual flow (see Qs 6.16 and 6.59):

2 *First insert long–handled Spencer-Wells forceps or equivalent into the endocervical canal.* In a recent (1992) MPC study of 400 women with 'lost threads', almost 50% of the IUDs were retrieved this way! Meaning that they had a wasted trip, since this could so easily have been done by the referring doctor.

If the threads are readily located and the IUD judged (perhaps after sounding) to be correctly located, no further action need be taken; but disappearance of the threads may be a sign of malposition. So it is often advisable – after discussion with the woman – to remove and replace the device. *An ultrasound scan may be helpful* here (see section 6 below).

3 *Try the use of thread–retrievers.* The most established of these in the UK is the Emmett retriever, which is available presterilized and disposable. It has a handle to which is attached a thin plastic strip with multiple notches designed to trap the threads, when the edge is used like a curette against each surface of the

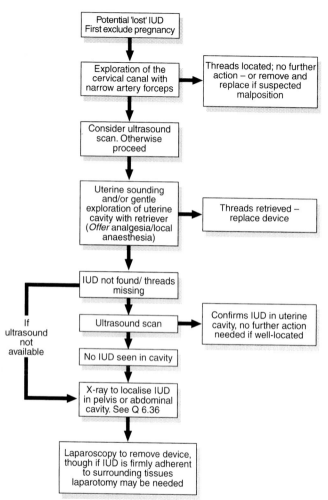

Figure 6.2 Management of 'lost' IUD threads. Q 6.36

fundus. There is also the Retrievette. The 'MI-Mark Helix' was found to be significantly less effective than either of these in the MPC study.

What about analgesia?

(a) Ideally a prostaglandin inhibitor such as mefenamic acid should be given about 30–60 minutes before any intrauterine manipulations.

(b) A few women, especially nulliparae, require a paracervical block with local anaesthetic (see Q 6.103). I have no personal experience of the instillation of sterile dental anaesthetic jelly, which is recommended by some authorities.

(c) Pretreatment with ethinyloestradiol (EE; 30 µg daily for 5 days) or, very simply, with one 100 µg oestradiol skin patch for 4 days may be given to soften and dilate the cervical canal. This would be appropriate if the cervix is not expected to be maximally oestrogenized (i.e. because the woman will be seen early or late in the cycle, or is peri- or post-menopausal). Oral HRT is another option (Q 6.117).

4 *Various resterilizable IUD retrieving forceps* (made by Rocket or Zeppelin), with short jaws opening wholly in the uterine cavity, may next be tried with success. Another option is suction using a Karman curette.

5 *Next try small, blunt IUD–removal hooks (Grafenberg pattern).* In skilled hands these metal devices can be used to hook down either a thread or part of the device itself. Excessive traction is dangerous (see Q 6.47).

6 *Arrange appropriate imaging.* If the facilities are available, an ultrasound (US) scan may be arranged at this point. This should be done earlier in order not to cause unnecessary discomfort, if the device was not readily located by sound or retriever at Stage 3 above. Confirmation of correct intrauterine location within a non-pregnant uterus can be helpful for a woman who wishes to continue using the same device; but if there is any suspicion that it is malpositioned (e.g. too low or rotated), appropriate steps should be taken for its removal as above.

Local anaesthesia is nearly always sufficient. General anaethesia should very rarely be required for any device which is in utero.

If the scan shows unequivocally that the uterus is empty, an X-ray is then required to differentiate between expulsion and perforation (see Qs 6.37–47).

7 *What if US facilities are not available?* It may then be useful to *arrange an X-ray with a uterine marker.* The most practical marker is another IUD, preferably of a different pattern from that originally fitted. There are three possible X-ray findings:

(a) Only the newly inserted device visible. This implies unrecognized expulsion of the first device.

(b) Two IUDs shown on the abdominal radiograph in close proximity. If a lateral view also shows that the IUDs are contiguous this means that the first device is actually in utero. This should be a rare finding if the X-ray is arranged only after stages 1–4 above. However, it is well worth removing the second IUD, as this may bring down part of the original device. More commonly curettage is necessary.

(c) The IUDs may be clearly separated on the X-ray. This establishes the diagnosis of complete perforation (translocation) (see Qs 6.42–47).

Expulsion

6.37 What is the frequency of partial or complete expulsion?

In most large studies this ranges from about 3 to 15/100 women at 1 year. The rates are influenced by:

1 characteristics of the woman (age, parity and uterine shape) – also the timing of insertion in relation to the menses (see Qs 6.15–6.17);

2 the size and nature of the device;

3 above all, the skill of the person performing the insertion.

6.38 When do expulsions most commonly occur?

During the menses, most particularly the first or second menstruation after insertion. About one-third of first year pregnancies among IUD-users occur after unnoticed expulsion. This should not happen if women are instructed to check for the presence of the threads (and the absence of any part of a partially expelled device), after each period and prior to relying on the device for that cycle. Among users for more than 3 years, the expulsion rate with most devices approaches nil. (See also Qs 6.35 and 7.18.)

6.39 What effect do age and parity have on the expulsion rate?

Nulliparous women have higher expulsion rates for all devices than do parous women. After the first child there is a negligible effect of increasing parity on the expulsion rate. However, IUD expulsion rates seem to decline in a fairly linear fashion with increasing age. In studies either of parous or of nulliparous women, the rates of expulsion are about half above the age of 30 as compared with women under that age.

6.40 What is the effect of the size and shape of the uterus?

If the cavity of the uterus is distorted, either congenitally or by fibroids, there will be an increase in uterine activity (and cramps) and an increased likelihood of both malposition and expulsion. Ideally, such women should avoid the intrauterine method. Careful sounding as described at Q 6.104 during the insertion may lead to a change of plan, but in practice quite gross distortions of the uterine cavity may be difficult to identify clinically. (See Fig. 6.5 and Q 6.87.) If in doubt a good preinsertion ultrasound scan is invaluable.

6.41 What is the effect of the size and shape of the device itself?

Different expulsion rates between devices certainly exist. For example, the rate for the now defunct Copper 7 (particularly for partial expulsions) was considerably higher than that for the Multiload IUDs even after controlling for other variables. However, expulsion rates are probably more correlated with the precise fit of the device within the uterus of different women. It is becoming clear that many IUDs are too wide for the uterine cavity at the fundus in vivo, particularly during menstruation; and also too long for the many nulliparae (see Q 6.89).

The Cu-fix (FlexiGard) solves the problem of fitting the uterus comfortably in a unique way (see Q 6.131) and so has a particularly low expulsion rate (3%).

Perforation

6.42 What problems are associated with uterine fundal perforation?

1 First, pregnancy. Most perforations first present as a pregnancy with 'lost threads'.

2 Secondly, if the device is bioactive (copper or progestagen-containing) it leads to adhesion formation or may penetrate the

wall of bowel or bladder. 'Closed' devices (e.g. rings) are particularly associated with bowel strangulation.

6.43 Should perforated devices be removed? Should it be considered an emergency?

In countries with developed medical services the benefits of removal always outweigh the risks. There are usually no specific symptoms so removal can be elective after diagnosis (see Q 6.36). However, while waiting for hospital admission the patient should be warned to use alternative contraception, and that any abdominal pain, particularly if there is associated diarrhoea, must be reported promptly. Serious complications involving the bowel have been reported (including one death from peritonitis in a Copper 7-user).

6.44 What is the frequency of uterine perforation following IUD insertion?

The true incidence is difficult to establish but is commonly quoted as around 1 per 1000 insertions. It is probably even lower for T-shaped IUDs that are positioned by a 'withdrawal' technique. Only one perforation in 1815 insertions of such devices was reported by Chi in 1987. See also Q 8.23.

6.45 What factors affect the perforation rate?

The rate is affected by the usual three kinds of variable.

1 *Features of the woman.* The main factor here is recent pregnancy. Puerperal insertion is notorious in this respect, particularly if the woman is *breastfeeding*. See Q 8.23. This means extra care!

2 *Features of the device.* Linear devices such as the Lippes Loop, which were inserted by a 'push' technique (rather than the 'withdrawal' techniques now more commonly used) were more likely to perforate. An important safety factor is to avoid loading any IUD into its inserter too far ahead of the insertion, so that the plastic loses its 'memory' (see Q 6.106).

3 *Features of the inserting clinician.* This is by far and away the most important factor. As Lippes himself observed: 'IUDs do not perforate. For this to happen we need a practitioner.' Almost all perforations are produced at insertion even though the diagnosis may be long delayed (and frequently emerges only when the empty uterus permits a pregnancy). Perforations are commoner when the operator is inexperienced; when the position of the uterus is misdiagnosed (especially unrecognized retroversion)

and probably when a holding forceps or tenaculum is not used to steady the cervix. See Q 6.104.

6.46 What is the best way to remove perforated devices?

This can often be done with minimal trauma by simple colpotomy (when the device is palpable in the pouch of Douglas); or at laparoscopy. If there are adhesions, the device can sometimes be grasped at one end or the other and pulled through its own 'tunnel'. However, great care is necessary as devices can be adherent to the actual wall of bowel or bladder. If in doubt, therefore, a minilaparotomy or full laparotomy may be safer, especially for bioactive devices.

6.47 Are there any special points about embedding and partial perforation?

If part of a partially translocated device can be grasped within the uterus, it may be possible to remove it transcervically. However, this should be done with great gentleness. It is possible for the part of the device which is through the uterine wall to be adherent to bowel or bladder. Removal under ultrasound or laparoscopic control may occasionally be much safer. See also Q 6.116 and Figure 6.9.

Pelvic infection

6.48 Do IUDs cause or aggravate pelvic inflammatory disease (PID)?

There can be little doubt of this being an associated hazard. But to what extent if at all is the association causal? Studies have repeatedly shown an increased risk of such infections in IUD-users as compared with controls, though there are major problems with selecting the latter (see Q 6.49). When they occur, in some studies, attacks appear to be of greater severity than in cases without the associated foreign body.

Now according to Westrom, one severe attack of laparoscopically diagnosed PID of any type carries a 1 in 8 risk of infertility due to tubal occlusion; two attacks, a 1 in 3 risk; and three attacks a 1 in 2 risk. So this has rightly become the greatest single anxiety about the IUD method, particularly for use by nulliparae.

6.49 What is the frequency of PID among IUD-users?

The absolute risk varies enormously according to the background rate of (sexually transmitted) PID in the population studied. The problem is that in most comparative studies the controls have been themselves *protected* against infection, either by using barrier methods or the combined pill. Oral contraception approximately halves the risk of PID (see Q 4.37).

Westrom studied all women aged 20–29 in the town of Lund, Sweden and found the incidence of PID per 1000 woman-years to be 52 for IUD-users, as compared with 34 for sexually active users of no contraception, 14 for barrier method-users and nine for pill-users. This suggests that the effect of IUDs as compared with 'true' controls (i.e. at equivalent societal risk of PID but not protected by their contraception) would be an increase between 50% and 100% in the rate of clinical disease. Even this may be too high an estimate of the real IUD-attributable risk. The main effect of IUDs seems to be to worsen any attack of PID (which is in reality a 'self- or partner-inflicted wound'), or make it more likely to be clinical rather than subclinical.

Several studies have shown low or absent risk in women claiming only one sexual partner. Even more convincing, in the study described below, *among 4301 women fitted with IUDs in China, where monogamy is the norm, there was not one single case of PID reported!*

6.50 What light is thrown on this PID problem by the review of 12 international WHO studies published in *The Lancet*, March 1992?

22 908 women (almost all parous) had one of ten types of IUD inserted, and there are no less than 51 399 years of follow-up. The overall rate of PID was low, 1.6/1000 woman-years of use (cf. Lund in Q 6.49). The most important findings were:

1 PID risk was more than six times higher specifically during the first 20 days after insertion than later; the risk was constant and relatively low thereafter for up to 8 years, with no evidence of being any higher than the local background rate.

2 Rates varied by geographical area, highest in Africa and nil in China, and were inversely associated with age. This mirrors exactly the background risk of sexually transmitted diseases (STDs).

3 Whether considered individually or grouped by type, the PID rates for copper-bearing, hormonal and inert IUDs were statistically indistinguishable. For all these devices this makes a specific IUD factor in the attacks very improbable, especially as

previous studies were readily able to show that one device, the Dalkon Shield, did specifically increase PID risk (see Q 6.54).

6.51 What factors affect the rate of PID in IUD-users?

The usual three categories must be considered – features of the woman, the device and the insertion process.

6.52 What features of the woman can influence the PID rate?

First age, as a marker for the risk of sexually transmitted infections. The risk is highest in young women and declines in a linear fashion as age increases (Fig. 6.3). In a study at the MPC in London, the incidence of infection was 10 times greater below the age of 20 than it was above 30 – although the 871 women were all nulliparous, had received the same type of IUD (Copper 7), at the same centre and all in the first 10 days of the cycle. Since:

1 there is no evidence that the uterus becomes more resistant to infection with age, and since:

2 the isolation of specific cervical pathogens and rates of PID in non-IUD-users show decline with age and correlate with sexual lifestyle;

it seems most probable that the vast majority of cases of PID in IUD-users are primarily sexually acquired. (Often, of course, the infection is transmitted to the relatively monogamous IUD-user by her partner who is less so. After the age of 30, fidelity by both partners is more common.) See Q 6.50.

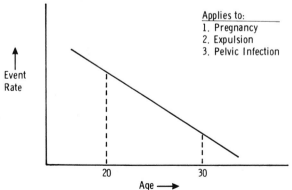

Figure 6.3 Effect of age on IUD performance. Qs 6.11, 6.39 and 6.52.

6.53 What features of the device can influence the rate of PID?

All IUDs are foreign bodies, and as such have the potential to facilate primary (sexually transmitted) infection, or to promote secondary invaders and the severity and chronicity of attacks. By definition, the foreign body effect of IUDs cannot be eliminated; however it may be reducible by device design, perhaps by:

1 avoiding embedding of part of the device in the myometrium;
2 elimination of the plastic carrier as in the FlexiGard (see Q 6.131);
3 release of progestagens or antiseptic substances into the cervical/uterine fluid, to hinder transfer of pathogens to the upper genital tract.

6.54 What is the effect of the threads traversing the cervical canal?

The thread of the now defunct Dalkon Shield was multifilament in design and this was shown to act as a 'wick'. Dalkon Shields should now always be removed on suspicion of their presence. Even when using IUDs with monofilament threads, however, elegant prehysterectomy studies by Sparks and Elstein have shown that symptomless bacterial infection of the lower part of the uterine fundus is almost invariable. However the uterus was always sterile if the threads were excised prior to insertion (even from Dalkon Shields).

This work may partly explain the short-term increased risk of PID in early days following insertion (see Q 6.50). So:

6.55 Should we go back to using threadless IUDs?

On balance, I think not. An early study in 1967 by Professor Elstein (now in Manchester) showed more infections among users of Lippes loops (with threads) than in threadless Birnberg bows. A (randomized) comparison from Sweden reported in 1992 a lower risk of clinical upper and lower genital tract infections at follow-up if the threads of Multiload Cu-250 devices were deliberately pushed into the uterus at insertion, than in normal Nova T controls. A third report from Hungary similarly showed higher PID rates in the group with threadless devices. However, at least six other comparisons of threadless and threaded IUDs have shown no difference in infection rate. More importantly, the WHO studies (see Q 6.50) among others, have shown vanishingly low rates of important infections among threaded device users if they were at low risk of STDs. This evidence suggests to me that pending more data any adverse influence of the threads must be very small in practice, and more than outweighed by their usefulness during IUD follow-up and to simplify device removal.

6.56 What features relating to insertion may promote infection?

Since it is impossible to sterilize the endocervical canal, both specific and non-specific organisms therein can be introduced into the uterus when IUDs are inserted. Such contamination is nearly always asymptomatic, but as we have seen above most studies have shown a higher rate of pelvic infection in the first 3–4 weeks after IUD insertion, thereafter diminishing with increased duration of use. Some of these early attacks may represent the flaring up of pre-existing infection of the upper tract, but others might be caused by the insertion process.

6.57 What are the *practical* implications, especially of the WHO studies (Q 6.50)?

1 Monogamous parous women as in China may use IUDs without fear of PID.

2 The remainder need to be informed where the infection really comes from, as well as very vigorous treatment when it happens! Or as the authors put it: 'exposure to sexually transmitted disease rather than type of IUD is the major determinant of PID'.

3 Providers should minimize the number of (dangerous) reinsertions (i.e. long term use is best, see Q 6.125)

4 The first routine follow-up visit might best be brought forward also, perhaps to 1 week? (see Q 6.114).

6.58 And how can we minimize the risk, stressed by WHO, of IUD insertion introducing or flaring up infection?

Ideally, screening for STDs, or at minimum chlamydia, should be arranged first, for all clients at the initial counselling visit. Positive results mean full therapy and contact tracing, and a reassessment of the decision to use this method.

As a second best, a careful preinsertion inspection of the cervix should always be performed. If there is an obvious purulent discharge (irrespective of the presence or otherwise of a cervical 'erosion'/ectopy, which is irrelevant), then endocervical swabs should be sent for urgent culture. The choice according to circumstances must be between postponement until the result of the culture is known, and careful insertion, possibly with a full course of antibiotic cover (usually a tetracycline). As always, this would be only in complete absence of pelvic tenderness.

6.59 What if there is a healthy cervix, no relevant symptoms, no tenderness and no discharge?

There should be the most thorough, mechanical cleansing to remove mucus from the external os. It is not yet agreed in this country that *routine* full antibiotic cover for every insertion is appropriate, but a low threshold is sensible.

See also Qs 6.15 and 6.16 *re* advisability of avoiding insertion during heavy days of bleeding; there is not only a higher expulsion rate following insertion at that time but also the suspicion of an increased infection risk.

6.60 How should IUD-associated pelvic infection be treated?

Bearing in mind the high likelihood that this is a sexually transmitted infection (see Q 6.52), ideally full bacteriological screening at a genitourinary medicine clinic should be performed. If such detailed bacteriology is impossible, at least endocervical swabs should be taken into the appropriate transport media. The usual first choice of antibiotic would be a tetracycline (preferably for at least 2 weeks, in order to treat the most common and possibly most harmful pathogen, namely chlamydia), with 5 days of metronidazole to deal with the frequently associated anaerobes such as bacteroides.

6.61 Should the IUD be removed?

There is controversy as to whether it should *always* be removed. My own threshold for doing this at the outset of treatment is very low in young nulliparous women – with consideration of the possible need for postcoital contraception according to the menstrual and coital histories (see Qs 6.13 and 6.14). The device should always be removed if there is no response to treatment within 48 hours, not omitting to arrange with the woman concerned a new method of birth control.

6.62 Should there be any other action, after IUD-associated PID?

Ideally, though regrettably this is not often done, the sexual contacts of all such women should be traced and appropriately treated. Moreover, a very clear warning should be given about the disastrous effects of *recurrent* PID (reaching after three hospitalized attacks a tubal occlusion rate of one in two), along with advice about condom use to avoid the other risk she may also be running, of HIV infection. All this is not being judgemental, just good preventive medicine.

6.63 Is pelvic infection *always* a contraindication to an IUD?

If currently acutely or chronically present, this is an absolute contraindication. All women reporting deep dyspareunia, or exhibiting tenderness of the pelvic organs whether on palpation or caused by cervical excitation, should not receive an IUD until infection has been excluded.

6.64 What about a history of past pelvic infection?

If this was not severe, more than 6 months ago and there has been no recurrence, and currently the woman is free of any symptoms or signs, then (after full discussion and counselling) IUD insertion is only relatively contraindicated. It would still be preferable that such a woman should have at least one living child. There should be serious consideration of tetracycline 'cover' for the insertion, and the woman preferably advised to use condoms or spermicides at each subsequent intercourse (see Q 6.18). She should also be advised to return exceptionally promptly at the first sign of another PID attack.

Past infection always contraindicates the IUD in a case at risk of endocarditis (see Q 6.86).

6.65 What is *Actinomyces israeli*?

This bacterium is normally a harmless commensal in the mouth and gastrointestinal tract. In the lower female genital tract it is only detected by cytology or culture when a foreign body is present.

6.66 How often are *Actinomyces*-like organisms (ALO) found in the cervical smears of IUD users?

The frequency with which routine smears show these organisms appears to relate in a linear fashion to the duration of use of the device. The organisms are virtually never found in the absence of an IUD. After 1 year's use 1–2% of smears are positive, rising to 8–10% after 3 years and over 20% after 5 years. It was at first though that copper prevented the carriage of these organisms. It is now believed that the main explanation for the lower incidence is the shorter average duration of use of copper than inert devices (plus, in the past, frequent *changes* – see Q 6.69).

6.67 What is the most serious potential significance of the finding of ALO in the cervical smear?

Frank actinomycosis is an extremely serious condition: a fatal outcome has been reported once in an IUD-user, and other young women have been known to require pelvic clearance as a lifesaving measure. However, the incidence of this complication is extremely low, even allowing for underdiagnosis among women with severe IUD-related infections. It seems clear that *actinomycosis represents a very small part of the spectrum of pelvic infection associated with IUDs.*

6.68 What action should be taken when a cervical smear report showing ALOs is received?

The patient should be recalled without delay and carefully questioned about the occurrence of pain, dyspareunia or excessive discharge. If there is even mild tenderness on examination, in my view the knowledge that ALOs are present should markedly lower the threshold for IUD removal. Endocervical swabs should be taken and sent with the removed device (threads excised), plus explanatory labelling, for appropriate bacteriology. Arrange appropriate referral for women with marked symptoms, either to a department of genitourinary medicine or a gynaecologist. If the laboratory recommends antibiotic therapy, penicillin is the usual choice but *in high dose for many weeks.*

However in most such cases no further action will be required, apart from arranging another method of birth control.

6.69 What action should be taken if ALOs are reported and there are *no symptoms* or signs at all?

Here there remains a dilemma. If over 20% of long-term IUD-users carry ALOs, and so very few ever develop symptoms, more morbidity (through resulting pregnancies) could be caused by insisting on device removal than by simply monitoring the situation with regular smears. The woman should be taught the symptoms associated with pelvic infection and advised if they occur to return even before her next routine smear.

A popular alternative course of action is simply to remove the device, send it for *culture* if this facility is available, and replace it *immediately* with a new (copper) IUD. In 1984 a study at the MPC showed that this schedule – device removal, *with or without* immediate reinsertion, and without any antibiotic treatment – was followed by disappearance of the ALOs from the subsequent cervical smears. Although later experience shows that such clearance is not invariable, most women after counselling now elect to try device replacement. If successful (checked by a cervical smear at 6–12 months and then annually), this reduces both *her* mild anxiety about harbouring a potential pathogen and *our* burden of responsibility for long-term follow-up.

Pain and bleeding

6.70 What is the most frequent complaint of IUD-users?

In practice, the most frequent problem is increased bleeding, so frequently accompanied by cramp-like menstrual pain that the two are often considered together. However, it is a good working slogan that: *Pain plus bleeding in an IUD-user has a serious cause until proved otherwise.*

The serious causes are listed at Q 6.23 above.

6.71 What types of bleeding pattern are observed by IUD-users?

The loss at the menses may be heavier and/or longer: the latter typically because of light premenstrual bleeding or spotting, before and after the flow proper. There may also be intermenstrual bleeding or spotting, too light to cause anaemia, but mighty troublesome to the woman.

6.72 How often do IUD-users discontinue the method because of pain or bleeding?

About 5–20% of inert or copper IUD-users have the device removed because of bleeding and pain within the first 12 months. Of the remainder, approximately half will admit to annoying bleeding symptoms which they have learnt to live with, and some will subsequently discontinue the method for the same reason. (Measurement of the loss has shown that inert devices roughly double the measured volume of flow, whereas the smaller copper ones only increase the amount by about 50%, that is about 20–30 ml on average.) Nevertheless removal rates have not been dramatically improved by copper devices. This is doubtless because they continue to cause the problems of prolongation of duration of flow and intermenstrual spotting.

These last two problems are still features of at least the early months of use of progestagen-releasing devices, even though they positively reduce the measured volume of loss. Perseverance is usually rewarded by frank amenorrhoea or infrequent light bleeds (see Q 6.134).

6.73 Is copper a haemostatic agent?

Menstrual blood loss measurement studies of my own in the 1970s, comparing Lippes Loops with and without copper bands (but otherwise identical) showed clearly that the measured mean volumes were similar. Indeed the *duration* of loss in the copper-using group was slightly increased. Hence it is possible to be definite, that the reduced amount of bleeding with copper devices is a function merely of their smaller size and surface area (see Q 6.9).

6.74 What is the cause of the increased bleeding as an IUD symptom, with or without pain?

1 Various types of *malposition* can cause both symptoms.

2 The fact that the cavity of the uterus is *distorted* congenitally or by fibroids may be missed, causing pain as the uterus attempts to expel the device.

3 Especially in *nulliparae* whose cavities tend to be smaller (see Q 6.89), the fitting of a *device which is too long or too wide* may similarly cause cramping pain. The stem of a device which is too long projects into the sensitive isthmic part of the uterus, and pain may also result from penetration of the myometrium by the side arms.

4 *Perforation of the cervix* by the stem of the device may result from partial expulsion and also cause pain (see Fig. 6.9 and Q 6.116).

In all these cases following bouts of cramping, some at least of the observed intermenstrual bleeding (IMB) may be caused by mechanical trauma to the endometrium.

5 According to some X-ray studies, small *devices which float too loosely* in a large cavity may also cause some IMB but without pain.

6.75 What is the uterine mechanism for IUD-related bleeding and pain?

Insertion of IUDs leads to a high concentration of plasminogen activators which increase fibrinolytic activity and hence lead to more blood flow. Linked in some way with these changes are alterations in the prostaglandin responses of the endometrium during menstruation. Prostacyclin activity is increased and this causes vasodilatation and inhibition of platelet function. An increase in other prostaglandins probably explains the increased menstrual cramps, but not why some are affected so much less than others.

6.76 Are there any drugs that can reduce the menstrual flow and pain in IUD-users?

There is no very effective therapy for the problem of prolonged spotting. However, for the heaviness of flow at the menses antifibrinolytic agents are certainly effective. Tranexamic acid is available, but it is not certain whether the benefits of treatment outweigh its well-documented risks (see Q 5.122), particularly as it is not an analgesic.

The pain-relieving prostaglandin synthetase inhibitors (PGSIs) are therefore normally preferable, particularly mefenamic acid (1500 mg), indomethacin (150 mg) and naproxen (1500 mg). (Amounts in parentheses are totals for each day, to be taken in divided doses.) These drugs need only be taken from the onset of menstruation, for so long as the patient feels the benefit from treatment. Response is very variable (Fig. 6.4), but some women report that the flow diminishes rapidly within an hour of taking a tablet.

6.77 Do many women persevere for long with an IUD if they have to take drugs regularly to cope with bleeding and/or pain?

Not as a rule. Few women would be happy to continue for years taking powerful drugs with each menstruation and doctors too would be worried by possible long-term risks. Antiprostaglandin drugs are certainly very useful to reduce the cramps at IUD insertion, and both pain and bleeding over the first few cycles. In

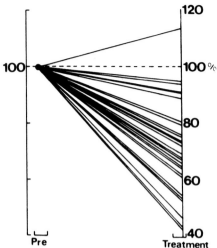

Figure 6.4 Percentage change in menstrual blood loss with mefenamic acid. Q 6.76. The figure shows the percentage reduction in menstrual blood loss with mefenamic acic 1500 g daily for a maximum of 7 days. The mean of two treatment periods is compared for each individual woman with the mean of two previous control periods expressed as 100%.
(From Guillebaud J 1978 Reduction by mefenamic acid of increased menstrual blood loss associated with intrauterine contraception. British Journal of Obstetrics and Gynaecology 85: 53–62, Figure 1)

practice, however, few women continue to take them (except intermittently for dysmenorrhoea) and the majority either live with their symptoms or eventually give up the IUD method.

Refitting, possibly with another design of IUD and perhaps after taking a 'break' for a couple of cycles, is sometimes beneficial.

SELECTION OF USERS AND OF DEVICES

Contraindications

Please see general discussion of this issue at Qs 4.101 and 4.102.

6.78 What are the absolute contraindications to IUD use?

These mostly relate to the side-effects which we have now considered. They can be classified into temporary absolute contraindications, which imply some variable delay before possible later insertion, and permanent contraindications.

6.79 What are the possibly temporary absolute contraindications?

1 Undiagnosed irregular *genital tract bleeding*. This is for fear of wrongly attributing postinsertion bleeding to the IUD, when in fact due to important uterine pathology, such as carcinoma of the endometrium.

2 Suspicion of *pregnancy*.

3 Current *pelvic infection* or pelvic tenderness/dyspareunia (see Q 6.63).

4 Recent exposure to *high risk of a sexually transmitted disease* (e.g. after rape) or marked purulent discharge. Ideally the insertion should be delayed until after full investigation; but in emergency situations such as postcoital contraception may be permissible with full antibiotic cover (after bacteriology arranged). See Qs 7.19 and 7.23.

5 *Immunosuppressive therapy*. See Q 6.83.

6.80 What are the permanent absolute contraindications?

6 Past history of tubal *ectopic pregnancy* (see Q 6.31) in *nulliparae*. Also past history of tubal surgery, or other very high ectopic risk, in those still wanting a child. In parous women these remain 'strong relative' contraindications.

7 Markedly *distorted uterine cavity*, or cavity sounding to less than 5.5 cm depth (see Fig. 6.5 and Q 6.87).

8 Known *true allergy* to a constituent (see Q 6.82).

9 Known *HIV infection or AIDS* (Q 6.83). Eventual interference with the immune system by the virus can be expected to increase the risk of severe infection.

10 *Wilson's disease* (copper devices).

11 Past attack of *bacterial endocarditis* or of severe pelvic infection in a woman with an anatomical lesion of the heart; or after any *prosthetic valve replacement* (Q 6.84).

6.81 What are the relative contraindications to IUD use?

These vary in their importance: the first is the nearest to being an absolute contraindication. Some are considered in more detail at

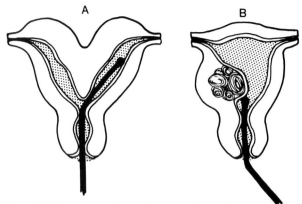

Figure 6.5 Uterine cavity distorted – congenitally or by fibroids. Q 6.80.
Note in A that it is easy to obtain a normal sounding depth despite a septate uterus.
Careful sounding will detect the abnormality, however, and will also identify a
submucous fibroid as in B.

subsequent questions. Nulliparity *combined* with 3, 4 or 5 would summate normally to produce an absolute contraindication.

1 *Valvular heart disease* with risk but no past history of bacterial endocarditis (see Q 6.84).

2 Any prosthesis which can be prejudiced by blood-borne infection, e.g. *hip replacement* (see Q 6.85).

3 Past *history of definite pelvic infection* (see Q 6.64).

4 Suspected *subfertility*. If the cause of the anxiety about future fertility is a tubal cause, this would come under 6 above (absolute contraindication).

5 Lifestyle *risking STD*.

6 *Nulliparity and young age*, especially less than 20. The reason here is both increased *risk* of infection and also the more serious *implications* thereof.

7 *Diabetes* (but IUD often acceptable, see Q 6.84).

8 *Fibroids or congenital abnormality without* appreciable distortion of the uterine cavity (see Q 6.87).

9 Severely *scarred uterus*, e.g. after myomectomy.

10 Severe *cervical stenosis*.

11 *Heavy periods* before insertion for any reason, including anti-coagulation.

12 Severe *primary dysmenorrhoea.*

13 *Endometriosis.* (There is no proven link, but part of the mechanism of endometriosis may be retrograde menstruation. Hence prudence dictates it might be preferable not to increase this. However a progestagen-releasing IUD ought to be ideal.)

14 *Penicillamine* treatment, whether for Wilson's disease or rheumatoid arthritis. (There are one or two anecdotes of in situ pregnancy occurring in penicillamine-treated copper IUD-users – possibly due to interference with the contraceptive action of the copper. This is unproven; inert or progestagen-releasing IUDs would not be affected.)

15 After *endometrial ablation/resection* – see *Qs 8.59–60* for more about this.

Note: When available, the LNG-IUD (Qs 6.132–6.135) will be the preferred device if almost any of the above relative contraindications apply. This device will also make some absolute contraindications into relative ones, e.g. past ectopic pregnancy in a nullipara. Also Wilson's disease and copper allergy will cease to be problems.

6.82 Can copper IUDs cause local or systemic allergic reactions?

Definite cases have been reported, though they are rare. For instance one case reported in 1976 presented with urticaria, joint pains, and angioneurotic oedema, and positive scratch tests showed a true copper allergy. There have also been reports of marked reversible uterine pain and tenderness plus vaginal discharge, with no evidence of infection, resolving immediately after removal of the device. Referral to a dermatologist for specific allergy tests may be indicated, though most contact allergies to metal bangles or rings are not due to copper.

6.83 Is there evidence that antibiotics, antiprostaglandin or immunosuppressive drugs might impair the efficacy of IUDs?

Since there is no evidence that the inflammatory reaction in the uterus and tubes of IUD-users is normally caused by any infective process, the few reports of pregnancy occurring during antibiotic use can be dismissed as coincidences. One study comparing pregnancy rates in IUD users with and without rheumatoid arthritis has shown no evidence that interference with endometrial prostaglandin metabolism can impair IUD efficacy.

There are reports that immunosuppressed transplant patients are more likely to become pregnant if they use IUDs. Probably more important is the risk of severe and silent *infection*. Hence if such drugs (including corticosteroids) must be used other methods of birth control should be advised.

6.84 What are the implications for IUD-users of anatomical lesions of the heart?

This is a rather 'strong' relative, approaching an absolute contraindication. It would definitely be preferable for such women to use another method – because of the increased risk of bacterial endocarditis. The main time of risk for this would be at insertion.

The fitting of an IUD should be avoided if there is a past history either of endocarditis or of pelvic infection; or of cardiac surgery for the lesion especially if prosthetic valve(s) were fitted. Intravenous drug-abusers are also at higher risk of endocarditis if they have a relevant heart lesion.

If the method were selected at all the fitting should be done by an expert, ideally in a hospital-based clinic, with antibiotic cover. Most cases with minor heart lesions may be given the Brompton Hospital regimen of an oral sachet of amoxycillin 3 g 1 hour before, repeated 8 hours after the procedure. Otherwise the more elaborate recommendations of the British National Formulary should be followed. Ideally spermicides should be used regularly (see Q 6.18), or a LNG-IUD selected if available (see Q 6.133). The patient would also need to be warned even more carefully than other IUD-users to seek prompt medical advice should she develop pelvic pain, deep dyspareunia, or excessive discharge. Any of these might herald a focus of pelvic infection and risk of bacteraemia, and such a case might indicate admission for urgent assessment and treatment.

Antibiotic cover for removal would only be indicated if it was difficult, and especially if intrauterine instrumentation were to be required.

6.85 A propos of prosthetic heart valves in the last answer: what if a woman has any other prosthesis which can be prejudiced by infection, such as a hip replacement?

This must also be a case for caution; definitely a new relative contraindication to insertion of IUDs in my view.

6.86 What are the implications of diabetes for a potential IUD-user?

It was suggested in a study from Edinburgh that diabetes rendered both inert and copper IUDs less effective. However, other workers, notably in Scandinavian countries, have completely failed to show this association.

More relevant is the fear that diabetes might make any pelvic *infection* more severe than it otherwise would be. However the IUD is a valid option, particularly for diabetics at low risk of STDs.

6.87 May an IUD be used by a woman with uterine fibroids?

The answer is yes, provided the cavity of the uterus is not distorted by any submucous fibroid, and (as will normally follow) she does not suffer from menorrhagia. After careful bimanual examination, and the usual discussion about future fertility, etc., provisional arrangements may be made for the device to be inserted. The woman should be warned that plans may have to be changed if, early in the insertion procedure, the uterine sound detects an obvious submucous fibroid – as in Figure 6.5.

Where the facilities exist, a preinsertion ultrasound scan is most useful (requesting specifically that the uterine cavity be checked for submucous fibroids).

Choice of device

6.88 How can one select the best IUD for each woman? What is uterine metrology?

Feet come in different sizes and shapes, and shoes therefore come in many different fittings. Uterine cavity sizes and shapes also vary. There is no fixed relationship between total uterine length as measured with a standard uterine sound and uterine cavity length which can comprise as little as one-third of the total (Fig. 6.6). Maximum fundal width also varies between individuals, and is less in vivo than when measured on hysterectomy specimens. The living uterus is a muscular organ, which contracts and relaxes, and whose tonus also varies with the menstrual cycle (Fig. 6.7). So why is there no routinely available method by which to measure the length and width of each woman's uterine cavity, and hence come to a rational decision as to the optimum size and shape of device to be fitted? The Hasson Mark II Winged Sound and the Kurz

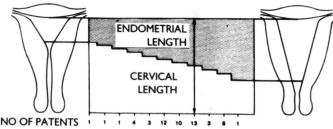

NO OF PATENTS 1 1 1 4 3 12 10 13 3 6 1

Figure 6.6 Measured endometrial and cervical lengths. Q 6.88.
Eleven different combinations were noted in a series of 55 patients, all with the same total uterine axial dimension of 7 cm.
(From Hasson H 1982 Uterine geometry and IUCD design. British Journal of Obstetrics and Gynaecology Supplement 4: 3, Figure 3)

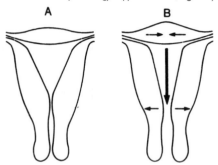

Figure 6.7 Functional changes in uterine shape. A, post-ovulation; B, at menstruation. Q 6.88.
(From Hasson H 1982 Uterine geometry and IUCD design. British Journal of Obstetrics and Gynaecology Supplement 4: 3, Figure 2)

Cavimeter have never become popular, partly because they may add to insertion discomfort. A non-invasive approach would be better: perhaps insertion under ultrasound control will one day be the norm.

6.89 If one could measure the uterus, would there be enough sizes to 'tailor' the IUD to the individual? (Fig. 6.8)

Clearly at present the answer is 'no'. What is more the available one-size option is often too big. Most copper devices are 32 mm in width and 32–36 mm in length (e.g. Copper T-380S, Nova-T). These dimensions are excessive for the majority of nulliparous uteri, especially during menstruation. Even for parous women, the devices are commonly too wide, so their ends penetrate the

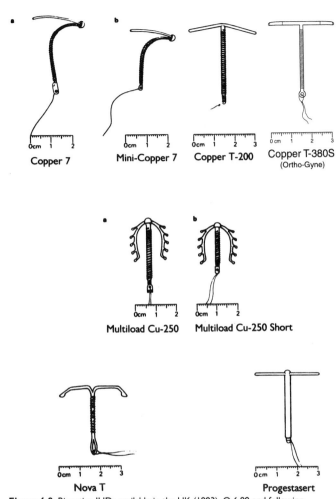

Figure 6.8 Bioactive IUDs available in the UK (1993). Q 6.89 and following. The Progestasert is being superseded by the LNG-IUD 20 (Q 6.132 and Fig. 6.11). See also Q 6.131 and Figure 6.10 for the Cu-Fix/Flexigard IUD.

myometrium. What is more, such penetration tends to be close to the uterotubal junctions, which are the trigger zones for uterine cramps.

The manufacturers should produce a wider range of sizes for each design shape. Otherwise we await the new FlexiGard (see Q 6.131).

6.90 Given the limited range of IUDs available in the UK, what is your normal first choice (Fig. 6.8) for a parous woman?

The current first choice lies between the Copper T-380S, Nova-T and the Multiloads (Cu-375 preferred).

The Copper T–380S: for most parous women I usually now (1993) start with this. It has one of the lowest cumulative pregnancy rates so far reported, and an *FDA–approved* lifespan of 8 years *minimum*: now (1994) also agreed in the UK. See Qs 6.10 and 6.124. This excellent device superseded the Ortho-Gynae-T-200, through the latter remains available.

The Nova–T has a narrower inserter tube (see Q 6.89) but has the following disadvantages by comparison with the copper T-380S:

1 It has definitely a *higher pregnancy rate,* in most studies above 1 and approaching 2/100 woman-years in the first year of use and still around 0.5–1 thereafter (contrast the copper-banded IUDs including the T-380S, see Q 6.10).

2 WHO studies suggest it is best *not* used for more than its approved 5 years life, by women under age 40.

3 The *ectopic pregnancy rate* is also higher than that of the T-380S. This suggests it may be less effective at blocking fertilization (see Q 6.29).

Multiloads tend to cause greater cervical discomfort (at removal as well as insertion) and are not so enclosed in a sterile tube while traversing the contaminated endocervical canal. There is little to commend the Standard Multiload Cu-250 version: it is better to use the Mulitload Cu-375 with its longer life, unless the Multiload Cu-250 Short is indicated (see Q 6.91).

6.91 Which IUD do you select for the nulliparous woman?

If the method is used at all (see Q 6.81), the choice among marketed IUDs lies between the Nova-T and the Multiload Cu-250 Short. Although the Nova-T is often first choice, it is too long and too wide for many nulliparae.

I have reservations about the Multiload devices for young nulliparae, chiefly related to their potentially traumatic shape and unsterile passage through the endocervix at insertion (see Q 6.56). However, the Multiload Cu-250 Short appears satisfactory, allowing for the minor insertion problem of needing a paracervical block and possibly cervical dilatation (see Q 6.103). It did well even, in one study, among women whose actual cavity length as measured by the Hasson Sound (see Q 6.88) was less than 35 mm.

Synthetic progestagen-releasing IUDs which actually reduce the risk of PID (and ectopics) will be the obvious first choice for nulliparae in future (see Q 6.135), provided they are available in small as well as standard sizes.

6.92 What became of inert IUDs and the Copper 7 devices?

All the inert devices have now been removed from the UK market for lack of demand, though any woman still using one may continue to do so until removed 1 year past the menopause (see Q 6.116). Loss of the inert devices poses no problem: the Copper T-380S appears to have a similar almost indefinite life, especially in older women.

The Copper 7 devices are also not missed, except for the Mini-version; no adequate substitute has been marketed for its particular function as a device suitable for uteri sounding to between 5.5 and 6.5 cm.

6.93 Which device do you choose for women who have expelled a previous IUD?

Usually a Multiload. But the same kind of device as just expelled may be used if it is otherwise the best choice and there are reasons for believing there was less than ideal placement of the first IUD.

INSERTION PROCEDURE

6.94 What is the importance of correct insertion?

This cannot be overstressed. A good 'revision test' is to check for yourself how it can be true that poor insertion technique is capable of producing every one of the eight IUD problems listed above (see Q 6.22).

6.95 When should IUDs be inserted following a full-term delivery?

See Qs 6.15-6.17 and 6.59 for discussion of the optimum time in menstruating women, which is *any time* from the *end* of the main menstrual flow through to day 19 of a 28-day cycle, or even later if no conception risk (e.g. if there has been abstinence since the last menses).

Postpartum, normal policy in this country is for IUD insertion to be delayed until the postnatal visit, i.e. at about 6 weeks. This is fine for lactating women, but if they are not breastfeeding, the woman will need to use another method of birth control from the fourth week onwards (see Q 4.37). Hence insertion during that fourth week might well be a better policy, depending on the amount of lochia and satisfactory uterine involution. See Q 8.21.

Immediate postdelivery insertion with careful fundal placement, manually or using a spongeholder or ring forceps, and directly after delivery of the placenta, has been shown in several studies to have acceptable subsequent expulsion rates. The FlexiGard (see Q 6.131) is expected to be particularly useful here.

6.96 What is the optimum insertion time after caesarean section?

The device can be sutured to the fundus with chromic catgut, by way of the lower segment incision. The offer of an IUD to a woman who is still in the delivery room is thus a realistic possibility. In my view it should be so offered to all women wishing to use the IUD where there are doubts as to whether they will return (in time) for a routine postpartum insertion. (However, efforts should still be made to follow such women, to replace expelled devices and often to shorten the threads, as appropriate.)

After a caesarean, normal practice is to defer insertion at least to 6 weeks (some would say 8 weeks) to be sure of complete healing of the lower segment scar. Since after involution this potential weakness finishes up very low, at the level of the internal os, there would in fact be no objection to the insertion by an experienced, careful clinician at the same time as for other women (i.e. even at about 4 weeks).

Puerperal infection (with or without operative delivery) would of course indicate postponement – if indeed an IUD insertion were ever to be appropriate.

6.97 When should IUDs be inserted following any kind of abortion?

Careful studies have shown that immediate insertion at the time of evacuation of the uterus – whether for legal induced abortion, or following an incomplete miscarriage – can be good practice in selected cases. Surprisingly to many, no statistical differences with respect to subsequent infection were found between two groups of women, one receiving and the other not receiving an IUD at the time of uterine evacuation.

Having said this, the studies were performed by experts. In routine practice there is the fear that a fragment of products might be retained. The presence of a foreign body, with a transcervical tail, might then both facilitate infection and render such infection more severe. In my view, therefore, in young nulliparae it is often better to postpone the IUD insertion for 2 weeks; and to proceed then only after excluding infection by a careful history and examination. However, in many individual cases, and perhaps routinely in parous women, insertion at the time of the evacuation is good practice.

6.98 What are the minimum practical requisites?

1 A firm couch at a convenient height.

2 A good adjustable light.

3 Sterile equipment, ideally from a central sterile supply department:
   (a) bivalve speculum;
   (b) Stiles or Allis holding forceps, preferably *not* a toothed *tenaculum*;
   (c) sponge forceps;
   (d) uterine sound;
   (e) kidney dish;
   (f) galley pot plus swabs for sterilizing solution;
   (g) scissors;
   (h) sterile gloves;
   (i) Spencer-Wells forceps.
   (j) elbow taps(!).

4 In reserve:
   (a) local anaesthetic, needles and syringes;
   (b) small cervical dilators up to 6 mm diameter;
   (c) an emergency tray (see Q 6.111).

5 *An assistant* in the room – not necessarily a qualified person, but *someone* (to aid sterile technique and reassure the patient).

6.99 What are the characteristics and qualities of a good IUD doctor, whatever the devices, wherever inserted?

1 First and foremost, the clinician should be really well trained, which means excellent bimanual and speculum technique for a

start, followed in the UK by the theoretical and practical training organized by the Joint Committee on Contraception (JCC) or its successor Faculty. This is now in two stages, with after the basic certificate a special advanced course in intrauterine contraception techniques (including management of 'lost threads').

This brief apprenticeship training with a good instructing doctor beats any amount of book learning (just like for cap fitting, see Q 3.34).

2 Before attempting insertion in any patient, some initial practice with the same devices using a small plastic model and working through the manufacturer's instruction sheet is, in my view, *essential*. Such a 'dry run' should also not be omitted whenever a new device arrives on the contraceptive scene.

3 Initial competence with any device should be *maintained* by continuing experience, and this cannot be by the insertion of only one device every month or two.

4 During both examination and insertion gentleness as well as competence should be the rule in all manoeuvres, especially when the sound or loaded inserter enter the uterine cavity. (Such gentleness is not the same as hesitancy or being excessively slow.)

5 Last but not least, the clinician should be a good communicator, able to use plenty of that 'aural valium' whose route of administration is the ears!

6.100 How does the insertion process begin?

Preferably by a good relationship developed during earlier counselling (see Q 6.112). Ideally the result of screening for STDs especially chlamydia should be available (see Q 6.58).

1 First, make yourself known to the woman. Even a brief initial conversation helps, followed by a matter-of-fact and informative commentary throughout the insertion procedure.

2 Make it explicit that *she is in control, and that you are primarily her agent*. During the procedure give warning of any actions which might cause discomfort, e.g. the needle for paracervical block or the application of the Allis or Stiles forceps (*not* a toothed tenaculum) to the anterior lip of the cervix.

6.101 How important is the initial bimanual examination (BME)?

This is essential. It has two main purposes:

1 First, to ensure that there is no uterine or adnexal tenderness especially on moving the cervix. (Check verbally that there is also no dyspareunia.) Positive findings mean that the insertion should be postponed.

2 The second essential purpose is to identify the size, shape, mobility and *position* of the fundus.

6.102 Which is the best position for the patient to adopt during the insertion?

Most insertions in the UK are performed with the patient in the dorsal position. Sometimes it radically improves access to use the left lateral position, which after all is equivalent to lithotomy rotated through 90°. This is of particular value if the cervical canal is very flexed and the cervix points directly either anterior or posterior.

The left lateral does lead to loss of eye contact with the woman, which must be replaced by better-than-average verbal communication.

6.103 What are the indications for preinsertion analgesia or local anaesthesia (LA)?

Most parous women questioned after an uncomplicated IUD insertion without LA reckon that the needle would have caused more discomfort than it would have removed. However, that is often *not the view of the nulliparous*.

At the MPC it is the norm that *all women* are *offered* premedication with a PGSI such as mefenamic acid 500 mg, half an hour to an hour before the procedure (checking first for contraindications). If they are unusually anxious a benzodiazepine may be added.

A sizeable proportion, especially of nulliparae, are also helped by a *paracervical block* (about 5 ml of 1% lignocaine injected under the skin of the cervix, at about 3–4 o'clock and 8–9 o'clock, high in each lateral fornix). After training, this is not a difficult nor time-consuming addition to the procedure.

Another possible and 'non-needle' option is 2% lignocaine antiseptic gel, which usefully also contains 0.25% chlorhexidine. Sufficient is injected to fill the cervical canal up to the internal os, but there must then be a minimum wait of 3–5 minutes for it to act.

> Note: that there are *two distinct pains*: the PGSI treats the (delayed) fundal cramps while LA is for the earlier somatic, cervical component.

6.104 Should tissue forceps be applied to the cervix, and should the uterus be sounded?

Normally yes: Stiles or Allis forceps cause minimal discomfort, reduced to nil if a little LA is injected at 12 o'clock. X-ray studies have proved that gentle traction straightens the canal and very much assists in passing the sound. The latter is also essential:

1 to confirm the direction and patency of the cervical canal;

2 to estimate the length of the uterine cavity (see Q 6.88);

3 to exclude obvious intrusion of any submucous fibroid or uterine septum. *This should be done in all insertions by gently rotating the handle of the sound through a small arc.*

The sound should be passed with minimal force, rested between the finger and thumb like a loosely held pencil. Note that the anatomy of the cervical canal is variable. Be prepared to repeat the BME, or to withdraw and reinsert the sound if it does not pass readily.

6.105 What about antisepsis?

The cervix should be first carefully inspected and, if there is a purulent discharge, swabs (re-)taken, and the insertion postponed (see Q 6.58). Otherwise the cervix should be thoroughly cleansed with a gauze swab dipped in aqueous antiseptic, concentrating on mechanical removal of any mucus at the external os. Using a non-touch technique, throughout, I teach that every object (sound, device or loaded inserter) which enters the uterus through the inevitably contaminated endocervical canal should also first be dipped into the aqueous antiseptic.

6.106 What other practical points should be considered?

1 Only at the last minute, and after satisfactory sounding, should the device be loaded into its inserter, for fear that it should lose its sterility or its 'memory'.

2 Some devices (e.g. Multiloads) are primarily pushed into the uterus; others are inserted primarily by a 'pull' technique in which the plunger is kept stationary and the inserter tube pulled back over it.

3 Take care that the device finishes in the *right plane*, by observing the marker wings on the inserter, and also in the correct high fundal position. This is confirmed by repassing the sound to just above the internal os. If in doubt the device should be removed and a new one inserted.

6.107 What about the prevention of the rare IUD insertion 'crises'?

1 First, so far as possible, they should be *prevented* by the presence of an assistant, a calm and relaxed atmosphere, combined with obvious competence and teamwork.

2 During the insertion, gentleness and accuracy while passing both sound and loaded inserter along the cervix canal reduce the incidence of vasovagal reactions.

3 Above all, starting at an earlier stage, good counselling and selection of cases, combined with a low threshold for premedication with an analgesic and perhaps a sedative, with or without paracervical block during the insertion – these are the essential prophylactic measures.

6.108 What if a vasovagal attack follows despite every precaution?

The patient becomes white and may sweat with a slow pulse. Rarely is there no warning – heed it!

1 The first thing to do is to abandon the procedure, stop any cervical stimulation, and remove a partially inserted device (but *not* one that is well placed).

2 The woman's head should be lowered or her feet elevated and, if available, an airway inserted.

All this takes a bit of time and occupies anxious bystanders, which is excellent because the majority of attacks are self-limiting.

3 At this point, 500 mg of mefenamic acid should be given, if not used as a premed, along with a non-PGSI such as dihydrocodeine, or equivalent.

6.109 What should be done if the woman continues to suffer severe dysmenorrhoeic pains?

I have no experience of the use of 0.3 mg sublingual glyceryl trinitrate for severe uterine cramps, but it is said this may help.

If they continue with pallor for 30 minutes after the insertion, in my view even a fully inserted device should be removed. The chances of long-term successful use of the IUD in this situation are too low. If ultrasound scanning were routinely done (see Q 6.88), most such cases would be explained by malposition or because of an unexpectedly small uterine cavity for the IUD selected (see Q 6.89). In an occasional case one might also be avoiding the later problems of an incipient perforation.

A subsequent attempt with local anaesthesia, an expert practitioner, and perhaps using a smaller device (such as the Multiload Short) may be successful. Consider also using preliminary exogenous oestrogen to soften the cervix (see Q 6.36(3)).

6.110 What unusual complications of IUD insertion may occur?

1 *Persistent bradycardia.* If the pulse is persistently less than 50 beats/minute, the slow intravenous injection of atropine 0.6 mg may help. If the pulse is absent a vigorous thump to the praecordium is more in terms of cardiopulmonary resuscitation than most clinicians will be called upon to do in a lifetime of inserting IUDs. (Though any competent doctor should also be prepared to deal with more prolonged cardiac arrest.)

   Beware of vomiting and the risk of inhalation of fluid when consciousness returns.

2 *Asthmatic attack* or other allergic reaction. Treat with 1 ml of adrenaline 1 : 1000, subcutaneously.

3 *Grand mal attack.* This may occur even in the absence of any history of epilepsy or the subsequent development thereof. It is usually self-limiting. Diazepam should be available. A good presentation for this situation is Stesolid rectal tubes; one 10-mg dose is administered rectally, repeatable once if there is no response after 5 minutes.

   Epilepsy needs to be distinguished from:

4 *Alkalosis* due to overbreathing, and causing carpopedal spasms. Treatment is by reassurance, and instruction in (supervised) breathing in and out of a plastic bag.

6.111 In summary, what should be available in the emergency tray?

1 An airway – the Laerdal pocket mask is recommended;

2 diazepam 10 mg either for rectal (Stesolid tubes) or intravenous injection;

3 atropine 0.6 mg for intravenous injection;

4 adrenaline 1 ml of 1 : 1000 for subcutaneous injection;

5 mefenamic acid oral tablets – dose 500 mg;

6 dihydrocodeine tablets – dose 30 mg;

7 Short-acting benzodiazepine tablets (Temazepam 20 mg) for premedication;

8 Syringes, needles, etc. as appropriate

Note: that this is all that is required, and most will never be used.

PATIENT INFORMATION AND FOLLOW-UP ARRANGEMENTS

6.112 What main points should be made in counselling any prospective IUD user?

As usual, a balance has to be struck between creating unnecessary fears which may impair the woman's acceptance and satisfaction with the method, and the need to help her reach an informed and valid decision based on the likely benefits and risks for herself. During counselling, often rightly delegated to the family planning trained nurse:

1 Mention first the many advantages of the method (see Q 6.19). Let her see and ideally handle the device she is to receive.

2 The possibility of failure should always be discussed, since it is higher than that of the combined pill in the young. A pregnancy which is known to be possible is less of a catastrophe . . .

3 Attention should be drawn to *pelvic infection* and *ectopic pregnancy*. Explain how both are linked with sexual transmission of infections. Elicit a careful history of past PID or treatments at a genitourinary medicine clinic. Under age 30, early (under 16) coitarche has been shown to be an excellent surrogate measure for having multiple partners.

It may be a little embarrassing to both parties, but is it not just good medicine to go on to say something like:

You know better than I can possibly know, what your likely risk of infection might be. This depends mainly on you and *also* your partner: stop and think, might he sometimes go with other women? Stress also the importance of returning promptly to the clinic should relevant symptoms occur (see Qs 6.23 and 6.115).

4 Arrange at least a chlamydia screen if at all possible.

5 In my view it should also be pointed out that some discomfort is common during insertion, and the use of premedication or local anaesthetic considered in the light of the woman's own views.

6 Problems like perforation are of sufficient rarity that they need not necessarily be mentioned proactively by the counselling nurse or doctor; but they are rightly in the leaflet (see 7). Honest and accurate answers should be given to all questions (see Q 4.96).

7 Finally, counselling should be backed up by a user-friendly leaflet, such as the one from the Family Planning Association,

'to be read now before the insertion, but also for you to keep for future reference.'

6.113 What instructions should be given to the woman after IUD insertion?

1 She may be reminded that the method is effective immediately.

2 If she is nulliparous and not in a very stable relationship, in my view she should always be encouraged to use a barrier and/or spermicide as well (see Q 6.18), thereby reducing both the risk of failure and of infection.

3 She should be carefully instructed in the palpation of her cervical threads, and advised that this check should be done postmenstruation in each cycle before the device is relied on. If she becomes unable to feel the threads, or palpates the hard end of the device, she should be told to take additional contraceptive precautions and arrange an early examination.

4 Intermenstrual bleeding should also be reported and not assumed by patient or doctor necessarily to be due to the IUD.

5 Finally, she should be encouraged to return promptly at any time should a disturbing symptom develop, notably pelvic pain, deep dyspareunia and excessive discharge – especially if with an unexplained pyrexia.

6.114 When and for what purpose should the first follow-up visit take place?

About 6 weeks after the insertion is usual, on a date planned to avoid the expected menses, or 1 week after insertion at termination of pregnancy. However the important data discussed at Qs 6.50 –6.57 suggest that making the first visit routinely at about 1 week would be preferable. Alternatively the woman should at least be advised to attend as an emergency is she has *pain* during the first 20 days. Infections are so much commoner in this postinsertion phase that such policies would permit more prompt, possibly tube-saving, antibiotic treatment.

The patient should be asked to report all symptoms as at 4 and 5 in Q 6.113 above. She should be asked whether she can feel her threads, and retaught as indicated.

On speculum examination the threads should be seen. As a general rule, in my view, but especially if the threads have apparently lengthened, the *lower* cervical canal should be sounded. This can be done with a sterile sound, or very simply using the omnipresent throat swab. In this way partial expulsion may be detected and the device replaced before an avoidable intrauterine pregnancy occurs. The BME is to detect tenderness and adnexal or uterine enlargement.

6.115 How frequently should subsequent visits take place?

If the first visit is at 1 week, another about 6–8 weeks is logical, since expulsions are commonest in the early months of use. Thereafter, in women without symptoms an annual routine visit is quite sufficient.

1 More important than any routine pelvic examination is *an IUD programme which makes it really easy for a user to obtain medical advice and help at once should a new problem occur*: notably an attack of pelvic infection or an ectopic pregnancy or 'lost threads'. *She should therefore be fully taught about symptoms which require prompt action.*

2 Iron deficiency anaemia is very easy to miss in long-term users with heavy bleeding. This should be excluded (in non blood donors), or treated if present.

6.116 Are IUDs always easy to remove by simple traction on the thread(s)?

Not if the threads are missing (see Q 6.36). But without that the device may be malpositioned or embedded, or there may be a type of partial cervical perforation (Fig. 6.9). In such cases it may sometimes be possible under local anaesthesia to grasp the devices and push it in a cranial direction to disimpact it first. Excessive traction at removal must always be avoided especially under general anaesthesia, for the reason noted at Q 6.47.

Upon discovery, any Dalkon Shield device must always be removed (see Q 6.54). Here discomfort is minimized by not being too tentative; its strong thread should be pulled along the correct axis of the cervical canal.

6.117 Do you have any tips for removal of IUDs which are a bit stuck after the menopause? Must they always be removed at all?

This is mainly a problem when removing inert IUDs or Multiloads, 1 year after the last period. A solution is to prescribe natural oestrogen, e.g. one cycle of Premarin 1.25 mg daily beforehand. This will soften the cervical canal. Mefenamic acid 500 mg as a premed also helps. See Q 6.3(3).

It is actually a matter of debate whether devices which are very 'stuck' after the menopause or after endometrial ablation do necessarily have to be removed. The postulated risk of a pyometrium is small and can be dealt with in the individual case. I

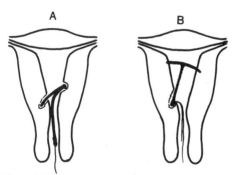

Figure 6.9 Two varieties of partial cervical perforation. Q 6.116.
Both of these could cause difficulty in removal. Both are best treated under appropriate anaesthesia by grasping the end of the device, and pushing in a cranial direction before traction.

would, personally, not now feel the risks of a general anaesthetic were justified for removal of an IUD postmenopausally, and would simply warn the woman to seek advice at the time if she were to develop an offensive discharge.

6.118 Are IUDs a genuine cause of male dyspareunia?

Certainly, above all if a device is partially expelled so that its end just protrudes from the external cervical os! More commonly, some men notice the threads of the device.

If this problem is not resolved by slightly altering positions of intercourse, the threads should be trimmed – but not to within a few millimetres of the os. This can actually worsen the situation . . . . Rather, if necessary, they should be shortened to lie wholly within the cervical canal. Ensure that this is noted in the records and that the woman will report the fact to any future doctor.

6.119 Is short-wave diathermy treatment contraindicated in IUD-users?

This treatment is now rarely given to patients with chronic pelvic pain, in whom removal of the device would normally first be tried. However, if there is an IUD present there is certainly a theoretical possibility that the copper wire might heat up. Experiments with devices in recently excised hysterectomy specimens have shown no obvious damage or charring to the endometrium, and the devices have merely become pleasantly warm. So this treatment is relatively contraindicated, a need for caution.

6.120 Are modern methods of imaging dangerous for the IUD-wearer, specifically nuclear magnetic resonance (NMR)?

Ultrasound is harmless, X-rays have no added risk, and provided the device is non-ferrous NMR would cause no problems. However, with steel devices (e.g. the M-device and Chinese rings) there would be the potential hazard of internal trauma, caused by movement of the ferrous metal caused by the magnetic field.

6.121 Are IUDs containing copper affected by any vaginal preparations?

There is no clear evidence that material from the vagina reaches the copper or affects the biochemical processes which cause the contraceptive effect (see Q 6.5).

6.122 Do the white deposits on IUDs removed after varying durations within the uterus have any clinical significance, particularly in copper IUD-users?

These deposits have been studied intensively. They contain organic material along with calcium, sulphur and phosphorus and other inorganic elements. They are not now thought to be linked with IUD failure. Many women's devices never develop this deposit. When present, if the IUD is copper bearing it seems that sufficient copper can pass through the deposit to continue the contraceptive effect. It is not an important factor in the rate of copper elution (see Q 6.124).

The explanation for failure of modern IUDs is, primarily, less than ideal placement within the uterine cavity (see Qs 6.11 and 6.12).

6.123 How often should inert IUDs be replaced?

In the few women who still retain these: without special cause they should never be routinely replaced.

6.124 How often should copper IUDs be replaced?

All the marketed devices have an officially approved duration, normally 3, 4 or 5 years. The reason for any limit is anxiety that the amount of copper available for release from the device might decline to a level at which the pregnancy rate would increase. Yet no study with any copper IUD up to 5 years of use has shown any such increase, rather the reverse.

With copper *wire* IUDs there may be a problem beyond about 5 years in the under 40s (see Q 6.129(a)), but not with the banded devices.

6.125 What are the benefits of long term use of IUDs?

Long-term studies (especially the WHO study, see Q 6.50) have repeatedly shown a steady reduction with increasing duration of use in:

1 pregnancy rates;

2 expulsion rates;

3 infection rates (overall);

4 bleeding/pain removal rates.

Exceptions which show a positive link with duration of use are carriage of ALOs (see Qs 6.64–6.69) and ectopic pregnancy (see Q 6.29) – but the latter association is probably confounded by increasing age.

6.126 What are the explanations for the apparent improvement with duration of use of IUDs in the risks of pregnancy, expulsion, infection, and removal for bleeding or pain?

It is too simple to interpret this as a genuine improvement due to the device 'bedding down'. The main point is that the long-term population of IUD-users is highly selected, and in all studies is only a small proportion of those who originally had devices inserted. They are the 'survivors', so to speak. Their success in long-term use has less to do with the passage of time as such, than with selection for features of the individual women themselves as compared with others earlier in the study:

1 They are likely to have been well fitted with an IUD, which was well matched to the particular shape and size of their uterus.

2 They are obviously well distanced in time from insertion-related expulsion, infection and bleeding/pain (see Q 6.23(a)).

3 *Much the most important factor*: the women with any side-effects or complications severe enough to have their device removed are by definition no longer in the study. For example, the most fertile become pregnant within the first year and have their devices removed, hence the reported pregnancy rates in later years are based on observation of a subgroup of the relatively infertile. Similarly those whose partners are less likely to transmit a sexually transmitted infection to them are overrepresented among long-term users.

4 They are also a little older – see Q 6.23 (g), 6.52.

6.127 What therefore is the view of the UK FPA and the National Association (now the Faculty) of Family Planning Doctors regarding long-term use of copper IUDs?

A statement published in *The Lancet* on June 2 1990 remains substantially in force:

> For routine management the modern copper-bearing IUDs . . . should be assumed to have an active lifespan of 5 years . . . Be-

yond that interval, an experienced doctor or nurse should discuss with the client the option of changing the IUD or leaving it in (it is wise to record this discussion in the notes).

> **Note: One thing specifically to record is that no promise was made that the device could not possibly fail; only that the failure rate is believed to be no higher than during the preceding years of successful use.**

In a supplementary letter, it was also stated that *any copper device* (even one of the non-banded ones discussed in the next question) *which was fitted above age 40 may remain in situ until the menopause.* This is acceptable because with diminishing fertility IUDs so very rarely fail above 40.

The Lancet statement, like the later WHO report (see Q 6.57), points out that less frequent replacement would have enormous health advantages, in reducing the risk of insertion-related PID (the main time it ever happens!), perforation, expulsion and malposition; not to mention inconvenience, pain, upset and cost for the woman.

What is now needed is a change to all the relevant IUD Data Sheets in the UK.

6.128 What about long-term use of the older, copper wire IUDs?

Studies in Manchester showed that standard (200 mm) copper wire devices begin to lose copper at an accelerated (and linear) rate from an average of 27 months onwards. The rate of copper release was greater than average if the women complained of heavy uterine bleeding. After 4 years' use 28% of removed IUDs show fragmentation of the wire. Silver in the core of the Nova-T wire prevents that occurrence but would not otherwise reduce the rate of copper release. Indeed it might even eventually increase it when silver become exposed, by a 'battery effect'.

Clinical studies now begin to correlate well with this laboratory work. A review of all the studies of copper wire IUDs *including the Nova-T* suggests that use beyond about 5 years might start to raise the pregnancy risk above the low rate which that (by now highly selected) woman should have. But this is not true of the copper-banded devices, whose upper duration limit is not known but certainly exceeds 8 years (see Q 6.10).

6.129 What does this all mean in practice? – Faced with (a) a Nova-T user or (b) a Copper T-380S user, both aged 30 without symptoms and 4 years since insertion? And what if (c) the Nova-T user was aged 48 and had it fitted at aged 41 or (d) any of these IUD-users have ALOs on their most recent cervical smear?

(a) Suggest replacement next year some time.

(b) Suggest she continues until at least 8 years, by which time the data may well suggest indefinite use (like the old inert IUDs).

(c) Suggest she continues use until 1 year after her final menstrual period.

(d) Suggest she considers having the device removed and immediately replaced (see Q 6.69).

6.130 How reversible is IUD contraception?

All prospective studies of the return of fertility after elective removal of IUDs have shown that the subsequent conception rates are indistinguishable from those to be expected in that population. The Oxford/FPA study found that within 2 years 92% had given birth, a similar delivery rate to the ex-diaphragm users.

Clearly, the women whose fertility might be impaired by IUD use are more likely to be those who drop out because of medical complications such as ectopic pregnancy or pelvic infection. Two American case-control studies reported in 1985 that past IUD use was significantly commoner in primary tubal infertility cases than in controls. The effect was less for copper-bearing IUDs and not significant if monogamy was reported. But so far there has been no successful prospective study following up a total (large) population of IUD-users and taking account of removals for medical reasons as well as for intention to conceive.

For the vast majority of acceptors the IUD is a fully reversible method of contraception. Among those who suffer tubal infertility due to PID or ectopic pregnancy, the main responsibility does not lie at the door of the IUD itself (see Qs 6.29 and 6.50). The frequency of this catastrophic outcome can be minimized by careful selection (see Qs 6.79–6.81); careful IUD insertion (see Q 6.105), with screening and consideration of antibiotic cover; and the rigorous follow-up of fully informed women.

6.131 What is the FlexiGard IUD (Fig. 6.10)?

Also known as the Cu-Fix 390, this is the result of some good lateral thinking by Dirk Wildemeersch of Belgium. It is simply a single monofilament nylon thread, bearing six copper bands similar to those on the Copper T-380S. A small loop and knot at the fundal end are inserted a measured distance of precisely 1 cm into the myometrium by a special stylet.

Initial results are very promising:

1 no extra insertion pain;
2 pregnancy and expulsion rates 0.3 and 0.9 at 1 year;
3 no increase in dysmenorrhoea pain (because no plastic frame);
4 similar bleeding problems to other copper devices;
5 no evidence in a very preliminary study of either endometriosis or of more than a very localized inflammatory reaction at the site of the anchoring knot.

It also shows so far a low expulsion rate following postplacental insertion. Watch this space!

6.132 What is the Levonorgestrel IUD/LNG-IUD 20 (Levo Nova)?

This Nova-T-shaped device, developed by the Population Council, slowly releases levonorgestrel (LNG) from a capsule in its vertical stem at a rate of 20 μg per day (see Fig. 6.11).

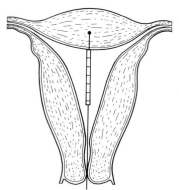

Figure 6.10 The Cu-Fix IUD or Flexigard. Q 6.131

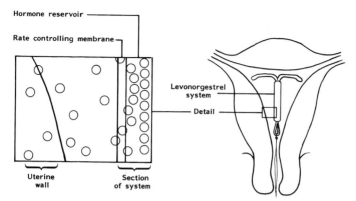

Figure 6.11 The levonorgestrel device (LNG-IUD 20). Q 6.132.

Early trials including one at the MPC showed great promise. Considerable delay in its development was then caused when the manufacturer withdrew the silicone 'Elastomer 382' from which the progestagen was released. However it is now marketed, using polymer from a new source, in several countries, and is expected in the UK before long. Other systems (devices, or intrauterine threads) releasing 3-keto-desogestrel and other progestogens are also awaited.

6.133 What are the advantages of the LNG-IUD 20?

1 Initial studies have shown it to be highly effective (failure rate 0.1–0.3/100 woman-years).

2 The *very low* ectopic pregnancy rate (nil in the Population Council study, see Q 6.29) contrasts favourably with the old Progestasert.

Note: Lower than in women using no method.

---

3 Like all progestagen-releasing devices, it makes the menses *less heavy*, leading to oligomenorrhoea or amenorrhoea. Also Hb rises.

4 Menstrual pain is said to 'disappear'.

5 It appears to *reduce* the risk of pelvic infection.

6 Its duration of action is at least 7 years.

7 Return of fertility is rapid after removal.

6.134 What are the disadvantages of the LNG-IUD 20?

1 The inserter has a relatively wide diameter of 4.5 mm; hence there may, especially in nulliparous women, be the requirement for paracervical block and slight dilatation of the cervical canal.

2 More importantly, rather more women than with copper or inert devices complain of intermenstrual spotting and bloodstained discharge in early months of use. However, these problems are not as marked as with the Progestasert, and the number of days of bleeding and spotting per month decline after the third month to less than with the Nova-T device.

3 Amenorrhoea, due to the development of an atrophic endometrium and not always with suppression of ovulation, is reported in over 10% of users.

Note: This can be acceptable to many women after counselling.

---

4 Some of the progestagen is absorbed, so there is the potential for systemic effects. However, the mean plasma concentration with the LNG-IUD 20 is very low – 60 pg/ml. In neither case have significant metabolic effects been described to date.

6.135 Which women might particularly consider a LNG-IUD?

It could be selected for almost any IUD-acceptor, but it would appear particularly suitable at the extremes of reproductive life. Indeed for young, nulliparous women this device may overturn all previous teaching – chiefly because of the reduced risk of pelvic infection (if confirmed) and of dysmenorrhoea.

In older women with heavy periods the LNG device may avert the need for a hysterectomy even among those who are anaemic. Moreover, in those with climateric symptoms requiring hormone replacement therapy using natural oestrogens, the device could be used instead of systemic progestagens, to protect the endometrium from the risk of hyperplasia and carcinoma (see Q 8.51).

CONCLUSIONS

6.136 What are your ten commandments about IUD insertion?

See Qs 6.98–6.106 for more details.

1 Thou shalt never insert any IUD without training, and without first having practised each step of the insertion procedure on a plastic pelvic model – and keeping in practice.

2 All manipulations of the cervix and uterus shall be performed gently – but not tentatively.

3 Thou shalt always consider and *discuss the option* of extra analgesia/anaesthesia – and even if not required, always use 'aural valium, and vocal local'.

4 Thou shalt ensure the best position of the patient for insertion (consider left lateral), always have an assistant, and use good equipment with a good light.

5 A preliminary BME will never be omitted.

6 The insertion will be postponed, pending diagnosis and treatment, whenever there is the slightest pelvic tenderness or other evidence suggesting infection.

7 The cervix will be thoroughly cleansed by repeated swabbing, and antiseptic technique followed for all objects passed through the endocervical canal into the sterile uterine cavity.

8 Careful sounding of the uterus will not be omitted – to check the direction and patency of the canal and to assess the uterine cavity.

9 The device will be loaded into its inserter at the last possible moment – to preserve its asepsis and 'memory'.

10 The correct technique will be used to deliver the IUD in the right plane to the correct high fundal position (checking subsequently by sounding of the canal).

6.137 What are your ten resolutions for the conscientious IUD doctor?

1 Remembering that one of the main times of action of IUDs is the last 9 days of the cycle I will follow the 7-day rule for elective IUD removal (see Q 6.14), to avoid 'iatrogenic pregnancies'. I will also be prepared to proceed with IUD insertion up to 'day 19' in selected cases (see Qs 6.15, 6.17 and 7.11).

2 Since the main IUD hazards and contraindications relate to threats to fertility, I will always make this the main point when counselling the *nulliparous*.

3 Since the rates of *in situ* pregnancy, expulsion and pelvic infection are inversely related to age, I will always make these

potential risks the main element when counselling the *young*.

4 Since incorrect insertion/malposition can cause every category of IUD problem, I will strive to ensure that my own insertions are correct, competent, careful and gentle.

Subsequent to fitting the right device in the right woman using the right technique, I will remember and (as appropriate) teach my patients the following:

5 That pain and bleeding are serious symptoms until proved otherwise, especially if sustained and intermenstrual.

6 More specifically, that any woman with menstrual irregularity and pelvic discomfort has an ectopic pregnancy until proved otherwise.

7 That 'lost threads' means the woman is pregnant or at risk of pregnancy until proved otherwise.

8 That in any continuing pregnancy the IUD should be gently removed in the first trimester if feasible, to reduce the risks of abortion and preterm delivery.

Moreover, there are two equally important but opposite slogans:

9 'Leave well alone' (often, after counselling, in asymptomatic long-term users – see Q 6.129).

10 'When in doubt take it out' (contrariwise): when the woman does have troublesome symptoms, and also for her own reasons upon her request 'so she knows she is boss in the matter!'

But then I must not forget to ask about any intercourse in the preceding 7 days, as well as about her plans for future contraception.

6.138 What problems of IUD use in Britain should be reported to the Committee on Dental and Surgical Materials (CDSM, a committee of the CSM)?

Any problems of complications whether or not in the list at Q 6.22, especially:

1 extrauterine pregnancy;

2 perforation/translocation;

3 severe pelvic infection – most especially actinomycosis (see Q 6.67) or bacterial endocarditis (see Q 6.86);

4 apparent true allergy to any constituent of IUDs (Q 6.82);

5 apparent interaction with a drug or imaging technique (see Qs 6.119–6.121);

6 severe insertion reactions (Q 6.110);

7 any unusual *possibly* related event.

QUESTIONS ASKED BY PROSPECTIVE OR CURRENT IUD-USERS

General questions

6.139 How does the IUD work? Is it often causing an abortion?

The answer depends on the definition of when pregnancy begins, see Qs 6.7, 7.2 and 7.3. If your own beliefs make you feel that contraception must never operate after fertilization, then this method is not for you.

6.140 Can the copper be absorbed from copper devices into the body?

A tiny amount is absorbed, but very little so it is only just detectable in the blood. By far the majority of the small amount of copper which is lost over the years goes out in the vaginal fluid.

6.141 Why does the IUD have a tail?

Mainly to check that the device is present, but also to remove it when required.

6.142 Which is safer, the IUD or the ordinary pill? Can a woman die from using an IUD?

Overall, the risk of death or life-endangering disease is very low with both methods, but even lower with an IUD. Deaths have been caused but they are extremely rare.

IUDs are a bit like that girl with a curl in the middle of her forehead – 'when they are good they are very very good, but when they are bad they can be horrid'. Even then, the problems are focused in the pelvic area and not all over the body, and they can be minimized, see Qs 6.136 and 6.137. The main problems have to do with future fertility (see Qs 6.23, 6.79 and 6.80).

6.143 Does the IUD cause any kind of cancer?

There is no evidence for this even for copper or hormone-releasing varieties (see Q 6.22).

6.144 If I get pregnant, will the baby be harmed?

Again there is no evidence of this, even if the pregnancy occurs with the device still in position. It should normally, however, be removed in early pregnancy (see Q 6.25).

6.145 What has using the IUD got to do with the number of sexual partners I have?

A great deal, since the main problem with IUDs is an increased risk of pelvic infection, and most IUD-linked infections are caught sexually. Also relevant is the number of sexual partners of your own partner, even if you are entirely faithful. *See also the question at Q 6.112.*

Counselling and fitting of IUDs

6.146 Do I need my partner's/husband's agreement to have an IUD?

No, the device can be inserted without his agreement. However, clearly it is always best if the couple are both agreed, whatever method of family planning is chosen.

6.147 Should I ask to see which IUD I have before it is fitted?

Yes, most certainly. Ideally you should also write down its name in case you move to the care of a different doctor or clinic.

6.148 I think I am allergic to copper; what should I do?

First, report the matter to your doctor. It may be possible to do special patch allergy tests. Since most people who think they are allergic to copper turn out actually to be allergic to another metal, it may be right then to insert the device and see how you get on over the next few days. If you get marked discharge and pain within a very few days of insertion, you should return most promptly for advice (see Q 6.82).

6.149 I am told I have a cervical erosion (ectopy)/a tilted womb/ a very tiny womb – can I have an IUD fitted?

If these are the only problems (i.e. there is no infection, or the womb is not distorted congenitally or by fibroids) a device can normally be fitted (see Qs 6.58 and 6.91). The Multiload Short can often be fitted to a small womb.

6.150 I have heard you get very bad cramp-like pains when an IUD is fitted? What causes this and what can be done about it?

The pain people feel at insertion varies a great deal, from nothing to quite a bit. Part of this is caused by the release of substances called prostaglandins, and you can ask your doctor for a specific painkiller that opposes their action. You should also discuss with him/her the possibility of having a local anaesthetic.

6.151 Does an IUD always have to be fitted during or just after a period?

No – not only *may* it be inserted later, there may even be certain advantages (see Qs 6.15, 6.16 and 6.59).

6.152 Does being an epileptic increase the chance of my having a fit during the insertion?

Yes it does, and your doctor should arrange to have available the treatment to prevent/stop an attack.

Instructions after fitting

6.153 How soon can I have sex after having the IUD fitted?

The protection is immediate, but it is recommended that you wait until the small amount of bleeding caused by the insertion itself subsides.

6.154 If I use a spermicide as well as my IUD, will it reduce the chance of infection as well as pregnancy?

Yes, there is some evidence that spermicides are also germicides, so this may well be a good idea if your lifestyle or that of your partner puts you at risk (see Q 6.18). A condom will be even more protective.

6.155 Can an IUD fall out without my knowing?

Yes, this is certainly possible (see Q 6.38). The most likely time is during a heavy period, in which case it may be hidden within a large clot or on a tampon which is then flushed down the toilet.

6.156 How often should I feel for the strings?

Once a month is sufficient; best right at the end of a period. This is so that you do not begin to rely on the method each new month, until you have checked that it is still in position.

6.157 How do I feel the strings of the IUD? What should I do if I now can't feel them?

Either squat down or put one foot on the bathroom stool. Insert both your index and middle fingers into the vagina and feel more in a backwards than an upwards direction until you come across the cervix. This feels rather like a nose with only one nostril, and you should then be able to find emerging from the opening one or two little threads feeling like ends of nylon fishing line. If that is all you feel, well and good. If, however, you feel something hard like the end of a matchstick, this could mean that the device is on its way out. In that case, or if you can no longer feel the threads at all, you must assume that you are no longer protected and start using another method of family planning. Contact your family doctor or clinic urgently in case the 'emergency pill' is required (see Q 7.18, also Q 6.113).

6.158 Can my IUD get lost in the body (perforation)?

Extremely rarely. It is 999 : 1 against this happening in your case. It is a rare cause of the problem of lost threads (see Q 6.46). Should it happen, the most that is normally required is a minor operation called a laparoscopy to retrieve it.

While your lost threads problem is still being sorted out, and you are perhaps waiting for a hospital appointment, make sure that you use another method of family planning (since the womb itself may be empty) and also take immediate medical advice if you get any pain in the abdomen.

6.159 Can I go back to using an IUD after a perforation?

This depends on the cause; but an IUD can often be reinserted with success, since the tiny hole in the womb heals up so completely.

6.160 Do women have more vaginal discharge with an IUD?

Sometimes the discharge has a specific and treatable cause, so it should always be reported to your doctor. If testing shows nothing specific, like anaerobic vaginosis or thrush, then it is probably caused by an increase in the usual vaginal fluid (which includes mucus, the fluid of sexual arousal and even semen). This needs no treatment.

6.161 Someone has told me the IUD can break into pieces inside you, is this so?

Years ago there was one rather bad batch of Lippes Loop devices which were distributed worldwide and were liable to fracture. No modern device will break up, except very rarely if removal is difficult. In that case a 'D & C' may sometimes be necessary to retrieve the missing portion.

6.162 My last period was very late and heavy, does this mean I might be miscarrying an early pregnancy?

Most probably not – heavy periods are not uncommon in regular use of an IUD, and the period could have been late just because your egg was released late in that cycle. However, you should visit the clinic for an examination, both to check that you do not need a 'D & C', and also in case your device was dislodged by the heavy flow.

6.163 Can my partner really feel the IUD during lovemaking as he says, and what can be done about it?

Some men notice the threads, depending on which way the cervix points and perhaps on the position of intercourse. Many couples just adapt their sex lives accordingly, but otherwise it is possible to have the threads cut right off (see Q 6.118).

6.164 Can I use a sunbed with an IUD in place, or have vibromassage?

Neither of these can affect your IUD in any way.

363

6.165 If my IUD contains metal, will it make an embarrassing 'bleep' when I pass through security devices at airports or large department stores?

Despite rumours, this does not appear to be a problem either with copper-bearing or steel devices – presumably because the amount of metal is too small. Another rumour which can be discounted is the one that was started by the woman who accused the magician Yuri Geller of causing the failure of her copper IUD. She claimed that the pregnancy was conceived when she made love on the hearthrug during a television demonstration by the above-mentioned showman of his metal-bending skills!

6.166 Can I cause my IUD to be expelled by vigorous aerobic exercises or intercourse in any unusual positions?

There is no evidence for this, and plenty of ordinary and sexual athletes use the method with success.

6.167 May I use internal sanitary protection after being fitted with an IUD?

The usual advice is to use only a sanitary towel at first, for the bleeding which follows immediately after IUD insertion. Subsequently sanitary protection can be entirely at a woman's choice. However, prolonged use of the same tampon (12 hours) is inadvisable, for fear of toxic shock syndrome (TSS) and also the possibility of promoting infection via the threads (see Q 6.50).

6.168 Are there any drugs that might interfere with the action of my IUD?

Tell your doctor about the IUD if you are to receive any treatment. Should this be a corticosteroid or other drug which may interfere with immune responses, it may be better for you to transfer to another method of birth control. However, there is no current concern about either antibiotics or painkillers (see Qs 6.81(12) and 6.83).

6.169 Do I really have to have my copper IUD changed at a set time, when it is suiting me well?

Nowadays this is becoming less and less necessary, and definitely not if your device was fitted above the age of 40. See Qs 6.122–6.129 for a full answer to this most important question.

6.170 How is an IUD removed? Is it ever difficult?

Normally there is no problem; there is much less discomfort than having the device fitted in the first place. However, there are some situations in which it is more tricky and uncomfortable (see Qs 6.36, 6.116).

6.171 If my IUD is removed so that I can try for a baby, should I wait, using another method for a set time?

It is recommended that you wait for one period to 'clear the womb' first. But this is not vital. Even women who conceive immediately the device comes out (so it was still in place during the last period before the pregnancy) seem to be as likely as anyone else to have a normal baby.

7

Emergency (postcoital) contraception

BACKGROUND AND MECHANISMS

7.1 What is the definition of postcoital (PC) contraception?

In current usage this is any female method which is administered after intercourse, but has its effects prior to the stage of implantation. The latter is believed to occur no earlier than 5 days after ovulation. Any method applied after intercourse which acts after implantation, even if this is before the next menses, should properly be called a *postconceptional* or *contragestive* agent.

The lay term 'morning after pill' should no longer be used, since it may actually cause pregnancies by preventing women from presenting many hours later than the 'morning after' (see Q 7.5). We now prefer to say 'the emergency pill' (see Q 7.42).

7.2 Is it ethical to use PC contraception?

Yes, if the prescriber and the woman concerned are happy to accept the modern view that 'conception' is a *process*, which begins with the fusion of sperm and ovum, but is not complete until implantation.

The ethical situation is clarified by considering the *status of the unimplanted blastocyst* (Fig. 7.1). If it stays where it is in the cavity of the uterus it is in a 100% 'no-go' situation – unless and until it can stop itself being washed away in the next menstrual flow by secreting enough human chorionic gonadotrophin (hCG) into the mother's circulation to maintain the corpus luteum. The menses cannot be prevented without successful implantation. As has been well said, if there is not yet 'carriage' how can application of any method of birth control be 'procuring a miscarriage'? Secondly, there seems little logic in putting a high value on something with which Nature itself is so prodigal.

Prescribers must respect the views of their patients, and PC methods should not be used for any who are unhappy with the above interpretation. They should then, however, also understand the implications in relation to other methods (see Q 7.3).

7.3 What are the implications of rejection of PC methods on ethical grounds?

In the main, this means that the woman concerned should also not use either the intrauterine device or the progestagen-only pill (see

369

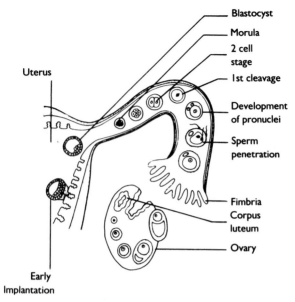

Figure 7.1 Ovulation, fertilization and early development to the stage of implantation. Q 7.2 considers the *status* of the unimplanted blastocyst, labelled above.

Q 5.74). Both these methods may operate sometimes, in rare cycles, by blocking implantation.

7.4 What is the history of PC contraception?

This is probably almost as old as the first recognition that semen is in some way responsible for pregnancy. Douching has been used since ancient times and remains in use today; 25% of women presenting for PC treatment in one UK study had first used a shower attachment, flannel or paper tissues, with or without a spermicide or household germicide. These methods are doomed to frequent failure, because sperm have been found in cervical mucus within 90 seconds following ejaculation.

The Persian physician Al-Razi suggested: 'first immediately after ejaculation let the two come apart and let the woman arise roughly, sneeze and blow her nose several times and call out in a loud voice. She should jump violently backwards seven to nine times.' Jumping backwards supposedly dislodged the semen, while jumping forwards would assure pregnancy.

A range of PC pessaries and douches have been described over the years, including wine and garlic with fennel, used in Egypt as early as 1500 BC; ground cabbage blossoms in the fourth century; and culminating in Coca-Cola in some developing countries even today.

The modern history begins in 1963 with trials of diethylstilboestrol (DES) at Yale University (USA). Because of the risks to any pregnancy should the method fail, DES has now been firmly rejected in favour of ethinyloestradiol (EE) or other oestrogens. Since the mid-1970s the Yuzpe method (devised by a Canadian gynaecologist) has increasingly become the first-choice method, using much less EE in combination with levonorgestrel (LNG).

Immediate insertion of a copper intrauterine device (IUD) is an alternative method first reported in 1972 and appropriate in some cases (see Q 7.27).

7.5 What are the currently accepted regimens of PC treatment?

See Table 7.1.

1 *Immediate insertion of a copper–bearing IUD*, not more than 5 days from the most probable calculated date of ovulation, even if there have been several acts of unprotected intercourse.

2 *The Yuzpe method.* This is commenced within 72 hours of a single unprotected intercourse, its efficacy declining thereafter. Two tablets of a contraceptive containing 250 μg of LNG with

Table 7.1 Methods of postcoital contraception – a brief summary

	Pill	IUD
Method	PC 4 or Ovran 2 pills stat 2 pills 12 hours later	Nova-T, Copper T-380S or Multiload
Timing after intercourse	Up to 72 hours	Up to 5 days after calculated date of *ovulation*
Efficacy	98%	Almost 100%
Side-effects	Nausea and vomiting	Pain, bleeding, infection risk
Contraindications	Pregnancy + those relating to oestrogen	Pregnancy + as for IUDs generally

50 μg of EE (PC 40 or Ovran) are given at once, followed by a further two tablets 12 hours later.

3 *Use of LNG 0.6 mg alone.* One study showed an acceptable failure rate (about 3/100 women treated) compared with the Yuzpe method, using this fairly high dose of this progestagen, alone, within 12 hours of intercourse. This is therefore an acceptable alternative to the IUD where there is an absolute contraindication to oestrogens. In this country it means taking the LNG as 20 Microval tablets in one stat. dose. It can be tried later than 12 hours also, but there are no efficacy data with that usage.

4 *EE,* again within 72 hours of a single exposure. This appears in a comparative study to be slightly more effective than method 2 above. The dose, however, is 2.5 mg bd for 5 days, or no less than 25 000 μg of EE. On the pocket calculator this works out at more than 3 years' worth of a standard 30-μg pill! Nausea and vomiting are extremely common, and prolonged.

5 *Conjugated equine oestrogens* (Premarin) in a dose of 10 mg tds for 5 days has also been used with some reported success. Once again this is a worrying megadosage regimen, equivalent to 8 months' daily hormone replacement with 0.625 mg.

Hence methods 1 and 2 above are normally preferred (Table 7.1). See also Q 7.7 for variants and Q 7.41 *re* methods being researched.

7.6 What is the mechanism of action of PC contraceptive methods?

The IUD operates here mainly by blocking implantation (see Q 6.7), though early in the cycle it might also block fertilization. The action of the hormonal methods will depend on when in relation to ovulation they are administered. It is important to remember that this could happen to be sufficiently early to prevent or *postpone* ovulation in that cycle (hence the requirement to use a method such as the sheath until the next period). It is probable that the uterine fluid/genital tract mucus may also be rendered hostile to sperm or blastocyst.

If, however, the hormones are given after ovulation, the method relies mainly on blocking implantation. The precise mechanism is uncertain, but desynchronization of the histology of the secretory endometrium has been observed along with blockage of oestrogen and progesterone receptors. The agents may also operate indirectly by impairing luteal function.

7.7 Might other regimens work?

A very wide range of alternatives has been proposed and there are anecdotal reports of success. These are very difficult to assess, because pregnancy is certainly not inevitable after a single act of intercourse, even if the woman were untreated (see Q 7.9). However, the following variants may be considered even though their efficacy has not been established in rigorous trials.

1 *Immediate insertion of a non-copper-bearing IUD*. One would expect a very low failure rate for almost any IUD design, including progestagen-releasing types, since they all share the same major mechanisms of action (see Q 6.7).

2 *Modifications of the Yuzpe hormonal mechanism*:
   (a) Since there is as yet no clear evidence that the delay of a few hours (within 72 hours) after exposure impairs efficacy, selected women seen in the afternoon may be allowed to delay their first dose until the evening. This will remove the need to set an alarm for the early hours of the morning. Alternatively:
   (b) The first two tablets could be given on presentation, and the subsequent ones could be given in appropriate divided doses, once again to avoid the patient being woken at night.
   (c) Clearly there are other ways of giving almost exactly the same doses of EE and LNG. For example, seven tablets of Microgynon 30/Ovranette will provide 210 μg of EE (instead of 200) and 1050 μg of LNG (instead of 1000).
   (d) A little less certainly, other progestagens might well be effective, such as desogestrel or gestodene; but neither their efficacy nor the best dose have been fully evaluated.

EFFECTIVENESS

7.8 What is the overall efficacy of the two most commonly used PC methods?

1 *For the IUD method* the failure rate is very low indeed. We have reported one failure with the device still in situ at the Margaret Pyke Centre (MPC), and there was another, with partial expulsion of the device, reported from elsewhere. This represented two failures in about 1300 insertions reported in the literature to that date. Considering that in this context the risk of pregnancy only applies for the cycle of insertion, this is a rate

of 1–2 failures/1300 cycles; entirely compatible therefore with the usually quoted failure rate of the IUD of 1–2/100 woman-years (100 woman-years equals 1300 cycles).

2

Reported failure rates for the Yuzpe regimen vary enormously, depending very much on factors such as the likely fertility of the women, when they were exposed and completeness of follow-up. Rates range from 1% for cases with exposure at any time of the cycle, to 2–5% for exposure at around midcycle. The MPC method-failure rate was 2.6% for women exposed between days 9 and 17 (corrected for cycle length variation from 28). However, if one could consider in the denominator only those who would actually have become pregnant even without treatment, the failure rate would be considerably higher. A useful estimate by Professor Trussell of Princeton is that the Yuzpe method prevents about 75% of conceptions.

7.9 What is the likelihood of pregnancy after a single act of intercourse in the absence of PC treatment?

This is discussed in more detail with Figure 1.1 at Qs 1.14 and 1.15. If a single exposure is around mid-cycle (days 10–14, corrected) the risk is roughly 20%, peaking at about 30% on the day of maximum risk. At other times during the cycle the risk is somewhere between 0 and 10%. The probability of conception is lowest in the days before the expected date of the next menses; though the possibility that the cycle in question might be unusually long must always be considered. There is a significant risk from day 7 to about 17 of a 28-day cycle — or the equivalent after correction for cycle length.

7.10 Should one be prepared to withhold PC treatment?

This can be a tricky decision. Although the risk of conception is very low if exposure was actually during the menses, or during what are believed to be the last 7 days of the cycle, the decision to treat depends on many factors: not least the amount of anxiety present. The treatment is very safe, if not entirely risk free.

In future it may be possible to discover, simply and accurately in the clinic, what stage of the menstrual cycle the woman has reached. At present, although treatment is not always indicated, it is not easy to be sure that ovulation will not occur on an atypical day in that particular cycle. So when in doubt, treat.

7.11 What are the time-limits for successful treatment?

1 *The IUD method*. Here the time limit of 5 days relates to the *most likely* expected day of ovulation. This is calculated in good faith from the menstrual data given by the woman, and applies irrespective of the number of earlier acts of unprotected intercourse. Five days is well within the time limits from intercourse to implantation, according to the consensus of medical opinion. It will not be construed in law as possibly procuring an abortion. Though some would play safe and say that the calculation should begin from *the earliest* calculated day of ovulation, my view is that, depending on the woman's own views about the ethics of the situation, it should be the *most likely* day. This is strengthened by a recent judgement which gives at least one day of legal leeway (day 20 rather than day 19 of a 28-day cycle) and hints at more:

Regina v Dhingra, 24th January, 1991. Mr Justice Wright did not convict a general practitioner accused of illegal abortion achieved by inserting an IUD 11 days after intercourse, because it was day 18 and thus prior to implantation. 'I further hold, in accordance with the uncontroverted evidence that I have heard, that a pregnancy cannot come into existence until the fertilized ovum has become implanted in the womb, and that stage is not reached until, at the earliest, the 20th day of a normal 28-day cycle, and, in all probability, until the next period is missed.'

2 *The Yuzpe method*. The early studies have been confirmed recently: there is an increase in the failure rate if treatment is initiated more than 72 hours after exposure (see also Q 7.12). This does not mean that the method is *absolutely* contraindicated any later than that.

7.12 Is it always preferable to treat at the earliest possible moment?

1 *The IUD method* is so effective that delay (up to 5 days after ovulation) is unlikely to lead to failure, but would give no advantage.

2 *The Yuzpe hormonal method*. Here the answer may be different according to whether the mechanism of action is by the blocking of ovulation or of implantation.

   If ovulation is imminent it is presumably important to treat as soon as possible. On the other hand, in view of the 5-day time lag between fertilization and ovulation, some delay in initiating treatment might actually enhance the anti-implantation effect. This is entirely theoretical, and in our own studies at the MPC we could demonstrate no significant difference in failure rate if treatment was initiated in the first, the second or the third 24 hours following exposure.

It remains normal practice to start treatment as soon as the women presents. But there may certainly be some flexibility, for the convenience of the woman herself or the clinician (especially with respect to the second dose; see Q 7.7).

7.13 What reasons may account for 'failure' of the oral preparations?

1 Treatment initiated *more than 72 hours after intercourse*.

2 *Multiple exposure*. This is one of the most important reasons. It is therefore essential to question each woman most closely about the possibility of inadequate contraception during intercourse at any time *earlier* than the index event.

3 *Vomiting within 3 hours of tablet-taking*. In practice this is a relatively rare cause of failure. Some authorities argue that there is no need to replace the second two tablets if are vomited back, since the occurrence of vomiting implies a particularly strong pharmacological effect. Again, there are no data to support or refute that view.

   In practice women should always be instructed to contact the clinician for consideration of some action, particularly in a high pregnancy-risk case. Such action could be the provision of a further two tablets (as appropriate these can be given in advance), or sometimes the insertion of an IUD.

4 *Non-compliance* leading to inadequate dosage. For this reason some clinicians prefer to see the first two tablets swallowed in their presence.

5 *Unprotected intercourse* subsequent to the treatment (see Q 7.6).

2 and 5 are the most common explanations, aside from the true method failures.

7.14 What are the risks if the PC treatment fails?

This is a vitally important aspect of counselling, dealt with here and in Q 7.15.

   Ectopic pregnancy should be mentioned. Whenever either method operates at the uterine level, if the woman has pre-existing tubal damage (known or unknown), tubal implantation will clearly not be prevented. Additionally, there is the possibility that the hormonal methods might interfere with tubal transport. This is disputed: Qs 6.30, 5.33 are relevant to this discussion.

Out of 715 women treated at the MPC before March 1983, one ectopic pregnancy occurred among 17 failures of the Yuzpe regimen. Other studies have similarly reported an ectopic pregnancy rate of up to 10% when other hormone methods were used, but the MPC case had a clear previous history of salpingitis.

In by far the majority of cases the association of an ectopic with PC treatment will not be causal. But any woman may have tubal damage and since she will be at risk with or without treatment, it is safest to warn her to seek prompt advice if any pelvic pain occurs.

7.15 If the pregnancy is in the uterus, will it be harmed in any way?

A small teratogenic risk cannot be ruled out since insufficient pregnancies have gone to term after hormonal PC treatment failure. In a series collected by the UK National Association of Family Planning Doctors, prior to going to press there had been 50 full-term pregnancies whose outcome was known. Among these the only major abnormality detected was an absent kidney (one case). The woman may be told:

> The risk of a pregnancy being harmed is believed to be extremely small, less than that when the ordinary pill is inadvertently taken in early pregnancy – but no one can ever be promised a normal baby. Research so far looking at babies born after failure of the emergency pill has shown up no harmful effects. The risk is so low that an abortion should never be recommended solely on these grounds.

Moreover, if the Yuzpe hormonal method is used very little of the artificial oestrogen and progestagen could reach the blastocyst via the uterine secretions since it is not yet implanted. Also it is very resistant to partial damage by noxious agents. Research in animals suggests that the blastocyst is either destroyed or else, since its cells are 'totipotent', it can recover and develop entirely normally.

It is very much accepted clinical practice for women to continue to full term when they have taken the ordinary pill for several weeks during organogenesis. Yet if anything there is then more risk of teratogenesis amounting to an increase of much less than 0.1%, on top of the background risk of important birth defects, which is 2% (see Q 4.205).

The circumstances of the failed postcoital conception mean that in practice most women request a therapeutic abortion. If a woman wishes to continue to full term, very detailed records should be kept to the effect that she has fully understood the arguments presented here and realizes that no guarantee can be given that the baby will be normal.

In the ultra-rare event of continuing pregnancy following PC insertion of an IUD, management should normally include removal of the device as discussed at Q 6.25 (see also Qs 7.30 and 7.32).

INDICATIONS AND ADVANTAGES OF POSTCOITAL CONTRACEPTION

7.16 What are the advantages of PC contraception?

1 It provides a way of escape from an unwanted pregnancy at a time of high motivation after (for whatever reason) unprotected intercourse has taken place.

2 By definition it is non-intercourse-related.

3 Both methods are effective; the IUD more so.

4 The methods can be applied well after exposure to the risk with a good chance of success: 3 days after if the hormone method is used, and in an extreme case up to 12 days (after exposure on, say, day 7), if an IUD is employed.

5 The methods are safe, though sharing the potential hazards of hormonal/intrauterine contraception respectively. No deaths have been reported.

6 Presentation for the PC treatment gives a welcome opportunity to discuss future contraception; in the case of the IUD, solving the woman's immediate problem can also provide for her long-term needs.

7 The method is under a woman's control (i.e. its use cannot be prevented by her partner, if she can find a sympathetic doctor).

8 The method can be prescribed in advance in selected cases: for example, a young woman about to travel abroad and anxious about rape or other circumstances of unprotected intercourse in foreign parts.

> **Note however: The present hormonal method is not appropriate for regular ongoing use, for several reasons (see Q 7.38).**

7.17 What are the indications for the treatment?

On presentation, depending on time of the cycle that exposure took place (see Q 7.10), whenever the clinician feels that the small risks of the method are outweighed by the risks of pregnancy and other relevant factors such as the woman's level of anxiety.

7.18 How do women present for treatment?

1 *No method used*
   (a) *'Moonlight and roses'* summarizes the commonest presentation in this category, where intercourse was unpremeditated. It is often with a new partner, especially first-time ever intercourse or extramarital affairs (e.g. where the husband has had a vasectomy). Or there could have been an unexpected reconciliation with an ex-partner. Bound up in these situations is that saying 'sex is hot but contraception is cold'; something which if discussed would, the woman feels, make her out to be unromantic at best and at worst a slut. Even today and worldwide, far too few men consider that birth control is any of their business what so ever.
   (b) Intercourse under the influence of *alcohol or drugs.*
   (c) Total misunderstanding of the *'safe period'* approach can be another way that, effectively, no method was used.
   (d) *Special situations*:
      Rape and sexual assault. Here counselling and management must be even more sensitive than usual and continuing emotional support is likely to be required. Involvement of the nearest Rape Crisis Centre and the local police force may be necessary. Avoid destroying forensic evidence if an accusation is to be made, and arrange tests for STDs.
      Incest.
      Certain sufferers from mental handicap.
      Recent use of teratogens – drugs, or live vaccine such as polio or yellow fever.

2 *Contraceptive failure (of the method or of its use)*
   (a) The commonest category here is the *split* or *slipped condom.* In a study from the West Midlands no fewer than 48 out of

80 women reported a broken sheath. In more than one case a fragment of rubber was retrieved from the upper vagina, proving that not all such reports are fictions to appear respectable in the eyes of the doctor.

Note: In such cases always discuss whether the condom might have been exposed to any mineral or vegetable oil (see Q 2.20)

(b) Complete or partial *expulsion of an IUD*, identified mid cycle. Here careful reinsertion of another IUD is preferable, especially if there has been repeated intercourse since the last menstrual period. But occasionally the Yuzpe method might be preferred.

(c) If there has been recent intercourse and deliberate *removal of an IUD* at midcycle is essential as part of therapy for infection (see Q 6.14).

(d) *Errors of cap use* – e.g. the discovery after intercourse that it was in the anterior fornix – or its too-early removal.

(e) Gross *prolongation of the pill–free week* in a COC-user. Normally when intercourse has continued and pills are missed the woman should simply follow the 7-day rule at Q 4.16. However, if the pill-free week has been extended to 9 or more days, *or the equivalent, due to missed pills during the first 7 days of a new pack*: it is probably wisest to recommend the full Yuzpe regimen, followed by immediate return to pill taking; and also the use of a condom for the next 7 days. (See Qs 4.15–21.)

   Hormonal PC treatment is usually redundant for mid-cycle pill omissions, provided at least 7 tablets were correctly taken; though it might be given empirically if 4 or more tablets were missed.

(f) *In a POP–user*: exposure any time from the first missed tablet until the mucus effect is expected to be restored justifies the Yuzpe treatment, followed by 7 days' condom use. But not during full lactation (Q 5.23).

(g) *Other contraceptive accidents* involving, for example, the contraceptive sponge, spermicides or the POP. Also if injectables have to be given slightly late. See Q 5.128.

DISADVANTAGES OF POSTCOITAL CONTRACEPTION

7.19 What are the disadvantages?

1 *The Yuzpe hormonal method.*
   (a) Nausea, and vomiting in up to a quarter of cases.
   (b) Failure rate (1–5%).
   (c) The method is usually avoided if there is an absolute contraindication to *oestrogen* therapy (e.g. past thromboembolism). Note, however, that most of the other contraindications to the combined pill can be disregarded, with such short-term use. *There is no age limit.*
   (d) Further unprotected intercourse following therapy must be avoided, in case of postponement of ovulation (see Q 7.6).
   (e) The next menses may sometimes be delayed (see Q 7.37).

2 *IUD*
   (a) 'A surgical' procedure involved – when what the woman is primarily requesting is a quick medical 'fix it'.
   (b) Pain may be caused to the woman at insertion or subsequently.
   (c) Risk of causing or exacerbating pelvic inflammatory disease (PID). Where the method must be used and the risk is high because of past infection or the circumstance of exposure (e.g. rape), then after the relevant tests antibiotic cover should be considered.
   (d) There is a risk of causing all the other known complications of IUDs, since these are so often insertion related (see Qs 6.22 and 6.94).

7.20 What is the incidence of nausea after the hormonal methods?

After the EE method some nausea is practically invariable lasting at least for the 5 days of treatment, and marked in 50–70% of women.

With the Yuzpe hormonal method the frequency is less, but disappointingly it was reported in 60% of 168 women studied at the MPC, though it was only slight or moderate in three-quarters of those with the symptom. It was also never prolonged beyond 36 hours, and usually lasted for less than 24 hours.

The incidence of vomiting in the MPC study was 24%, most commonly occurring once only.

7.21 What can be done to minimize the nausea problem? Should one give antiemetics?

1 In the first place, forewarned is forearmed, and most women in this situation are happy to accept the side-effect.

2 Where the timing of intercourse and presentation permit, the second dose should be followed by sleep if possible.

3 Some authorities have recommended the use of antiemetics (Hyoscine is now proposed). However, the use of such drugs adds to the risk of side-effects (e.g. oculogyric crises in young woman given metoclopramide (Maxolon), and to the complexity of counselling about any possible effect on a pregnancy should the PC treatment fail (see Q 7.15). Moreover, it may not successfully eliminate the symptom. Hence at MPC antiemetic treatment is given selectively, not routinely.

4 Since the COC has been shown to be absorbed from the vagina, if vomiting is a problem one possibility to consider (which has *not* as yet been formally studied in this context) is to give repeat doses into the vagina, retained by a tampon. NAFPD suggests 4 tablets of PC4 by this route, to replace any one dose.

7.22 What other symptoms are associated with PC treatment?

The only common one is breast tenderness, though this is less frequent than after the EE regimen and usually of short duration. A range of other symptoms have been reported including dizziness, headaches, eye symptoms, etc., but the association with therapy is not necessarily causal.

A few women report a 'withdrawal bleed' following treatment and the woman should be instructed not to assume that this is her next period (unless she was treated very late in the cycle), but to report it at the follow-up visit.

PATIENT SELECTION AND CHOICE OF METHOD

7.23 What are the absolute contraindications to PC contraception?

1 *Pregnancy.* The presence of an early implanted pregnancy may be difficult to eliminate; but every effort should be made by taking a careful history, doing a vaginal examination and where indicated the most sensitive pregnancy test available.

2 *Absolute contraindications* of the method to be used:

(a) *To hormonal methods* (i.e. normally use IUD instead). The absolute contraindications to oestrogens are usually held to apply (especially past thromboembolism (NAFPD Guidelines (1992) classify this as a *relative* contraindication but I consider it to be '*strong*') or a current focal migraine attack). Absolute contraindications which relate to long-term use of hormones, or specifically to arterial disease (atherogenesis) – and hence primarily to the progestagenic component – need not be considered as contraindications to any hormonal PC method. *There is no upper age limit* (if there is sufficient risk of conception).

(b) *To the intrauterine device* (i.e. normally use a hormonal method). The majority of both the temporary and permanent contraindications listed at Qs 6.79–6.81 would be held to apply. However, it may be acceptable practice in selected cases to insert a copper IUD with full antibiotic cover (see Q 7.19) when PID has not been excluded; or in women at high risk (especially after rape).

If the IUD method is thought inappropriate for long-term use (e.g. in a nullipara who has had a previous ectopic pregnancy), it can always be removed following the next period.

3 In the case of a patient who defines any treatment which might act after fertilization as 'inducing an abortion', and the latter is ethically unacceptable to her.

7.24 What are only relative contraindications to the use of the hormonal method?

1 Presentation *more than 72 hours* after unprotected intercourse. But it is still an option since self-evidently the hormonal method's efficacy does not disappear precisely at 72 hours.

2 *Previous ectopic pregnancy.* Ectopic pregnancies have been described after both types of treatment (see Q 7.14). However, the cause of those tubal implantations is most commonly pre-existing tubal damage. Hence if the PC treatment is timed to prevent implantation, the ectopic risk will be the same with or without treatment. Indeed if exposure were early in the cycle a hormonal method could be beneficial, since it might prevent fertilization.

3 If a woman accepts that PC treatment is family planning, but can neither accept the minimal risk of teratogenesis nor an induced abortion were the method to fail, the very much more effective option – insertion of an IUD – would clearly be preferable.

4 *Post partum*. If there exists an ovulation risk, there need be no worries about thrombosis (see Q 4.45). The woman can be reassured that the Yuzpe method will not impair *lactation*. If she is concerned to avoid the vanishingly small but unquantified risk through the artificial hormones entering her breast milk, this can be done by expressing the breast milk and bottlefeeding the infant for 24 hours.

7.25 What if a woman taking an enzyme-inducing drug should require emergency contraception?

See Qs 4.31-3 for a full discussion of this important question in relation to regular use of the COC. The solution here according to Professor Orme is simply to double the doses given. In other words, 4 tablets of PC4 or Ovran would be taken stat., followed by 4 more 12 hours later.

7.26 What are the relative contraindications to PC IUD insertion?

1 All the relative contraindications listed at Q 6.81 might apply if it is intended that the method will be used long term, but some (e.g. history of dysmenorrhoea or menorrhagia) are irrelevant to short-term use, until the time of the next period (see also Q 7.23).

2 *Past ectopic pregnancy*. This is a slightly stronger relative contraindication than it is to the Yuzpe method (see Q 7.24), but does not preclude very short-term use in selected cases (Q 7.23).

7.27 Since the majority of women presenting for PC con traception prefer and expect oral treatment, when should the intrauterine method be offered instead?

As the question implies, the Yuzpe hormonal method is the normal first choice *except* where there are the following special reasons for an IUD:

1 Where she desires the *most effective* available option.

2 Where there is an *absolute contraindication to oestrogen* (unless the LNG 0.6 mg method at Q 7.5 is deemed appropriate). This includes the case of a woman with *focal migraine* who has a migraine at presentation.

3 Where there has been *multiple exposure*, and the clinician inserts the device in good faith no more than 5 days after the most probable calculated ovulation date (see Q 7.11).

4 Where presentation is *more than 72 hours* since a single episode of unprotected intercourse (the upper time-limit being as at 3).

5 The woman's desire to use *the IUD as her long–term method*. However it is always permissible and sometimes to be recommended that the device is used purely to solve the immediate problem, and removed at the next menses.

6 Rarely, *after vomiting of the tablets* when Yuzpe's regimen was initially selected. IUD insertion is only indicated if she is a high pregnancy risk case and if the vomiting occurs within 3 hours of the woman ingesting a dose, especially the first dose. Otherwise additional tablets may be given, *along with an antiemetic* (or perhaps by the vaginal route? See Q 7.21).

COUNSELLING AND MANAGEMENT AT THE FIRST VISIT

7.28 How important is counselling for PC contraception?

From the doctor's point of view the treatment is simple. It is the counselling before treatment which can be both taxing and time consuming. Obviously if there has been a simple condom rupture or dislodgement occurring in a stable relationship the amount of emotional support required will be far less than in cases of rape or incest – although the availability of such support should always be made clear. Every woman in this situation is under some stress, and needs information and clear instructions sympathetically given. In practice much of the counselling can be delegated to a family planning-trained nurse.

7.29 In summary, what aspects should be covered in taking the medical history?

1 Date of the last menstrual period, and whether it was in any way abnormal.

2 Details of the patient's normal menstrual cycles – shortest, longest and most unusual lengths.

3 The calculated date of ovulation.

4 The day(s) in the cycle of all unprotected intercourse.

5 The number of hours since the *first* episode of unprotected inter-course.

6 The current method of contraception.

7 Any contraindications (from the history) to either type of PC treatment. (See Qs 7.23–7.27.)

It should be stressed that the whole 'contract' to give this kind of treatment depends on mutual good faith and honesty, especially concerning the menstrual/coital history.

7.30 What are the ten main points to cover in counselling for emergency contraception?

1 Assess the menstrual and coital history in Q 7.29, and hence whether any treatment is necessary.

2 Discuss the methods available and their mode of action and medical risks.

3 The failure rate of each method, and the implications: i.e. the (low) risks of fetal abnormality (see Q 7.15) and of ectopic pregnancy (see Qs 7.14 and 7.24).

4 Explore her attitudes to possible failure of the regimen and con-tinuance of the pregnancy.

5 Discuss the consequential importance of follow-up – and the possibility that her next period might require medical assess-ment. Suggest that she brings an early morning urine sample if it is surprisingly light or absent.

6 Make the final decision about whether to use PC treatment, and which method, only after full discussion with the woman.

7 If the Yuzpe method is selected advise her regarding nausea and vomiting. She should telephone the clinic or surgery for advice if she vomits within 3 hours of either dose. (Or she may be given two extra tablets in advance.)

8 Discuss contraception in the current cycle (see Q 7.6) – not a problem if the IUD is used.

9 Discuss long-term contraception. See Q 7.33 for the advice to be given if the combined pill is selected.

10 Keep an accurate record, written at the time, dated and signed.

7.31 Should these women always be examined vaginally?

In my view the answer is *normally* 'yes', as for a routine first visit contraceptive consultation, unless there are special reasons for not doing so: a good example being anxiety in a young teenager presenting after her first-ever sexual experience.

Otherwise this first examination is valuable because:

1 It can exclude a concealed clinical pregnancy.

2 Pelvic tenderness or a purulent discharge suggestive of infection may be discovered.

3 Microbiological samples can be taken, especially for chlamydia.

4 Suitability for an IUD can be assessed (in case it becomes indicated).

5 Finally, *a baseline is established*: e.g. if an irregular outline of the uterus is noted (suggesting small fibroids) this will assist any follow-up examination. The latter is only required if clinically indicated (see Q 7.36).

Women receiving a hormonal method should normally also have their baseline blood pressure measured.

7.32 Should the woman be asked to sign any type of consent form?

This is held to be unnecessary provided accurate contemporaneous records are kept, the clinician asserting that the woman gave verbal informed consent. It is most helpful to supplement the counselling with an appropriate leaflet (see Q 4.97). Unusually, the leaflet provided by the manufacturer (of PC4) is acceptable, as is that of the FPA.

In the MPC experience, if women sign to the effect that it is their responsibility to return, the follow-up rate is much higher.

FOLLOW-UP

7.33 If the woman selects an oral contraceptive subsequent to PC treatment, when should she take the first tablet?

It is now routine that both the COC and the POP are commenced on the first day of the menses. However, there is sometimes a light (and not relevant) withdrawal bleed just after the Yuzpe hormones, and a light 'threatened abortion' loss may also occur very early in pregnancy. I used to teach, therefore, that both the COC and POP should be started on about the second day, when the woman was convinced that the flow was within her own normal range. This slight delay still allowed the woman not to be required to use extra contraceptive precautions (see Q 5.25, Table 4.4).

I am now convinced by colleagues who argue that the pill is so unlikely to lead to any diagnostic problems that allowing women to start as usual on the first day is simpler and preferable. They should be told to take urgent advice first before starting the pill if there is only a slight 'show' and they would plan to continue to term if pregnant.

7.34 Might she be instructed to start the combined pill immediately following PC treatment?

Except as in the next paragraph, this is not generally thought to be good practice, for an obvious medicolegal reason. If the woman were to conceive, and the baby have an important fetal abnormality (as occurs in 2% of cases), a claim that the abnormality was caused by the extra packet of combined pills being given after implantation would be difficult to resist. It would, of course, be highly unlikely that such an abnormality was truly caused by the COC (see Q 4.205). However, it would be less unlikely than teratogenesis caused by the Yuzpe regimen alone (Q 7.15).

There are certain circumstances in which this may be acceptable management, provided there has been a thorough and documented discussion of all the implications with the woman concerned; especially in a case where the risk of PC treatment failing is considered to be particularly low. One example would be where the pill-free week has been extended, and this has already been mentioned (see Q 7.18).

7.35 What should be done if a woman has already received PC treatment and returns 3 or 4 days later reporting condom rupture during the latest intercourse? May one use the Yuzpe hormone treatment more than once in a given cycle?

Yes. Since in clinical practice we cannot be sure when ovulation occurs, and it may have been postponed by the earlier treatment, it may well be right to represcribe, for a second or even a third time. The only problem may be assessing any irregular bleeding which follows.

IUD insertion might also be reconsidered, in a case at exceptionally high pregnancy risk.

7.36 How important is it to follow up PC women after treatment?

A defined follow-up visit is important, normally set for 3–4 weeks post-treatment. Equally important, the woman must be clear that she should return earlier should any untoward symptom arise, particularly low abdominal pain or heavy bleeding.

At the follow-up visit (*or telephone contact*), ensure that:

1 The woman is not pregnant, either in uterus or tube. A pregnancy test may sometimes be necessary and, if there is any clinical doubt, a pelvic examination.

2 She now has an effective method of contraception. Those who were fitted with an IUD may normally retain the device. But beware of the pressure that there may be to 'leave well alone' in circumstances in which the IUD is a poor choice for long-term use (see Qs 6.78–81 and 7.23), and the original and better plan was to transfer to another method.

   Users of hormonal contraception should already have started their tablets. Users of a barrier method should be taught or retaught as necessary.

3 If the method has failed, good pregnancy counselling should follow. There is no real difference in the content of this counselling from that when any other method of birth control has failed (see Q 7.15). Unless the woman is having a termination, if she is pregnant with an IUD in position the device should be gently removed (see Qs 6.25 and 6.26).

7.37 What is the usual time of onset of the next period after PC treatment?

This is variable with the Yuzpe regimen. Among 45 women treated successfully at the MPC, the next period began on the expected date (± 1 day) in 22% and was up to or more than a week early in 62%. Only in 16% of women was the next period 2–6 days late. It is believed that late onset is more likely when treatment was early enough in the cycle to postpone ovulation. When it acts to block implantation the method tends to bring the next period on early, whether or not there is withdrawal bleeding immediately after the treatment (the latter being quite uncommon).

It is useful to be able to tell the woman that her next period is likely to be on time or early, so she will not need to be in suspense for too long.

No obvious impact on cycle length has been reported following postcoital IUD insertion.

7.38 What are the objections to the Yuzpe method being prescribed in advance for use on a regular basis?

1 The treatment would have to be given after each act of intercourse and many women could finish up having taken more hormones than if they simply took the COC daily for 21 days. But repeating the regimen is acceptable as a short-term expedient (see Q 7.35); also advance prescription of one-off treatment may sometimes be justifiable (see Q 7.17).

   Most women who request regular emergency contraception are those who have intercourse once a month or less, on a rather unpredictable basis. There are still two objections however:

2 The incidence of nausea is high (see Q 7.20) and relatively few women would find this acceptable on a regular basis as the 'penalty' for intercourse.

3 More importantly, the existing Yuzpe method is simply not effective enough to be used on a regular monthly basis. This is because its failure rate is about 2% of those treated, and higher among those who would have become pregnant (see Q 7.8). Taking the 2% monthly figure, this means very roughly that at the end of 1 year of treatment, once every 28 days, the *cumulative* annual risk of pregnancy could be as high as 26/100 woman-years.

7.39 What would be the features of an ideal PC contraceptive?

These would be similar to those of any reversible birth control method (see Q 0.10), but the following aspects would require particular emphasis. The ideal PC treatment would:

1 be so effective each month that on a cumulative basis the annual rate of failures was less than 1/100 woman-years (cf. Q 7.8);

2 be effective for the remainder of each cycle as well as in relation to the particular act of intercourse (see Q 7.6);

3 require only a single dose;

4 have a very low incidence of side-effects, whether dangerous or annoying (such as nausea);

5 cause no disturbance of the menstrual cycle;

6 be free of teratogenic effects.

With these features, a PC method could be realistically prescribed in advance for use on a regular basis. Women with an 'erratic sex life' could then use a non-intercourse-related method for application only when required, thereby reducing their exposure to medication.

7.40 What are the prospects for the future of PC contraception?

A really reliable postovulatory contraceptive agent with the features in Q 7.39, coupled with a simple and reliable method of determining whether intercourse had taken place before or after ovulation, would be a considerable advance. Indeed, in the distant future it might be possible for regular release of a PC agent (e.g. from an implant) to be actually triggered by a biological event such as the LH surge.

Another potential approach, though one fraught with ethical and legal difficulties, is the regular use of a postconceptional or *contragestive* agent to be administrated only when the woman is overdue her period. This approach would of course be a regular method abortion, but it would mean exposure to the potential systemic risks of the agent only on a few occasions each year. This is because, even among fertile couples having regular intercourse, implantation is only successful once in every two or three cycles.

7.41 Specifically what agents are being studied?

1 The greatest current interest is in progesterone receptor blocking agents, such as *RU 486 (mifepristone)*. Using the usual criteria for PC treatment, there were no failures among over 400 women treated, in a study from Edinburgh comparing this with the Yuzpe hormonal method (which failed at the usual rate).

2 *Danazol* alone shows some promise in studies from Italy (though unconfirmed), and like mifepristone it does not cause the nausea problem.

3 *Luteolytic agents and methods involving immune mechanisms* are also under study.

QUESTIONS ASKED BY PROSPECTIVE USERS OF POSTCOITAL CONTRACEPTION

As with the POP, too few questions are asked because there is still remarkable ignorance among the general public that this option is even available. Most of the likely questions have already been answered above.

7.42 Is the 'emergency pill' the same as the 'morning after pill'?

Yes, it is. The reason for the new name is that the treatment can be given much later than the morning after (at least 72 hours, and after many days if the IUD method is chosen), so the old name was extremely misleading. It should now be abandoned!

7.43 Is the emergency pill the same as the contraceptive pill?

It contains the same two hormones as one type, but it is given in a different way, i.e. in two larger doses, 12 hours apart, following intercourse.

7.44 If it is so similar, why do doctors keep the treatment hidden away? If my sex life is erratic, why can I not be given pills in advance for use on a regular basis?

The answer to this common question is given at Q 7.38. The existing method is really not effective enough for regular use, and causes side-effects, especially nausea and vomiting. In addition, there are some special reasons it should not be used at all by some women, or why the alternative IUD method would be medically preferable (see Qs 7.24 and 7.27).

There is a contrary view, that since the pill method is remarkably safe healthwise and there is such an epidemic of unplanned pregnancies in many countries, the benefits would outweigh the risks if it were much more available, e.g. over the counter, supervised by pharmacists. I have a lot of sympathy with this idea, given certain safeguards and the availability of medical back-up.

7.45 I shall be travelling alone in the Far East and South America for the next 6 months. Could I take a supply of PC treatment for emergency use?

In this situation, providing there are no contraindications for you to use the method at all, it would be very reasonable for you to be prescribed a supply in advance (see Q 7.38). You might, alternatively, consider arranging a regular method like the pill or even an IUD.

7.46 Can I wait a few hours for my own or the doctor's convenience, or should I be treated just as soon as possible?

There should certainly not be any undue delay, but the evidence available suggests that delaying a few hours so long as you remain within the 72-hour time limit is unlikely to affect the outcome. Certainly there is no need to disturb the doctor within a few minutes or an hour of intercourse!

7.47 Should I mention any earlier times when we made love (since my last period), when I attend the doctor for morning-after treatment?

Yes this is essential. The decisions as to whether to treat and how to treat successfully all depend on your being entirely forthcoming about every relevant fact. This also includes telling the doctor the correct date of your last period. The whole 'contract' between you and him/her depends on what is called 'utmost good faith'.

7.48 Will I need to be examined before PC treatment?

Normally yes, but it may be safe to miss this out if you are very anxious about examinations (see Q 7.31).

7.49 Why might the doctor decide not to treat me, if I attend for PC treatment?

The main reason might be that, after considering the time of the month and every other aspect, your doctor judges that there is an almost-nil risk of conception occurring; and that this does not justify the (small) risks of the PC treatment.

7.50 What should I do if I vomit within 3 hours of either of my doses, especially if I actually bring back some of the pills?

Take the urgent advice of your doctor. If he or she thinks that there is a high risk of conception in your case, it may be right then to insert an IUD; but sometimes it will be enough just to give you additional tablets, or even no special treatment at all (see Q 7.13).

7.51 Why did the doctor recommend an IUD for me when I really wanted pills?

For one of the reasons in Q 7.27. This could then be a good method for you to continue using long term; but remember that you can instead have it removed after your next period, if you then plan perhaps to transfer to another effective method such as the combined pill.

7.52 Why should I use another method of family planning between PC treatment and the start of my next period?

The reason is that sometimes the method may be working not by blocking the fertilized egg from establishing itself in your womb, but instead by blocking egg release. There is then the risk of fertilizing that later egg if your partner does not use another method such as the condom.

7.53 Should I expect a period immediately after using PC pills?

A few women get what is known as 'a withdrawal bleed' within a day or two of the treatment. This will not seem like a proper period and, unless you were due one, it is important to continue using the condom or any other effective method you were recommended to use, until you have a definite period – or until you are seen for follow-up at the clinic. Fortunately, your proper period normally arrives either on time or a little early. It is still essential that you keep your follow-up appointments, and this is even more vital if the next period is delayed or unexpectedly light (in which case take urgent advice before starting contraceptive pills).

7.54 For what reasons should I see the doctor sooner than arranged, following PC treatment?

The main reason would be because of any pain in your abdomen, because of the small risk of pregnancy in your tube (see Q 7.14).

7.55 Does morning-after treatment cause an abortion?

No, not according to the modern view of when pregnancy starts (see Q 7.2 and Fig. 7.1).

7.56 Must I have an abortion if PC treatment fails?

Not necessarily. It is thought that this treatment will not significantly increase the risk of an abnormal baby above the surprisingly high 2% risk that all women run. So the decision (always very difficult) about what to do about the unplanned pregnancy is really just the same as it would be if any other systemic method of family planning were to fail, such as the pill (see Q 7.15).

8 Conspectus: present and future

As intended, and mentioned in the Preface, this book has been primarily about how best to select and use the existing reversible birth control technology. *The rather brief discussion of related subjects does not imply that they are unimportant.* See Further Reading!

This chapter includes much that is useful revision of the information elsewhere in the text. I am particularly indebted to Toni Belfield, Head of Information and Research of the UK Family Planning Association (FPA). She has allowed me to use sections of her own text from a 1992 article, but much rearranged in this book's question-and-answer style.

8.1 What is meant by the term 'contraceptive dynamism'?

Please refer to Figures 8.1 and 8.2, along with Tables 0.1 (see Q 0.11) and 0.2 (*re* failure rates).

The relative importance of the two main factors – maximum *health safety* as opposed to maximum *effectiveness* and independence from *intercourse* – and hence the appropriateness of different methods, varies greatly according to all the factors shown in Dr Christopher's 'Factors Wheel' (Figure 8.1 and see also Appendix).

Choice, it seems, is seldom based on rational or objective information – the fact that a friend had a dreadful time with an IUD will weigh far more heavily than any amount of statistics that show this is not usually the case. It is also influenced by age and stage during an individual couple's reproductive lifetime. Decisions are made at specific times:

- At the beginning of sexual experience.
- After an accidental pregnancy or 'near-miss'.
- Life changes, e.g. career change.
- A planned birth.
- When there are problems with a particular method.
- When the family is complete.

Initially, while the relationship is being established, a high degree of efficacy may be considered most important. However if their sexual experience is infrequent or sporadic, barrier methods

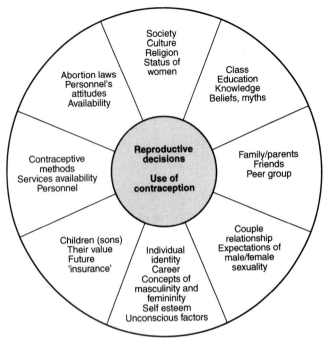

Figure 8.1 Reproductive decisions – The Factors Wheel. (Courtesy Elphis Christopher). See Q 8.1 and Appendix.

may be ideal provided they are used correctly, especially as they have the bonus of some protection against sexually transmitted diseases (STDs).

For child spacing, less efficient methods with reduced health risk may well be preferred. Once the family is established, but the couple are not sure whether it is yet complete, the IUD can have particular merit. These points are summarized in Table 8.1, which is derived from Table 15 of my book *The Pill*.

This changing pattern of reproductive desire, in the couple's total life situation, places a big responsibility on the doctor or nurse to be themselves flexible and fully informed about the whole range of methods available. *They must also be able and willing to spend time finding out who they are actually dealing with* under the headings summarized in Figure 8.1!

Table 8.1 The seven contraceptive ages of woman

'Age'	Suggested method – but there are other options
1. Birth to puberty	No method required. However, responsible matter-of-fact sex education is essential – principally from the parents. Schools can help. Discussion of RELATIONSHIPS more important than biological and medical details.
2. Puberty to marriage	Either (a) a barrier method (sheath or cap plus spermicide) or (b) the combined pill or an injectable, or (c) the 'best' oral contraceptive (i.e. saying 'no') Choice depends on factors like religious views, the steadiness of the relationship, and frequency of intercourse
3. Marriage to first child	First choice usually the combined pill, followed by a barrier method for 1 month before 'trying' for the first child. Sponge also usable
4. During breastfeeding	First choice: barrier method – could be the sponge until periods start. Second choice: (a) IUD (but a small risk to future fertility), (b) progestagen-only pill (but unknown effect of the minute amount of hormone transferred in the breast milk)
5. Family spacing after breastfeeding	Perhaps shift to combined pill at this time for greater effectiveness and a regular bleeding pattern
6. After the (probable) last child	First choice: IUD. Other possibilities: barrier methods or the oestrogen-free hormonal methods, according to choice
7. Family complete, children growing up and other methods unacceptable	Vasectomy: or female sterilization using clips or rings

8.2 Do not the words 'compliant' and 'non-compliant' sound rather 'bossy', and as though we prescribe and then everything else is those silly contraceptive-users' fault?

Yes: but if we can ourselves agree not to mean anything of the sort, there are no simpler words alluding to the user's responsibility in avoidance of user-failure. More on the provider's responsibility follows later.

Regardless of whatever professional hat we wear, we are all consumers when it comes to thinking about or using contraception. But *how* contraception is *considered, discussed* and, more importantly, *delivered* will determine just how well it is accepted and used.

8.3 How big is the problem?

Today contraceptive choices and services are freely available, and research shows that people have the facts (in their heads) about contraception. Yet unintended pregnancy and requests for abortion remain consistently high.

Abstinence, that most effective of all methods, applies in recent surveys to less than half of all girls who were 16 at their last birthday (just 48% claimed to be virgins in a 1991 study from the South-west of England, and only 12% by age 20). Given the potential emotional and psychosocial trauma, quite apart from the risk of STDs and cervical neoplasia, this group (and the boys too), should receive our encouragement, as providers, to continue resisting peer-group pressure; i.e. that it really is worth *waiting* for 'Mr or Miss Right'. They should not be labelled a *minority* group, since this has an implication of abnormality. Yet, in the real world, the remainder do need confidential and appropriate family planning services.

Although the under 16s achieve more publicity, the older teenagers and women aged 20–25 are together responsible for far more unplanned pregnancies. A 1991 study of recent mothers by Anne Fleissig showed that in the UK as many as one in three of the last pregnancies was unplanned. In the same year it was estimated in 'Population Trends' that one in five clinical pregnancies ended in legal abortion. Cumulatively, about one woman in three in the UK now has at least one termination before the age of 30.

In a 1991 study of teenage mothers 84% had no intention to become pregnant, but were using no contraception when they conceived ... Although in some studies where there *was* good compliance, the combined oral contraceptive (COC) has had failure rates which were well below 1 per 100 woman-years (Table 0.2), in typical use failure rates of 3% are commonly reported, rising to up to 20% in inner city areas. Worldwide, it has been calculated that if by improved pill taking we could reduce the failure rate of this one method by 1%, at least 630 000 fewer women would have accidental pregnancies each year.

8.4   What is the most important single reason for unwanted conceptions?

Sex! But not just in the obvious way.

1   Sex is embarrassing. Contraception is inextricably linked with emotional and sexual well-being, and it is impossible to talk about contraception without addressing sexuality – the two are inseparable. Research shows that contraception continues to be a source of considerable embarrassment and anxiety for both men and women, and this has implications for its uptake and usage. It can have an inhibiting effect on people's willingness to seek information and advice from professionals.

2   Also, in Elphis Christopher's memorable phrase (see p 441), 'sex is hot, and contraception is cold'. Snowden wrote in 1990 that while it may be argued that the prevention of pregnancy is beneficial, the use of contraception is not a pleasant experience for most people, which is a marked contrast to the sexual behaviour which prompts its need! Actual choice results from a negative process of 'seeking the least bad' among the options. The methods not chosen are even more disliked than the method that is chosen.

3   And sex is *now*, the possible problems seem unimportant at the time. Head knowledge can be superb without affecting behaviour in the heat of the moment.

> Risk-taking and AIDS are not unlike risk-taking and pregnancy. Neither AIDS infection nor fertilization are certain, the gambler often survives, and the penalty is remote: nine months in the case of pregnancy, maybe years in the case of AIDS. (Malcolm Potts, 1988)

So like safer sex the built-in problem of family planning is the *'planning* bit'.

This highlights the potential advantages of the postcoital methods. But the potential may not be realized. A 1992 study of unplanned pregnancies in Central London showed that more than half of those who could have sought such emergency help because they (a) knew about it and (b) knew there had been a contraceptive risk, did not do so! Asked why, the reason given amounted to that they 'had got away with it before'. . . . So strong in matters of sex is the gambling instinct! plus inertia. . . .

4 Finally, 'the fact that contraception has to do with sex seems to set up an environment where risks are exaggerated or misunderstood' (Malcolm Potts). So 'sex' even explains some of the risk illiteracy of our clients about (say) the pill . . . . ordinary, unprotected, sex seems so natural and safe by comparison!

8.5 In the many studies of compliance in developed countries, what are the *background* factors that have been shown to correlate with non-use or poor use or early discontinuation of contraceptive methods?

Here is a list, longish but doubtless not complete, relating mainly to the COC:

- Young, immature (youth also increases fertility, hence a greater likelihood of not getting away with any of the more frequent compliance errors. According to Jones and Forrest in 1989, failure rates of the pill in the first 12 months of use are more than five times higher in the under-20s compared with the 35–44 age group.)
- Unmarried.
- Nulliparous.
- Early coitarche.
- Multiple sexual partners.
- Previous contraceptive failure/abortion, or:
- Perception of low personal risk of conception (especially because of previous 'scares' which resolved).
- Erratic daily time-table

- Cultural or religious opposition to birth control.
- Poor social conditions.

- Parents not married.
- Lack of parental support.
- Low evaluation of personal health.
- Low educational attainment and goals.
- Feelings of lack of personal self-worth and self-determination.
- Feelings of *fatalism* (babies happen, rather like death, 'when your number comes up').
- Cigarette smoking (unplanned conception more likely, but in several studies of young teenagers *also* likely to start sexual activity younger).
- Alcohol drinking (53% of 16–24 year olds in a SW England study felt they were more likely to forget about the risk of pregnancy after drinking alcohol). The same must apply to other drugs of addiction.

- Media 'scare stories' and misinformation/myths.
- Fear of side-effects.
- Experience of side effects:
    above all, bleeding side-effects;
    also other side effects, perceived or real, especially weight gain, headaches, nausea, depression, breast tenderness, acne.
- Wrong or incomplete information (e.g. about missed or vomited pills).

- Poor service delivery /counselling/advice about the methods This is the (*preventable*) provider contribution to compliance problems! See Q 8.16.

> **Note: there is some considerable *overlap* between these risk factors, but more importantly and very usefully in practice, there is *synergism*. Ensure more time for counselling when combinations of the above apply! See also Appendix, pages 441–8.**

8.6 What situations/circumstances correlate with unprotected intercourse?

Here are a few which are well documented:
- First ever intercourse (or first with a new partner).

- Around the start or the end of any relationship – another good argument therefore for long-term relationship(s) since there will be fewer 'bust-ups'!

- Times of major life stress: e.g. bereavement, unemployment.

- On holiday, or trips away from home – indeed any situation where the individual or couple feel anonymous, a bit mad, and so liable to behave out of character.

8.7 What are the factors in non-compliance and discontinuation in the Third World?

Everything above, only more so. Wrong information, for instance. In Egypt in a recent (1991) survey the commonest error of *providers*, leave alone users of the pill, was the belief (as often in the UK, see Q 8.8) that the next packet of pills should be routinely started on the 5th day of the withdrawal bleed! Fatalism, and cultural and religious obstacles to good compliance are often very strong.

But the biggest single factor is the basic one of *non–availability of the actual methods*, or the drying up of supplies once a good method like DMPA has been initiated . . . If artificial contraceptives are seen as too expensive this can also apply in many poor communities of the developed world.

8.8 What do surveys show about more *specific* aspects of COC compliance?

A 1986 general practice survey in a mainly low social class (inner city) area showed that only 28% of women were taking the pill in accordance with the makers' instructions. Much of the confusion related (most crucially, see Q 4.15!) to when to start the next packet after the pill-free interval (PFI):

- 12% believed they should wait until the 5th day of the withdrawal bleed;

- 11% thought they should start the next packet only when the bleeding stopped, or after 1 week but only if the bleeding had stopped.

Starting late with the next packet was not perceived as anything to do with missing pills! (see Q 4.17). Two-thirds of the pill-takers in a similar GP study thought that the most contraceptively risky pills to miss were in the middle of a pack . . . .

By contrast, in 1988 in a semirural setting of higher social class, 89% were found to take their pills correctly. *But could this in part be because those women had much more personal attention from the providers, before and during a course of pills?* Rather than castigate users, we must admit that medical error can be a significant component of user failure (see Qs 8.15 and 8.16).

8.9 Do we expect a lot from pill-takers?

Yes.

Correct pill use means that a healthy woman has to take a pill daily for months or years at a time, whether her intention is to delay or prevent pregnancy, and whether she is consistently sexually active or not. She must know how long to wait between pill packets, how to make up missed pills, and when to use another method as a back-up. She then must have the back-up method available and actually use it. Finally, she must be confident about the pill's effectiveness and safety, despite frequent rumours and negative reports in the press. *In short, the pill is a more complex method to deliver and use than we previously thought.* (Linda Potter, Family Health International)

According to a NOP survey in the UK in 1991, 'on average women seem to forget a pill about eight times a year'! And young teenagers seem to be late with their pills up to three times per month.

8.10 Teenagers are mentioned a great deal in the context of compliance. What are the important medical and legal considerations when prescribing a medical method like the pill to girls before the age of consent (16 in the UK)?

1 *Medical.* Although early cycles after the menarche are assumed to be anovulatory, very early conceptions can still occur and are becoming ever commoner. Aside from that there is the risk of STDs, cervical neoplasia and much potential emotional trauma. *But it must be made clear that the risks are those of precocious sexual activity and multiple* partners, not of the pill or other contraceptive.

A modern low oestrogen, lipid-friendly, *combined pill* usually proves the most suitable method. As far as we know once periods are established it poses no special problems in teenagers, as compared with women in their 20s (including with respect to breast cancer or cervical cancer, see Qs 4.71 and 4.73).

Injectables are currently preferable to *IUDs* because of their protective effect against pelvic infection, though the latter are not absolutely contraindicated. The *ideal IUD* will probably be the levonorgestrel-releasing variety mentioned above, when available, since it likewise reduces the risk of infection as well as relieving dysmenorrhoea.

But since this age group may now be the most at risk of all sexually transmitted agents including HIV it is essential to promote *use of the condom in addition*, often, to the selected main contraceptive. Reliance on the condom alone for pregnancy prevention by teenagers usually gives poor results. If it is selected, take every opportunity to mention the *'emergency pill'*.

2 *Legal and socio–ethical.* Sexual intercourse before the age of consent represents a major category of technical law-breaking, not by the girl but by the male partner(s). Yet prosecutions are very rare if they are about the same age.

Any general practitioner faced with an under 16 year old needs first, as appropriate, opportunely and non-patronizingly, to raise the advantages – both psychological and physical – of delaying intercourse until later. Next, if this 'rings no bells', seek agreement by the young person that they will tell, or allow you to tell, at least one parent. This is vastly preferable.

8.11 But what if under-16s completely refuse the involvement of a parent/guardian?

In 1985 the House of Lords overturned an Appeal Court judgement in the celebrated case brought by Mrs Victoria Gillick. In the new ruling Lord Fraser of Tullybelton made the following points which are also in the revised DHSS *Memorandum of Guidance* (DHSS HC(FP)86).

It is good practice to proceed to prescribe a medical contraceptive without parental knowledge and consent if:

1 The girl although under 16 years of age will understand the doctor's advice.

2 She cannot be persuaded to inform the parents or allow the doctor to inform them.

3 She is very likely to begin or to continue having sexual intercourse with or without contraceptive treatment.

4 Her physical or mental health or both are likely to suffer unless she receives contraceptive advice or treatment.

5 Her best interests require the doctor to proceed without parental consent.

Whatever else applies, *at all times the young woman must have 100% assurance of confidentiality*.

8.12 How are compliance, side-effects and discontinuation connected?

In a complex way. To quote Linda Potter again referring primarily to pill-users in poor communities (in inner cities of rich countries as well as in the Third World):

> Poor compliance can lead directly to pregnancy. However, incorrect use can also contribute to discontinuation. Studies indicate that as many as 60% of new OC-users discontinue use before the end of the first year, most within the first 6 months, and most of these because of menstrual irregularities and other side-effects.
>
> The side-effects may be either the cause or effect of incorrectly taken pills, and may lead to either discontinuation or failure, making the relationship a complex one. For example, nausea in the first few months may lead to intermittent use, which in turn may provoke breakthrough bleeding, which in turn may lead to discontinuation.

8.13 According to the UK FPA's national information service, what in order to help them to use contraceptives well do potential consumers themselves consider most important?

Above all, information. Some professionals feel consumers cannot deal with 'too much information'. The FPA enquiries (about 200 000 per year) lead to the conclusion that consumers want *more* information, *not less*.

Sadly, in the FPA's experience too many professionals do not provide full information about the range of options, fully explain the side-effects or discuss risks and benefits of contraceptive methods.

Many professionals make assumptions, often underestimating a person's degree of motivation, ability or needs and 'censor' or limit information, and many use a variety of ways to pressure a woman to use certain methods. Because of this, women (quite rightly) express feelings of anger, frustration and powerlessness because they feel they are not listened to, not spoken to on equal terms and given neither time nor 'permission' to voice fears or anxieties.

Family planning professionals need to be aware of how far they might go in determining choice rather than influencing it, i.e. there is a need to consider the differences between informed consent and *informed choice*.

There are fears, worries and doubts about potential, perceived and currently known side-effects. What consumers consider important when choosing a method are:

- Effectiveness – will it work? (emphasis on failure rather than success).
- Suitability.
- Risks and benefits.
- How to use a particular method.
- How the method works.

8.14 How should the information be conveyed?

Verbally and by the written word. The onus is on providers to give information that is accurate. It should update, reassure and demythologise – all without embarrassment. Good information leads to empowerment, enabling more people to seek help as and if required.

Providing written information, and currently the best source in the UK is the FPA leaflets, offers privacy, anonymity and *time* to absorb information at leisure. People can remember only 20% of what they hear and only 50% of what they hear and see.

The length of the text is not a barrier to communication for consumers, provided the material is well organized, well laid out and well signposted. Indeed the more comprehensive FPA leaflets which are now available should be given with the words *'keep this in a safe place for reference'*.

By 1994 in the UK all drugs will contain patient information leaflets, and contraceptive manufacturers and family planning organizations are at last actively working together to standardize and simplify the information given. Providers can already choose, selectively, to offer some of the better manufacturers' literature, which has been much improved in recent years. Possibly even more important is creative packaging, whereby user-friendly design assists compliance and some companies' packets now convey valuable information like what to do in the event of missed or vomited pills. The increasing use of video and audio recordings is also welcomed as they can save time and be discussion openers, ensuring the ground is covered fully, especially the bits the provider may find 'boring' and so forget to mention at the crucial first visit.

8.15 As an overstretched but well-intentioned family practitioner, how might I improve my family planning service?

1 Generally, more people do attend GPs for contraception than community-based family planning clinics, but for a start you might lend support to the view that *availability of the choice* of service is paramount. Availability of complementary (not rival) and accessible services is important; at present, potential users of contraception may have to run an obstacle race in order to find the service that meets their specific needs. One of the most useful improvements that most health authorities could make would be to implement the recommendation of the 1991 RCOG Working Party on Unplanned Pregnancy, that there should be 'a senior specialist to oversee the provision of contraception and sterilization, both by community clinics and in general practice . . . .' – a coordinating community gynaecologist, in fact.

2 In your own service, set aside any illness-oriented style and adopt an information providing and counselling mode for these healthy couples.

3 There are a number of very practical questions you might consider:

Family planning, the scope — *In our practice, do we:*

- Provide a full range of contraceptive methods, on site or easily arranged, including postcoital contraception and condoms (discuss with the local AIDS budget-holder)?
- Provide pregnancy testing and support and counselling for unplanned pregnancy?
- Provide counselling and referral for male and female sterilization?
- Provide advice and help with regard to 'safer sex'?
- Provide help or referral for sexual and relationship problems?
- Provide advice, treatment or referral for STDs?
- Provide advice, help or referral for infertility?
- Provide comprehensive well-woman/well-man services?

Service provision — *Do we:*

- Work as a team (I include here receptionist, health visitor, school nurse, practice nurse, partners)?

- Provide flexible clinical services, with rapid access/walk-in facility for urgent first visits (postcoitally) and adequate support to those with follow-up problems (e.g. side-effects of IUDs or pills)?

- Provide *sufficient time* for all family planning consultations, especially the first or the postcoital visit? Have we fully thought through the pros and cons of a dedicated session?

- Provide an assurance especially to the young of *confidentiality* in visits, communications and record keeping?

- Provide (where possible) a choice of male or female doctor?

Training — *Do we:*

- Ensure all staff (including reception/clerical staff, but most especially nursing staff) are appropriately trained?

Information — *Do we:*

- Always provide standardized, complete, up-to-date and objective information? That is, the information we ourselves would expect to receive.

- Use suitable language that both enables and informs? Thus, *do not* talk about *coils, rhythm method or morning–after contraception*, but *do* talk about *IUDs, natural family planning and emergency (postcoital) contraception.*

- Make it clear during counselling for pills and barrier methods that there is a profound difference between the failure rates for perfect use and typical use?

- Always discuss risks *and* benefits?

- Recognize people are not always comfortable and may feel too shy to ask questions? (It may help to 'ventriloquize' some questions, and to ask certain others to check that the most important facts have been retained.)

- Always provide good *written information* that backs up and reinforces any verbal advice?

- Publicize our services so people know about them?

Ensuring compliance is, after all, not about professionals 'telling' consumers what to do – it is about enabling consumers to make informed choices through a partnership with health professionals.

IATROGENIC CAUSES OF UNPLANNED PREGNANCIES

8.16 How wrong can we, the providers, sometimes be? May a doctor or nurse be an accessory in causing 'iatrogenic' unplanned pregnancies?

Very much so. We have just been reviewing, in a contraceptive context, plenty of evidence for the saying: 'you can take the horse to the water but you cannot make it drink'. But is it not also clear already that we as providers may fail in the first place to 'take the horse to the water'?

Many 'sins of omission and of commission' by providers are obvious from Qs 8.13–5 above. The list which follows of about 30 more errors, primarily medical or prescribing errors in nature, is by no means complete. Indeed I should be interested to receive other examples, for use in my next edition! As it stands it already reveals many traps for the unwary FP provider . . . .

The prescriber may be an accessory to an unwanted pregnancy in any of the following ways:

1 First and foremost, by not allowing *enough quality time* for the contraceptive consultation, backed by good literature. This leads to one of the commonest, most basic errors, which is when the practitioner simply says 'you must stop the pill' without *any* adequate discussion of the future method (see 7 below).

2 When changing methods, by not ensuring an appropriate overlap between them. For instance, when changing from progestagen only pill (POP) or IUD to condom, failing to advise use of the condom for 7 days *before* the POP is discontinued or device removed. Or if a woman is transfering to a (for her) untried method like the diaphragm or Femidom (see Q 3.67), removing an IUD before she has found it to be satisfactory. And prior to female sterilization, failing to advise abstinence or extra care with barrier methods for the cycle leading up to the surgery risks a clip-induced ectopic *or* an intrauterine conception. (See also Qs 6.13, Q 6.14.)

3 Especially post partum, if any amenorrhoeic sexually active woman wants to start using a hormonal or intrauterine contraceptive, by insisting on waiting (a) for a 6-week postnatal visit (see Q 8.21) or (b) for the next period (*which then never comes because she conceives during the wait!*) – when there are ways of minimizing the risk of fetal exposure (see Qs 5.127–8 and 8.21).

Chapters 1–3

4 After a bad attack of pelvic inflammatory disease, overstressing that the woman may be infertile – so she is inefficient with subsequent contraception.

5 *Overstressing the ineffectiveness* of coitus interruptus (see Q 2.6) so it is not used when it would be a very great deal better than nothing in an 'emergency' situation.

6 Failure to warn about the 300 million sperm in each man's ejaculate, and the unpredictability of sperm survival in the female genital tract. Hence failure to explain the consequences: that a tiny 'leak' of semen may cause a pregnancy, and that the postmenstrual 'safe period' is of a completely *different order* of potential efficacy from the properly identified postovulatory phase (see Qs 1.4–1.17).

7 Failure to advise *re* effective condom use, and especially *re* common chemicals/prescriptions which rapidly damage rubber (see Q 2.20).

8 *Re* caps, giving such a profusion of other instructions about spermicide, etc. (most of which have never been validated), that the woman fails to get the most important message: namely that she should make a secondary check that her cervix is covered following every insertion of her diaphragm or cap, however comfortable it feels.

Chapter 7

9 Failure to inform male and female barrier contraceptive users about the existence of *postcoital (emergency) contraception*; and failure to offer it when appropriate (e.g. if an IUD has to be removed midcycle, see Q 6.14).

10 Use of the incorrect term 'morning after pill', and failing to stop its use by others (see Q 7.1)

11 Failure to inform women that the PC 'emergency pill' can be used up to 72 hours after exposure.

12 Not being prepared to insert an IUD postcoitally up to 5 days after *ovulation* as calculated in good faith (see Q 7.11). With exposure on day 7 this could mean, quite legally and ethically, insertion up to 12 days after unprotected intercourse!

Chapters 4 and 5

13 Giving erroneous starting instructions for the combined pill (see Q 4.38 for the correct ones).

14 Failure to explain the significance of the pill-free week (see Qs 4.15–24). Examples:
   (a) not stating that starting the new packet on time is critically important, and the first pill is the most 'dangerous' if missed;
   (b) not explaining that if pills are missed at the end of a packet, the next following pill-free break should be shortened or eliminated;
   (c) implicitly wrong instructions for subsequent packs, e.g. 'the doctor said (s/he probably didn't, but was the point clarified?) that I should wait until the 5th day of my next period – or until it is finished – before I restart each packet';
   (d) not amplifying the instruction to start a *new brand* of pill on day 1 of the withdrawal bleed (WTB). (If by chance the woman gets no WTB in that cycle, she may wait beyond 7 days unless otherwise instructed.)

15 Simply represcribing the COC (perhaps with a 'pep-talk' about compliance) after true pill method failures, or even when only one or two tablets missed. *Instead, the tricycle method should be offered* (see Qs 4.24, 4.28).

16 Inadequate explanations at pill discontinuation. Examples:
   (a) Failure to inform a woman that the second half of her pill-free week is *only a safe time for unprotected intercourse if she does in fact restart a new packet*. If she is discontinuing the method, it is very common for a woman to assume that the condom is unnecessary for the first week. In reality she might well ovulate early in the second week (see Qs 4.15 and 4.21).
   (b) Failure to explain that calendar calculations, of even the potentially safer second phase of the safe period, are completely invalidated during the first cycle following pill discontinuation, which can be very variably prolonged.

(c) Failure to dispel the myth: 'I heard that women often take a long time to get pregnant after stopping the pill, so I thought I would be safe'.

17 Failure to forewarn and explain that the occurrence of *breakthrough bleeding* should not be considered as a period (and the pill therefore stopped in mid-packet) – and that it may subside over time. Choosing brands which produce good cycle control is obviously helpful too.

Many studies have shown that confusion about irregular bleeding, and its nuisance-value as a side-effect, are among the most frequent causes of pill-taking errors, discontinuations and unwanted conceptions.

18 Failure to explain that *absent withdrawal bleeding* does not necessarily mean a pregnancy has occurred. (Some women become pregnant through failure to restart the pill after the first episode of absent WTB, and hence become unnecessarily pregnant solely because they thought they already were . . . .)

19 Ovulation induction in a woman who presents with oligoamenorrhoea but definitely does not (yet) want to be pregnant! (see Q 4.57). 'No-one ever asked me if I wanted my fertility problem treated!'

20 Unnecessarily avoiding the COC in cases of past secondary amenorrhoea from which there has been a complete recovery (see Qs 4.56 and 4.60).

21 Unnecessarily instructing the woman to discontinue/avoid the COC because of the *medical myths* in Qs 4.216, 4.234 and 4.235 including for minor surgery like laparoscopy (see Q 4.178).

22 Unnecessarily instructing the woman to stop the POP before any surgery, however major (see Qs 5.41, 5.71).

23 *Just telling the woman to stop the pill before major surgery (see Q 4.177) – or any other VALID reason – but failing to discuss with her and organize a suitable alternative such as DMPA!*

24 Failure to explain to a woman transferring to the POP that she should cease to take 7-day breaks.

25 Failure to discuss with a lactating POP-user that her chance of breakthrough conception will greatly increase whenever she begins weaning her baby. So if efficacy is very important to a woman, she should be advised to start the COC on the first day of one of the first of her returning periods (see Q 8.28).

26 Failure to advise appropriately (see Qs 4.31, 5.28, 5.89) when prescribing any of the hormone methods of Chapter 4 and 5 in the event of use of *interacting drugs*, whether short term (e.g. rifampicin just for 2 days!) or long term.

27 *Bad handwriting* (a real problem in practice). The most dangerous example of this is when Femodene is intended but Femulen is read by the person issuing the pills. I am aware of at least one pregnancy caused this way, as the woman continued to take routine pill-free breaks of a week's duration!

Preventive recommendation, as practised at the Margaret Pyke Centre:

Always write: Femodene 30
                Femulen POP

Also: Marvelon 30
                Mercilon 20 (these are easily misread too)

Chapter 6

28 Failure to observe the 'do not rely on the IUD for 7-days pre-removal rule' recommended at Q 6.14. Avoidable intrauterine *or* 'iatrogenic' extrauterine pregnancies in IUD-users following clip sterilization may also result. (I also warn barrier method users of the need to be exceptionally careful, or preferably abstain, during the same 7 preoperative days.)

29 Failure to insert an IUD on presentation around midcycle, if necessary up to day 5 following the most probable day of ovulation. As explained at Q 6.15, a much more generous interpretation of the phrase 'post-menstrual' could lead to a worthwhile reduction in the number of conceptions caused by clinicians who wait for the woman's elusive next period.

30 Failure to warn women that if they fail to feel the threads of an IUD, until proved otherwise, their uterine cavity is IUD-free (see Q 6.35).

CONTRACEPTION/STERILIZATION AFTER PREGNANCY

8.17 When should counselling start?

It should not be an afterthought: it should be initiated antenatally. Counselling should be non-directive, with the doctor or midwife acting as an adviser and facilitator but never making the decisions. It is true that most women are more motivated towards family planning just after childbirth than at any other time, and in many parts of the world postnatal follow-up is weak or non-existent. While it may therefore be correct to 'strike while the iron is hot', caution is necessary especially *re* sterilization, and all kinds of pressure are to be avoided. For all women this is a time of emotional turmoil as well as one of rapidly changing hormonal status.

8.18 What is known about sexual activity in the puerperium?

See the book by Esther Sapire, 1990. According to Masters & Johnson, writing in 1966, after delivery almost 50% of women have low levels of sexual interest for at least 3 months. In another study the same percentage had resumed sexual activity as soon as 6 weeks, but possibly with little enthusiasm on the woman's part. However that may be, the onset of sexual dysfunction reported much later can often be traced back to this time. Sleepless nights, exhaustion and limited time together may affect both partners. The man may resent exclusion from the intense bond between mother and baby, compounded by his wife's fatigue and diminished libido. In the woman, there may be multiple anxieties about the baby and about adjustment to motherhood. All these can be worse if there is a true postpartum depression.

Physical problems include breast and nipple tenderness, or dyspareunia due to pain at the site of perineal suturing, monilial vaginitis or diminished vaginal lubrication.

8.19 When does fertility return after pregnancy? What is the earliest postpartum day on which ovulation may occur, without and with breastfeeding?

Despite much research it remains impossible to predict this accurately for any individual woman. This is due not only to normal biological variation, racial or genetic factors, but also to the effects of:

1 The nutritional status of the woman.

2 The stage of gestation at which the pregnancy ended.

3 Whether indeed she is breastfeeding – and in that case the timing, frequency and duration of nipple stimulation, the amount of supplementary feeding and the time elapsed since delivery.

Although fertilization is the only proof that an ovulation is fertile, *research suggests that in the absence of breastfeeding fertile ovulation could possibly and very rarely occur on day 28, and contraception of some kind should therefore be started by then (see Q 4.45)*.

It is even more difficult when attempting to answer the same question for *lactating women*, because the variability in intensity of baby-induced nipple stimulation is superimposed on woman-to-woman variation. But avoiding all freak ovulation events is perhaps asking too much: a better question is 'For how long can lactation be expected to provide the same kind of contraceptive protection as other acceptable birth control methods, such as the IUD?' One answer is contained in the so-called 'Bellagio Consensus Statement' – see Q 1.32. The essential proviso is that (as should be the case with all methods) no promise of complete efficacy is implied.

8.20 Isn't there a two-way interaction between lactation and contraception?

Yes. *Lactation can affect contraceptives*, primarily by greatly increasing the efficacy of all non-hormonal methods like barriers and spermicides. Conversely, *the COC for example can affect lactation* by altering the quantity and constituents of breast milk. Perforation of IUDs is reported more commonly during lactation.

Breastfeeding should also be advocated and promoted by clinicians because of the strengthening evidence that it protects against *breast cancer*.

8.21 In an amenorrhoeic woman seen postpartum, say at 6 weeks, if contraception has been questionable how can one avoid starting a medical method (e.g. fitting an IUD) in early pregnancy?

Some doctors are so paranoid about this that they insist on the arrival of a period. But they thereby risk an iatrogenic conception (see Q 8.16 (3)).

One practical preventive of this problem is so obvious that it ought not to need saying – but it does: *Why aren't all postnatal checks arranged at or just before 4 weeks*, when the risk of a fertile ovulation having occurred is negligible (see Q 8.19), even if the woman has not managed to breastfeed?

Availability of one of the ultrasensitive slide pregnancy tests now marketed for use in the surgery is invaluable here, preferably sensitive to 50 IU/l of human chorionic gonadotrophin (hCG; e.g.

Clearview). On an early morning urine this will diagnose pregnancy at or before the 14th day after ovulation; but not of course one very recently conceived, due to fertilization within that time.

If that is a relevant possibility, one *useful protocol* is the following:

1 Request that the woman agrees to avoid all risk of conception – by abstinence, combinations of methods, whatever – for the next 10 or 14 days (depending on the sensitivity of the available test).

2 She then returns with an early morning urine. If it gives a negative result this can be interpreted as 'no' conception having occurred:
   (a) up to 10 (or 14) days previously (this by virtue of the sensitivity of the test), *plus*:
   (b) *since then also*, on her responsibility, as she had agreed to be 'safe' during that time.

3 After discussion (recorded in the case-notes) of the tiny risk that an early conception might yet be present, the COC could be started or one might proceed at once to a DMPA injection or IUD insertion. If hormones are to be used, for extra security the couple should use the condom for a further 7 days. And there *must* be a follow-up visit to exclude pregnancy after 3–4 weeks.

8.22 Can natural family planning be used successfully after childbirth (Aside from the Bellagio criteria Q 1.32)?

See Q 1.31. The fundamental problem of this approach, throughout reproductive life, is how to recognize fertile ovulation far enough in advance to allow for the capriciousness of survival of the very best among the millions of sperm deposited at intercourse.

The problem is compounded after pregnancy by the very variable effects of lactation, as discussed above.

With or without breastfeeding, postpartum the oestrogenic changes of increased quantity, clarity, fluidity, slipperiness, elasticity and good spinnbarkeit occur well in advance of the first fertile ovulation. Hence, if cervical mucus is used there are numerous false alarms.

Users of natural family planning who begin mucus observations from the cessation of lochia and who do abstain or switch to another method from the very first appearance of oestrogenic mucus onwards will most probably avoid pregnancy. But they will also be avoiding unprotected intercourse for an unnecessarily long time. Changes in the cervix – dilation, softening and elevation away from the introitus – may help (see Q 1.31).

To date newer techniques using various biochemical changes are equally disappointing for ovulation prediction – far enough ahead.

8.23 Do you recommend an IUD for family spacing?

Yes, and it is an even better choice when the family might prove to be complete but the couple aren't sure yet.

See Chapter 6 for more details. Particularly relevant points at this time are:

1 *Infection*. This can be caused by lack of care during insertion, or exacerbated if uterine tenderness due to postpartum endometritis is overlooked. The individual's risk of sexually transmitted conditions still poses the main threat for the future, however (see Q 6.50).

2 *Perforation*. This is a particular concern in relation to postpartum IUD insertion. Heartwell & Schlesselman (in a 1983 report) found this complication to be 10 times more frequent among lactating than in non-lactating women. However, *no* significant additional risk for T-shaped IUDs was shown by Chi in 1987 (rate 1 in 1632 during lactation) (see Q 6.44). Perforation in lactation seems to be primarily a problem of linear (e.g. Lippes Loop) devices and can be almost eliminated by withdrawal insertion techniques and by extra care by an experienced inserting doctor. Ideally, postpartum clinics should not be used routinely for training purposes, since lack of expertise markedly increases this risk.

8.24 What is your advice on the timing of postpartum IUD insertions?

See Q 6.95. Good results are reported whenever this is between 4 and 8 weeks after delivery. I favour 4 weeks to avoid all the 'hassle' discussed in Q 8.21 above, though the postcoital contraceptive action of the IUD method does provide some leeway.

After lower segment caesarean section (LSCS) the scar will have healed by 4 weeks, and is situated at the level of the internal os. So there is no need to delay insertion beyond say 6 weeks. After elective LSCS the cervical canal may require gentle dilatation, often with local anaesthesia, as for nulliparae. These insertions are not for beginners.

Immediate postplacental insertion

See Q 6.96. The new Copper-Fix IUD (Cu-Fix 390 or Flexigard – see Fig 6.10) is perhaps the best prospect for this, which has often been found advantageous in research projects with *unmodified* IUDs, but has yet to catch on as a routine option. Even if expulsion does occur, the risk of pregnancy is not as great during the puerperium as with the expulsion that follows interval insertion. Follow-up arrangements should be made so that those women who do attend may have their now elongated threads shortened, or a new device inserted if partial or complete expulsion is noted.

Immediate insertion after caesarean section

Modern IUDs may similarly be inserted via the lower segment incision immediately the placenta has been delivered, with superb results reported from China. Some researchers suture the device to the fundus with chromic catgut, but this appears to be unnecessary.

Postabortion insertion

See Q 6.97.

8.25 Are COCs suitable immediately postpartum?

Despite their efficacy, convenience and many other advantages, COCs should *not* be used during lactation. Most studies report some adverse impact on breastfeeding performance and milk volume composition. And in any case the COC cannot improve upon the near 100% efficacy of the POP plus full lactation.

8.26 When should the COC be started in women who do not breastfeed?

If a COC is started too late, some women will become pregnant before their first period. If it is started too early, there is the risk that the oestrogen content will increase the already increased risk of thromboembolism in the puerperium. So ideally COC taking should not begin until the similar changes induced by pregnancy have returned to normality. This starts dramatically with delivery of the placenta, but fibrinogen concentrations actually increase at first until a decline starts around day 5. Dahlman and others found that both blood coagulation and fibrinolysis were significantly increased during the first 2 weeks, but by 3 weeks both were in general normal.

This literature may be interpreted as implying that oestrogen-containing pills should normally not be commenced earlier than day 21 of the puerperium, and this would be the optimum time for those perceived as being at high conception risk (see Q 4.45). Selective delay beyond 4 weeks using an alternative contraceptive may be safest where known risk factors *for thrombosis* apply, particularly in combination. These factors are obesity, preceding severe pregnancy hypertension, operative delivery, especially caesarean section, restricted activity, age above 35 and grande multiparity.

8.27 What if the woman did have pregnancy-related hypertension?

It used to be thought that women with hypertension in a preceding pregnancy would be unusually prone to oral contraceptive-induced hypertension. This was disproved by Pritchard & Pritchard in 1977. It is definitely however a relative contraindication (see Q 4.103), meaning judicious use of the COC method with extra careful subsequent monitoring.

Why? Because the RCGP study showed that this past history is linked for unknown reasons with an increased risk of arterial thrombosis – and seriously so if they also smoke (risk ratio of over 40!). If pre-eclampsia was severe at the preceding delivery, COC taking should be delayed for at least 8 weeks.

8.28 Where should the POP fit into any scheme for postpartum contraception?

Very prominently. This is discussed in detail at Qs 5.54–7. Unlike the combined pill, POPs have not been found to impair the quantity or the quality of breast milk.

1 *Timing of postpartum use.* Since there is no anxiety about enhancing the risk of thrombosis, it is medically safe to start the POP in the early puerperium. However, studies have shown an increased risk of puerperal breakthrough bleeding in POP users, despite the expectation that they should have amenorrhoea during lactation. It is therefore now suggested that women (whether or not breastfeeding) should begin to take the POP after about day 21 following delivery.

Any amenorrhoeic woman in whom cyesis has definitely been excluded, if necessary by the routine described above (see Q 8.21), may start the POP at any time, with 7 days additional contraceptive precautions.

2 *Efficacy.* It is important to bear in mind that since there is the additional contraceptive effect of breastfeeding, less than perfectly compliant POP-takers will 'get away with it': until, perhaps, weaning and hence fertile ovulation commences (see Q 5.57). Two successive women in one of my own recent clinics (summer 1992) gave the history that their next baby came 'too soon' that way, because the suggestion that they might prefer to switch to the COC at weaning had not been made to them!

This point needs making in *advance*: if efficacy is very important to a woman, she should be advised to start the COC on the first day of one of the first of her returning periods (not rigidly the very first as the early bleeds may not relate to ovulatory cycles).

8.29 What about injectable contraception? Does the same apply as *re the POP (above)*?

Most studies of DMPA show either no change or an improvement in both quantity of milk and duration of lactation. Both DMPA and NET-EN and their metabolites cross from maternal plasma into breast milk, and to a greater extent than with the POP. It has been calculated that a child would have to breastfeed for 3 years to receive as much DMPA as the mother receives in 1 day. To date, no morbidity and no adverse effects on growth have been found.

1 *Timing of the first dose.* Since in some countries contact with medical personnel may be limited to delivery, the first dose of DMPA is often given within 48 hours of delivery. Injectables do not increase the risk of puerperal thrombosis; but this is much earlier than necessary for contraception and it has been noted that such early administration increases the likelihood of heavy and prolonged bleeding. Hence in the UK the first dose is now preferably (but not always) delayed to 5–6 weeks postpartum.

2 *Efficacy.* Here there is no concern that the method will become less effective as breastfeeding frequency diminishes. Instead, the

woman must be warned to plan well ahead if she wants another baby, because of the well-recognized delay in return of fertility (see Q 5.113).

8.30 What is the policy about hormonal methods if there was trophoblastic disease in the last pregnancy?

This is fully discussed at Q 4.69.

8.31 What considerations apply to male or female sterilization in the early puerperium?

It often appears convenient for all concerned if the woman is sterilized at this time, and if so the earlier the better. But Professor Robert Winston showed that the decision is more commonly regretted at this time of emotional instability for many couples. So there is a welcome trend to offering laparoscopic sterilization as an interval procedure about 12 weeks postpartum. A distinct minority, who decide during that time to keep their options open longer, reap the benefits.

There then still remains the risk of early death of the latest child (e.g. by the sudden infant death syndrome). Many vasectomy services therefore prefer to defer the procedure until the youngest child is 6–12 months of age. It is not clear why such admirable caution is less commonly observed by obstetricians with regard to female sterilization.

For more about sterilization, see Qs 8.56–60 below and the relevant chapters in *Contraception: Science and Practice*, and the *Handbook of Family Planning*.

8.32 How would you conclude this section?

By three important reminders:

1 The best time to discuss future plans for contraception/ sterilization is antenatally, and definitely not in a rush during labour or the early puerperium!

2 Delaying the start of contraception until the first menses or the postnatal visit risks in a minority the phenomenon of 'shutting the stable door after the horse has bolted . . .'.

3 Above all, a good doctor or nurse will neglect neither the particular, such as local physical healing after vaginal delivery, nor the general, such as the psychosexual aspects of the couple's relationship.

CONTRACEPTION FOR THE OLDER WOMAN

Background factors

8.33 What is the intrinsic fertility of older women, above age 40?

The available evidence suggests as shown at the bottom of Table 0.2, Q 0.13, that the intrinsic fertility of such women is reduced to about half what it was at the age of 25, with a further decline above 45. An unknown part of this is due to reduced frequency of intercourse. Whatever the explanation, the conclusion is that a method with an accidental pregnancy rate unacceptable in a younger woman may well be satisfactory for the use in the 40s. For example, the POP in the Oxford/FPA study has a failure rate (0.3 per 100 woman-years) which is indistinguishable above age 45 from that to be expected in a younger woman using the combined pill. Another example is the recommendation to use the contraceptive sponge above 45 (see Q 6.36).

Some older women, however, may have actual or potential gynaecological morbidity to weigh up against the risks of the combined pill (see Q 8.38) and so may be better off due to its beneficial effects although not really needing such a high efficacy method.

8.34 How may one normally diagnose physiological infertility after the menopause?

Occasionally women with many months of amenorrhoea, symptoms of the menopause and even elevated FSH levels subsequently ovulate and menstruate. As a rule of thumb, women above the age of 50 years who have had amenorrhoea for over 12 months, preferably also with vasomotor symptoms, may abandon alternative contraception. During the 1-year wait any simple method (e.g. sponge or foam) is adequate. Below age 50 there is a greater risk of spontaneous late ovulations, so 2 years' of amenorrhoea with extra precautions is recommended. Below 40 the secondary amenorrhoea needs to be investigated fully by standard tests.

The classical rule is as above; 2 years' amenorrhoea are required for the infertility diagnosis right up to 50. That age limit seems to have been arbitrarily chosen, without any hard data. Lowering it to

45 in recent years has made life easier for many women: minimally less safe, but perhaps acceptably so.

If FSH levels (preferably two) are performed it may be possible in some situations (see Qs 5.63, 5.121 and 8.45) to shorten the time of use of other contraception after the apparently last period. But it must always be made clear that the risk of a later fertile ovulation cannot be completely excluded.

8.35 What are the medical risks associated with pregnancy?

Although it may be easier to prevent, pregnancy at this age is in many ways a greater catastrophe. Both maternal and perinatal mortality are much higher. There is also a steady increase in the risk of chromosome abnormalities with maternal age. Hence while we should certainly avoid using too 'strong' a method, the woman needs to be reassured that any chosen method will in reality prove to be effective in her case.

8.36 What is the best method for women above 40?

There is no such thing as a single best method. Individualization is key, as usual.

Hormonal methods

8.37 Is the term 'the contraceptive gap' now applicable to smokers only?

Yes: with modern pills, available epidemiology and the relevant authorities suggest that we may now legitimately continue the ordinary COC at a woman's request to the menopause, if she is an entirely healthy non-smoker. *Age alone is no longer a contraindication.*

For smokers however, starting at age 35 we are left with a 'contraceptive gap' between that age and the menopause. It poses an acute problem for those many couples who have hitherto been 'spoilt' by non-intercourse-related methods. Many seek sterilization, some without being entirely ready for so permanent a step: yet it would be unnecessary if they were non-smokers.

8.38 What are the desirable features of contraception at the climacteric?

Table 8.2 summarizes the desirable features. It is clear that only some *appropriate* combination of oestrogen with progestagen is capable of providing all the first six features in that table. What is appropriate? That depends on the need for contraception, see Qs 8.39 and 8.40.

Over and above the reassurance of regular bleeds, it is now clear that there is often some symptomatic loss of ovarian function starting 5–10 years before the actual menopause. Women in these years would derive additional *non-contraceptive* benefits if (upon

Table 8.2 Desirable features of any contraceptive for use up to and during the climacteric

---

1. Effective in this age group.

2. Improves sex life by:
   (a) perceived effectiveness and reassuring period pattern;
   (b) not being an intercourse-related method;
   (c) oestrogenic slowing of skin ageing, improved body image and libido, and treatment of vaginal dryness.

3. Controls climacteric symptoms (especially vasomotor and psychological symptoms, and the urethral syndrome).

4. Controls symptoms of 'normal' cycle (especially the premenstrual syndrome, and irregular, heavy or painful periods).

5. Reduces incidence or manifestations of gynaecological pathology. This potential benefit applies to pelvic infection, extrauterine preganancy, fibroids, dysfunctional haemorrhage, endometriosis, functional ovarian cysts, and carcinoma of the ovary and uterus.
   [Consequent reduction in the risks of treatment for these conditions, especially hysterectomy]

6. Oestrogenic protection against osteoporosis.

7. Absence of masking of the menopause.

8. Absence of systemic adverse effects:
   (a) known serious conditions such as hypertension and arterial cardiovascular disease;
   (b) anxiety about possible effects on other serious conditions, for example, breast cancer, especially with long duration of use.

NB: Only a combination of oestrogen and progestagen is capable of providing all the above desirable features (*excepting* numbers 7 and 8). The remaining options chiefly act as contraceptives – without a positive benefit, and sometimes with a deleterious effect, on the conditions shown.

their request) they were allowed by their physicians to use some form of combined therapy. Many of the desirable features listed in Table 8.2 can be provided, at least in theory. There is the potential to improve sexual harmony by avoiding intercourse-related methods, and by preventing oestrogen deficiency with associated skin ageing, poor vaginal lubrication and loss of libido. The first manifestations of climacteric symptoms can be suppressed. Many women suffer preventable hot flushes and in some osteoporosis may begin before they see their last period. Symptoms of the *so–called* 'normal' menstrual cycle (premenstrual syndrome, heavy and painful periods) are often controlled.

Perhaps most important is the reduced risk of frank gynaecological disorders which are related to the menstrual cycle, listed at (5) in the table. It follows that use of an appropriate COC will reduce the risk of treatment for these conditions: such as prolonged use of high-dose progestagens (e.g. norethisterone in doses up to 15 mg per day) or danazol, which may markedly alter plasma lipids in a direction likely to promote atherogenesis.

8.39 Table 8.2 suggests that the benefits of the COC are greater in the older age group and so still outweigh the risks even if they are increased somewhat with age. But which pill should be used?

First, I must reiterate that this increased permissiveness applies only to risk-factor-free women. Ideally the minimum acceptable dose of any progestagen and the oestrogen should always be used, to produce the least possible metabolic effects on both lipids and clotting factors. At present Mercilon seems a good first choice.

8.40 Is it ever appropriate to give a cyclical hormone replacement regimen (HRT) before the menopause? And might this be for contraception?

Not for *contraception* – none of those giving oestrogen alone at some time in their cycle is reliable. There are new modalities being devised which do use natural oestrogens by various routes plus continuous progestagen and are contraceptive. But otherwise standard HRT products, although medically even safer (see Q 8.41), are best reserved (and then usefully) for those with oestrogen deficiency symptoms who are not at risk of pregnancy. They might be abstaining, relying on sterilization or vasectomy, or happily using some other contraceptive.

Cycle control may be a problem here, due to interaction with the woman's own hormones. So use of the COC may still be justifiable in some cases for its therapeutic benefits (Table 8.2) alone.

8.41 So what is the real difference between the COC and HRT? How is it we can recommend HRT to smokers of any age, whereas smokers must stop the COC at 35 for fear of exacerbating arterial disease?

In the past this was because higher dose combined pills were used and an important epidemiological hazard was demonstrated in those with recognized risk factors. The *progestagens* used in the combined pill were of a type which could adversely affect plasma lipids and hence further increase the smoker's risk of atheroma. Now we have the modern 'lipid-friendly' progestagens (desogestrel, gestodene and norgestimate), and for the other reasons listed at Qs 4.232 and 8.38, it has become medically appropriate for *non-smokers* if they so choose to continue to use the lowest-dose COC products until about age 50.

However even now there remains the problem of *synthetic oestrogen*. Ethinyloestradiol (EE), even at the lowest practical dose for contraception plus acceptable cycle control, does create pro-thrombotic changes in the blood. The fear is that these might facilitate superimposed arterial thrombosis in an important artery, if its wall has already been affected by atheroma. These arterial wall changes are much more likely among smokers, who also have enhanced platelet aggregation and impaired fibrinolysis. So: no COC for older smokers.

After the menopause – or leading up to it if birth control is not an issue (see Q 8.38) – the 'gentler' *natural oestrogens* are sufficient. Blocking ovulation is no longer an issue and along with intermittent progestagen they can and do give good control of endometrial shedding, especially when no longer competing with the woman's own hormones. Moreover they seem to have beneficial effects on atherogenesis. This is suggested by a reduction in heart attack rates in many studies. It is also biologically plausible because they seem to correct unfavourable menopausal lipid changes plus various non-lipid mechanisms involving arterial tonus, prostaglandins and fibrinolysis. Moreover there are either minimal or no changes in coagulation/haemostasis with oral HRT, and this may be even more true when using non-oral routes, which avoid a 'bolus' peak dose via the portal vein to the liver.

One study from the USA showed no significant difference in acute fatal myocardial infarction rates in heavy smokers given HRT and in controls. This certainly suggests that the beneficial effects of oestrogens on the risk of cardiovascular disease may be counteracted by smoking, but not necessarily totally cancelled, and even if they were, HRT need not be denied to smokers who also generally have an increased tendency to hypo-oestrogenism. Moreover in another American study, if women with actual angina or a previous history of heart attack took HRT they were surprisingly 50% less likely to suffer a later fatal attack.

8.42 Why then do we not use natural oestrogens for contraception in all women, with or without risk factors, before the menopause?

Mainly because of the need for contraception and cycle control, which EE does so well. Since natural oestrogens are less completely or predictably absorbed and have lower potency, they have so far not proved so effective in either capacity. This may change with further research.

Natural oestrogens can be used for women, especially smokers, using for example sterilization or vasectomy but needing HRT before the menopause: in synchrony with their own cycle, and with forewarning about breakthrough bleeding. But in risk factor-free women Mercilon with only 20 μg of EE is more effective, since it 'removes' the menstrual cycle and then replaces it with a (usually) well-controlled artificial cycle.

8.43 Why do we not use lipid-friendly progestogens after the menopause?

Why indeed? The answer at present is that, sadly, appropriate versions of desogestrel, gestodene and norgestimate have not yet been marketed, either alone (progestagen-only) or in a simple-to-take HRT combination. Dydrogesterone is available and appears better for lipids than the other progestagens used for HRT.

8.44 If the combined pill or cyclical HRT products are used in a woman's late 40s, will they not mask the menopause?

Yes. The 'standard' teaching has been to switch to a non-hormonal method and only discontinue all contraception after the occurrence of complete amenorrhoea for 12 months (or 2 years if under age 45). But this precludes use of HRT (whose withdrawal bleeds like those of the combined pill will indefinitely mask the menopause, and which is not safely contraceptive) at the very time when vasomotor symptoms may be most pronounced.

8.45 How then might in fertility at the menopause be diagnosed in COC- or HRT-users?

Arbitrarily at age 50 the woman switches to a simple method (Delfen foam or the Today sponge being adequate at this age) and records any subsequent bleeds and vasomotor symptoms. Hot flushes will follow in less than 1 month if she has been relying on the COC or cyclical HRT for her oestrogen (this is like suddenly losing ovarian oestrogen by oophorectomy). A high FSH result (above 30 IU/l), preferably repeated, after 1 month suggests final ovarian failure. Along with advice that the risk of later ovulation cannot be completely excluded, the woman may then discontinue contraception, whether or not she chooses to (re)commence HRT.

There are two useful variations which do not require the current treatment to be stopped. FSH level(s) may be done during the oestrogen-only phase in HRT-users and on the 7th pill-free day in COC-users. If results >30 IU/l are obtained, they strongly suggest the end of fertility. But the warning at the end of the above protocol should still be given.

If however the woman has a normal FSH result and/or menstruates while off hormones, she should assume residual fertility and use a simple method (e.g. foam), again whether or not she starts or continues HRT. Indeed, all who want more complete reassurance may if preferred continue a simple contraceptive method, as usual until 1 year after the last non-hormonally induced bleed.

8.46 Is it always important to establish precisely when the menopause takes/took place?

No, not in my opinion. If contraception is not an issue and the woman is on HRT with natural oestrogen, the diagnosis of the precise time of the menopause may be considered of academic interest only. The woman simply continues seeing artificial 'periods' for as long as she chooses to use HRT. The management of any irregular bleeding is the same.

But, for the reasons given at Q 8.41, the COC is not recommended after the menopause, or normally at all above age 50, since fertility is so low that a very simple contraceptive will suffice. Those who abandon non-hormonal contraception without having followed the strict rules of Q 8.34 above (with or without being on HRT), have to be prepared to take responsibility for their decision: a guarantee that ovulation will not occur again cannot be given.

8.47 Aside from a low dose COC, while we await new developments, what *contraceptive* forms of combination hormone therapy might be given – especially in smokers above age 35 who hate barrier methods?

This essentially means using natural oestrogens in some form. It is already not uncommon for some doctors to prescribe an *oestrogen preparation* by any standard route (e.g. percutaneously) in the years leading up to the menopause, and combine it *with a POP*. They could be said to be giving the progestagen to protect the uterus from oestrogen-induced cancer, but choosing to give it in such a way (i.e. daily) that the couple can also be told they need no longer use a barrier contraceptive. The failure rate is unknown, probably similar to that of the POP alone; though some have argued it might be higher due to interference by the oestrogen with the mucus effect of the POP.

The main problem before the menopause is that the prescriber and the woman do not have the reassurance of regular bleeding. Breakthrough bleeding and spotting are frequent. These may sometimes be suppressed by giving a second or even a third POP daily, but fear of endometrial overstimulation leads to the need for frequent endometrial biopsies.

8.48 Are not oestradiol implants adequately contraceptive at this age?

Yes: another option available now, for cautious monitored use by smokers, is the *oestradiol 17β* implant inserted subcutaneously every 6 months: normally starting with 100 mg and reducing after the first 6 months to 50 mg. After age 35, and after the first 3 months during which extra precautions are advisable, and given with only 12 days of a progestagen in each month to combat overstimulation and produce a withdrawal bleed, this has an acceptably low pregnancy rate: probably around 1 per 100 woman-years though the conception risk is very age dependent. This is also one of the few proven treatments for the premenstrual syndrome.

However there is the problem of tachyphylaxis, in which oestrogen-withdrawal symptoms keep returning each time the blood oestrogen levels fall, even though the plateau level after each implant has escalated to much higher than the normal premenopausal range. So the implants must not be given more often than every 6 months and oestradiol monitoring is advisable. Altogether this is a bit of a rigmarole for long-term use, and therefore normally reserved (without any need for progestagen) for women with no uterus.

Alternatives to the oestrogen/progestagen contraceptives

The main problem is that most of these are just that, simply contraceptives. They do not provide the gynaecological benefits, the control over climacteric symptoms nor the potential prophylaxis against osteoporosis, as given by the combined pill or the various HRT oestrogen–progestagen regimens. Some of the alternative contraceptives below can even exacerbate bleeding problems. Yet they remain valid options when COCs are not desired or are contraindicated.

8.49 What about the progestagen-only pill on its own?

This is highly effective and deservedly popular in this age group (see Qs 5.1–5.78). The problems (see Q 5.32) include worrying amenorrhoea with possible hypo-oestrogenism (see Q 5.65) and fear of pregnancy, and erratic bleeding patterns. Gynaecological disorders are not helped and may even be commoner (functional ovarian cysts). See also Q 5.63 *re* diagnosis of the menopause.

8.50 What about injectables, implants and rings (see Ch. 5)?

These have similar problems to the POP, related both to amenorrhoea and to irregular bleeding. Moreover, most women are looking for added oestrogen at this age, hence the ideal implant or vaginal ring from the symptomatic point of view should contain oestrogen as well as the progestagen. Implants and rings would always be preferable to injectables because of their more rapid and woman-controlled reversibility.

8.51 Is the IUD device underutilized at this age?

Yes, definitely, see Q 6.20. It is suitable not only because it is about as effective as sterilization, as a result of reduced fertility, but also because infection and expulsion rates decline with age and are lowest in the 40s. In the absence of intermenstrual or very heavy bleeding (which may lead to curettage and minor or major gynaecological surgery) it can be highly acceptable. There is no need routinely to change any copper intrauterine device fitted after the 40th birthday, until after the menopause (see Q 6.127).

8.52 How about the levonorgestrel-releasing IUD (see Qs 6.132–6.135)?

Currently undergoing trials in the UK, this is likely to be a most useful option. Not only could protection against most of the gynaecological problems be expected, especially menorrhagia, even due to fibroids, but also it should provide progestagen protection against endometrial hyperplasia and cancer. This would enable oestrogen hormone replacement to be given systemically while almost completely avoiding the risks of systemic progestagens. Alternative progestagens such as 3-keto-desogestrel are also being tried. The sooner this valuable delivery system is made available to women, especially older women, the better. Watch this space!

8.53 What about the condom and vaginal contraceptives?

These options are as appropriate at this as any other age, and have their own obvious advantages. But in my experience they (especially the condom) are not sufficiently 'user-friendly' to be accepted for the first time by couples who have not used them regularly earlier in their reproductive life. Many women introduced to the diaphragm however are surprised by its ease and convenience.

The use of spermicides alone is not recommended, except above the age of 50 and at any age for the year following the (probable) menopause. The Today contraceptive sponge is believed adequate from the age of 45, and it is usually very acceptable too (see Qs 3.55–66).

8.54 Can the methods based on fertility awareness be recommended leading up to the climacteric?

In the past it was standard teaching that these cannot be recommended owing to erratic ovulation past the age of 40. However, innovative techniques for predicting ovulation, provided these were capable of predicting it at least 5 days in advance (because of the capriciousness of sperm survival – see Q 1.8), might permit a change of policy.

At present for those with strict views, the mucus and cervical assessment methods (see Qs 1.24, 1.31) require a lot of unnecessary abstinence by older women, because there is an increasing amount of that kind of follicular activity which provides oestrogenic mucus from time to time without necessarily being followed by a fertile ovulation.

In an older woman who ovulates only (say) once every 4 months, a simple new way to predict each ovulation, far enough ahead to allow for sperm survival, would be most valuable. Just three short spells of abstinence per year and she could avoid all the risks of the artificial methods of birth control.

8.55 Isn't postcoital contraception (as in Ch. 7) best avoided in this age group?

Not so, it may be entirely justifiable. There should be no hesitation in using the Yuzpe method even above the age of 45, so long as there is actually a finite pregnancy risk (see Q 7.23). Only past venous thromboembolism or gross obesity would absolutely contraindicate this method.

8.56 Surely either male or female sterilization is the ideal answer?

It can be – for many. According to recent surveys around 50% of couples above age 40 in the UK rely on sterilization of one or other partner. It is effective, convenient and *female* tubal surgery is free of all proven long-term risks after the initial operation.

A 60% increase in prostate cancer incidence after *vasectomy* was reported (1993) in two USA cohort studies; although unproven, this possibility should be discussed proactively during counselling. But WHO deems 'unlikely' the (unconfirmed) finding in two studies of an increased risk of testicular cancer.

Most authorities consider any association of bleeding problems with *female sterilization* by tubal occlusion using clips or rings is coincidental, not causal.

Yet neither method gives any protection against gynaecological disorders – nor even against STDs.

There are many traps for the unwary clinician, above all now marriage breakdown is so frequent. Requests for reversal are more frequent after vasectomy because the man often remarries a younger woman. Careful counselling is mandatory, including an assessment of both the general and the sexual relationship of the couple, and a consideration of relevant aspects of gynaecology even if vasectomy is the operation proposed. Do not forget to warn of the (very small) risk of late failure, even after vasectomy with two subsequent negative sperm counts.

8.57 Are the alternatives to sterilization offered often enough?

I think not. Many couples would actually prefer to avoid surgery and there are plenty of ways of doing so, as outlined above. Before referral for sterilization, especially of relatively young couples, in my experience two important choices are far too often not even mentioned. The first is the injectable, DMPA (see Qs 5.86–130). The second is the IUD, and specifically the Copper T-380S – read all about its remarkable efficacy at Qs 6.10, 6.129.

Certainly another method would be preferable to sterilization when the woman is past the age of about 47, since sterilization will not provide 'value for money'. (The chance of pregnancy is so low and her 'auto-sterilization' by the menopause is imminent.)

8.58 A hysterectomy on request?

A hysterectomy may *sometimes* be appropriate and indeed may be recommended on gynaecological grounds. Hence the vital importance of diagnosing in the female significant menorrhagia, large fibroids, and stress incontinence before even vasectomy is arranged. The morbidity and mortality, however, greatly exceed that of sterilization.

8.59 Is transcervical resection or ablation of the endometrium for menorrhagia contraceptive?

Unfortunately, not so. After all, blastocysts can even implant sometimes in the ovary or on the peritoneum, so the absence of (most of) the endometrium is not enough. Younger women conceive with surprising ease. Moreover there are important risks emerging:

1 The pregnancy has a high chance of being a tubal ectopic.
2 The resulting fetus may have a major malformation.
3 There may be serious intrauterine growth retardation.
4 There may be varying degrees of placenta accreta.

8.60 So what contraception is recommended for a woman having endometrial resection/ablation?

It is normally preferable that laparoscopic sterilization is performed under the same anaesthetic. Otherwise one of the above effective methods may and should be initiated, not excluding an IUD.

However, according to Christopher Sutton of Guildford, IUDs are relatively contraindicated, and are probably best fitted immediately, with great care and antibiotic cover. Allowing 4 or 6 weeks for healing may make the fitting difficult because of (frequent) cervical stenosis. And it must be understood that the device can sometimes be almost impossible to remove, stuck among adhesions in a shrunken uterine cavity.

The levonorgestrel-IUD (see Q 6.132), of course, might prevent the need for this surgery in the first place!

8.61 So what is your conclusion – what practical guidelines are there regarding contraception for the older woman?

1 As usual, the choice will depend on the outcome of non-directive counselling, considering all the options discussed briefly here and more thoroughly earlier in this book. It begins to look as though no method is absolutely contraindicated on the basis of age alone.

2 *For contraception*, the very best option may soon be a progestagen-releasing IUD – *alone, or with oestrogen if needed for relevant symptoms (and then the IUD should protect against endometrial cancer).*

8.62 What else is important in discussing contraception around the climacteric?

It is important to remember that contraception is often a 'ticket' to see the doctor. In reality there may be many basic anxieties or problems concerned with sexuality, the woman's relationship to her partner, health, ageing, and low self-esteem with the 'finality' of the approaching menopause. Moreover, even if as so often the woman tries to assume sole responsibility, her partner's caring involvement should be sought, and promoted if found! See also Appendix, pages 441–8.

8.63 What should be the direction of future contraceptive research?

Figure 8.2 displays rather elegantly, though too simply, the primary sites of action both of the existing methods and those currently under study. Those which are most likely to become available within the next 10 years have been discussed in detail in the appropriate earlier chapters.

Inspection of Figure 8.1 confirms an obvious fact: that the major scientific interest in birth control research has been directed at relatively high-technology, interventionist methods which have the potential or the reality of systemic side-effects. Returning to a theme with which we began the book (see Table 0.1, Q 0.11), the main choice for women is between the efficacy and convenience of systemic methods like the COC but the associated risk of both

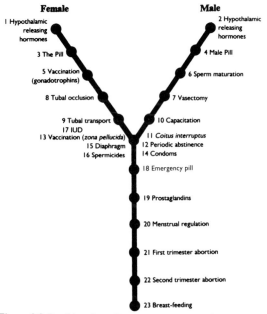

Figure 8.2 Possible points of intervention to control fertility. Q 8.63. For existing methods, the figure shows the *main* sites of action of each. Updated from People (IPPF) 1981 8(4): 6–7.

437

annoying and serious side-effects; and the relative lack of efficacy and inconvenience of methods like the diaphragm, coupled with their virtual absence of risk. ('Inconvenience' primarily indicates that the method is coitally related.)

Regrettably, most contraceptive researchers have concentrated on attempts to improve the existing pill and devising similar systemic agents; but they are always trying to make the effective, convenient but *potentially dangerous methods safer*. It is in my view – and one that is shared by the majority of the women and their partners that I meet – that the researchers would do better to concentrate their resources on making the *safe methods which also help to protect against STDs* more effective and more independent of intercourse. This indeed is the orientation of the research programme at the Margaret Pyke Centre.

It is impossible to contradict the following statement: 'no chemical can be devised which, whether given to women or to men, and whether used by the oral, nasal, retinal, cutaneous, subcutaneous, rectal or vaginal route, will be totally free of all risk'. Try as we will (and indeed must, since the urgency of world birth control demands research along every possible avenue) with new steroid compounds by slow-release and innovative routes, or using releasing hormone analogues, immune methods, or whatever; anything that gets into the bloodstream gets everywhere in the body and must therefore be capable of causing harmful effects, somewhere.

This is the heart of the problem to which Carl Djerassi drew attention in his classic book *The Politics of Contraception*. How do we prove that the unwanted effects of a systemic agent are acceptable or (hopefully) do not exist? It is because this process is so difficult, so expensive and so time consuming that Djerassi was so pessimistic about the future of contraceptive research.

Perhaps we should be starting somewhere else. Far more research should concentrate on producing a method, empowering women and acting probably at the vaginal or cervical level, which is as effective and 'user friendly' as the levonorgestrel IUD but as medically safe and STD protective as the condom.

Concentrating on improving these methods is surely at least as important as the conventional wisdom of the scientific establishment, which starts with current or innovative systemic methods which are effective and convenient, and then strives diligently towards making them risk free. Success down that road – though it must be travelled as well – will be nearly as impossible to prove as it ever will be to achieve!

And even if it is, in view of the world shortage of monogamy . . . . for safer sex many couples will still need to use a condom or equivalent as well . . . .

Appendix: Factors to be considered in giving contraceptive advice

Some notes in a handout prepared by Dr Elphis Christopher for the Margaret Pyke Centre Doctors' Courses in Basic Family Planning, edited and used here with her kind permission.

THE FACTORS WHEEL (Fig. 8.1, Q. 8.1)

Introduction

Although divided into equal segments in Figure 8.1, the different factors are not compartmentalized but rather overlapping and interlocking. Some factors are obviously more important than others for individuals, couples and societies and will vary over time: changing with increasing knowledge and experience both about contraception and abortion and the reality of pregnancy, child-rearing and population pressures. Altered socioeconomic circumstances and changing relationships (separation, divorce) will also have differing consequences for the use of contraception. Running like a leitmotif through all the aspects of family planning is the *status of women* and how their role is perceived: whether they are seen principally as child-bearers and -rearers.

Attitudes towards sexuality and its expression – e.g. whether regarded mainly for procreation or pleasure – can have profound consequences for the sustained use of contraception and the planning of families.

Sexual activity is often impulsive and not planned for, tied up as it is with powerful and often overwhelming drives and emotions (*sex is hot*) whereas the use of contraception requires forethought and conscious effort (*contraception is cold*).

At some level most couples would prefer *not* to be bothered about contraception.

I SOCIETY, CULTURE AND RELIGION

Societal attitudes towards reproduction, fertility, sexuality and family planning are important in so far as they create the general climate in which arise the decisions about whether to have children, how many, and whether to use contraception.

All religions are pronatalist and antiabortion. Some may allow a pregnancy to be terminated for specific reasons, e.g. where the woman's life is at risk.

Religions may not be adverse to planning or limiting one's family but may be divided as to the means to do it, e.g. abstinence or natural family planning for Roman Catholics.

Orthodox Jews: the man must not impede the sperm hence male methods are not used though the woman may use contraception.

For *Muslims* both husband and wife must agree to the use of birth control; abortion may be allowed to prevent a handicapped child. Strict Moslem women can only be examined by female doctors and touch their own vulva with the left hand.

Cultural factors rather than religious ones appear more significant among *Caribbean* women. Birth outside of wedlock is not considered a social stigma. Fertility (or the proof of it) is considered very important.

How seriously people take their religion and their perception and knowledge of what it actually says with regard to family planning obviously varies. Thus in giving contraceptive advice it is essential to ascertain the particular person's views and to avoid making assumptions about their beliefs and attitudes.

Note: Treat the person not the culture.

Some aspects of 'subculture'

Feelings of – Apathy
Fate
God's Will

Those for whom birth control is anathema may feel they have little control over other areas of their lives. Their sexual relationships are the one free area of their lives

Especially among the socially deprived (of whatever ethnic background) in the inner cities, such vulnerable individuals find it difficult to seek advice about sexual or contraceptive matters due to fear of professional attitudes; they are highly suspicious about loss of confidentiality. Sex however is free and available within a relationship. It is private and satisfying. Sex may provide a positive counterbalance to the idleness of unemployment and low self-esteem. Motherhood may seem the only source of fulfilment in an otherwise gloomy picture.

They often lead chaotic disordered lifestyles with frequent change of partners and may be poorly motivated to sustain their use of contraception and need much support, e.g. by a domiciliary family planning service.

2 CLASS, EDUCATION AND KNOWLEDGE

Generally speaking those in long-term education and from a higher socioeconomic class tend to have similar family sizes, regardless of cultural/societal/religious influences, and are more motivated to use contraception.

Included in education is *sex education*. For years there has been a belief that teaching teenagers about contraception will be giving them a licence to have sex. Sexual ignorance is seen as bliss. The adolescent is often caught in a double bind. There is a loss of face for a teenager to admit to ignorance on sexual matters though he/she may desperately need help.

There is considerable anxiety about sex education and its effects among certain ethnic groups in Britain, particularly the *Cypriot* and *Asian* minorities.

3 FAMILY, PARENTS, PEER GROUP

In patriarchal cultures such as *Asian* and *Cypriot,* marriages are arranged or semi-arranged. A marriage is not considered a true one unless there are children, especially sons, who increase the status of women within those societies.

Peer group pressure can be significant among certain teenage groups especially girls who have been in local authority care.

4 THE COUPLE

The balance and quality of the relationship can effect the use of contraception.

Consider:

- Trust, mutuality, sharing good communication.
- Humour.
- Consideration and care can cope with the vicissitudes of contraception.

Erratic use of contraception:

- Anger, disappointment, resentment with the partner: the woman may stop the pill and try to withold sex.
- The question of who is in *control*, who is in charge, can get acted out in whether contraception is used and who is the one who uses it.
- Resentment of the other's sexuality demands/needs.
- Conflict *re* pregnancy: where one partner wants a pregnancy but the other does not and sabotages the use of the method (pills thrown away, IUDs removed without telling the partner).
- A pregnancy may be 'arranged' to hold on to the partner.
- When relationships are beginning or ending this often leads to erratic or non-use of contraception.

The sexual relationship – attitudes to sex itself

Whether attitudes are positive or negative can be revealed at the contraceptive consultation and whether there is sexual self-confidence. *Vaginal examination is very pertinent here, reveals much.*
Sexual problems can present *covertly*, and can be shown by:

Ambivalence towards contraceptive methods:

- Nothing is suitable; reluctance to be examined.
- Sex is really for procreation.
- Giving in to sexual desires – losing control – may not fit in with image of nice clean upright woman.
- Inability to give oneself permission to enjoy sex.

Sexual abuse may lead to:

- Promiscuity ('acting out').
- Masochistic behaviour.
- Repeated terminations.
- Repeated sexually transmitted infections.
- Cold, unresponsive.
- Vaginismus.
- Avoidance of vaginal examination.
- 'Sex made good by having babies.'

Sexual problems can influence the use and choice of contraception. If the man has premature ejaculation or the woman has no sexual desire or if there is infrequent sex, the couple may feel the use of contraception is pointless.

Or the methods themselves may cause sexual problems, e.g. man may lose his erection with the condom.

5 THE INDIVIDUAL

Attitudes to concepts of male/female, femininity/masculinity. Equated with possibility of having children. Obtain sexual identity and self-esteem from that. Pertinent for teenage girls with nothing else in their lives. For the man who feels inadequate and unable to compete with other men, getting a woman pregnant may satisfy a need to prove himself.

Unconscious factors:

- The need for a baby.
- Testing the relationship.
- Unresolved conflict about the future of the relationship.
- Sex is 'disgusting' though consciously saying it is a good thing.
- After birth 'mothers can't be lovers' (altered body image; real and imagined damage).
- Bad birth experience ⎫ exacerbates sexual and
- Abnormal birth, stillbirth. ⎭ contraceptive problems.
- Post abortion – grief and dismay about the need for a termination may lead to erratic use of contraception despite consciously saying do not want to get pregnant.
- Post diagnosis of sexually transmitted disease or abnormal

cervical cancer (feelings of anger, grief, shame, past secrets, sexual abuse may all be revealed; woman may not want to continue with her sexual relationship but be unable to talk about it, she may complain of loss of libido, blaming the pill).

6 CHILDREN

Importance and value of children. Confer adult status, carry on the family name, insurance for old age, keep you young, ensure some kind of immortality, keep the marriage or relationship together, prevent boredom and loneliness, provide interest/entertainment, satisfy the need to be needed, define a role in life and provide stability.

- They can be used as a bastion against an unfriendly world 'me and my baby' (certain teenage mothers), or as creating one's own tribe (can be seen in families with many social problems).
- Can lead to non-use or poor use or fault finding with all contraceptive methods.

7 METHODS THEMSELVES AND SERVICES

Truism – we do not have the perfect method = MAGIC.

8 ABORTION SERVICES

Need for good abortion service as supplement to family planning services because methods fail, couples fail to use methods conscientiously and women should not have to have a child they feel they cannot care for properly. But abortion interacts in many ways: e.g. with conscientiousness of use of methods, effects of guilt feelings, etc.

How are emotional factors revealed?

1 Ambivalence *re* methods.

2 Dissatisfaction with methods.

3 Reluctance to be examined – psychosomatic examination, vaginismus, *always* menstruating.
Vagina   private area, frightening, vulnerable
              dangerous, dirty, messy, blood and discharge comes from it

not owned as a nice pleasurable place
symbol of messy sexual desires
exposed is shameful

4 Reluctance to involve partner.

5 Not keeping subsequent appointments.

6 Running out of supplies.

Vulnerable groups who need special support:

1 The young.

2 The young single mother.

3 Where different fathers for pregnancies/children.

4 Chaotic lifestyle, unstable relationships.

5 Mentally and physically handicapped.

6 Mental illness.

7 Families with children 'in care' and/or on the non-accidental injury register.

8 Women who have repeated abortions.

9 Women with five or more children especially with poor spacing and achieved by a young age.

Some defences:

1 Chaos creator in waiting room. Diverts you from the problem. Patient wants you to get rid of her at one level; at another, cry for help.

2 Hostility, aggression, hides anxiety.

3 Chatty, friendly, doesn't let you get a word in, de-doctors you.

4 Jokiness.

5 Tears. Real/imaginary. Hostile 'keep out'.

6 Sexualizes interview. 'Easier to relate to me sexually than work with me as a doctor.'
   Denial
   Avoidance
   Hidden communication. Secret code you need to decipher. Non-verbal clues.

Treatment:

1 Awareness on part of doctor about problems and how they present.

2 Listen carefully (what lies behind patient's words) – overt, covert.

May need to *confront* – 'nothing on offer seems right for you. Perhaps angry that you have to take responsibility, prefer partner to.'

3 Use of doctor's own feelings with this patient provides powerful clues, for example:
Anger
Sympathy, or seduced
Feeling put down
On a pedestal, preening with pride 'only you can help, doctor'.

ABOVE ALL:

4 Reactions to suggestion of vaginal examination and to the actual examination.

Further reading

Note: The majority of references and quotations in this book will be found in the first five titles of this list.

Filshie M, Guillebaud J 1989 Contraception: science and practice. Butterworths, London.
Loudon N (ed) 1991 Handbook of family planning, 2nd edn. Churchill Livingstone, Edinburgh.
McPherson A (ed) 1993 Women's problems in general practice, 3rd edn. Oxford University Press, Oxford.
Potts M, Diggory P 1983 Textbook of contraceptive practice. Cambridge University Press, Cambridge.
Sapire E 1990 Contraception and sexuality in health and disease. McGraw-Hill, Isando.

Djerassi C 1981 The politics of contraception: birth control in the Year 2001, 2nd edn. Freeman, Oxford.
Ehrlich P, Ehrlich A 1991 The population explosion. Arrow Books, London.
Guillebaud J 1990 The pill. Oxford University Press, Oxford.
Whitehead M, Godfree V 1992 Hormone replacement therapy: your questions answered. Churchill Livingstone, Edinburgh.

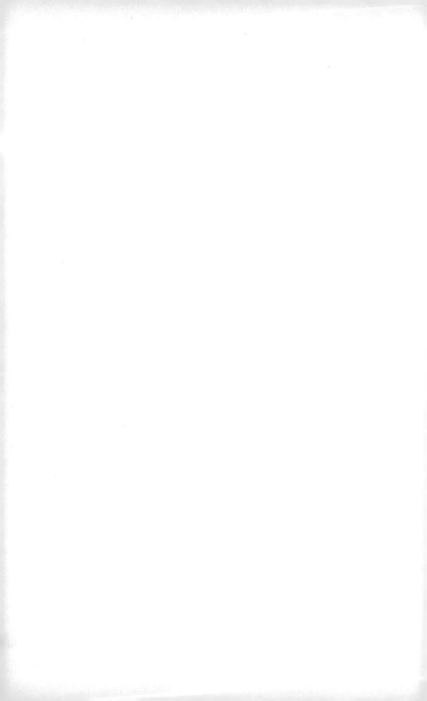

World Directory of Pills — Equivalent Brand Names

Below are listed details of some equivalent brand names used worldwide, identical with or very similar to currently marketed UK products. It is based, with permission, on the *Directory of Contraceptives* published by the International Planned Parenthood Federation, 1992, edited by Ronald Kleinman. The pill brands which are available in Britain are in *italics*.

> **Note: Beware that sometimes the same or a very similar name is used in different countries for quite different formulations, e.g. Noriday, Ovysmen.**

Abbreviations

Oestrogens		Ethinyloestradiol	EE
		Mestranol	MEE
Progestagens	Group A	Norgestimate	NGM
	Group B	Gestodene	GSD
	Group C	Desogestrel	DSG
	Group D	Levonorgestrel	LNG
	Group E	Norethisterone (in N. America called norethindrone)	NET
There are also pro-drugs for NET:		Norethisterone acetate	NEA
		Ethynodiol diacetate	EDDA

+ means that the pill also contains (non-contraceptive) dextronorgestrel. Numbers given with abbreviations refer to dosage in µg.

Group A (norgestimate, NGM)

EE 35   NGM 250   *Cilest*, Ortho-Cyclen

Also a Triphasic product is in prospect (1993), called Ortho-Tri-Cyclen, Tri-Cilest.

Group B (gestodene, GSD)

EE 30   GSD 75   *Femodene, Femodene ED*, Femodeen, Femoden, Femovan, Ginoden, Gynera, Gynovin, *Minulet*, Minulette, Moneva, Myvlar

Triphasic formula

EE 30 + GSD 50
EE 40 + GSD 70   }   Milvane, Phaeva, *Tri–Minulet, Triadene,* Triodena, Triodene
EE 30 + GSD 100

Group C (desogestrel, DSG)

EE 30   DSG 150   Desogen, Desolett, Frilevon, *Marvelon*, Marviol, Microdiol, Ortho-Cept, Planum, Practil, Prevenon, Varnoline

EE 20   DSG 150   *Mercilon*, Microdosis, Myralon, Securgin, Segurin

Group D (levonorgestrel, LNG)

EE 50 + LNG 250   Anfertil + , Anulette + , Anulit + , Contraceptive HD, Daphyron + , Denoval, D-Norginor, Duotone, Dystrol, Euginon + , Eugynon 0.25, Eugynon + , Eugynon 50 + , Eugynona + , Evanor + , Evanor-d, Femenal + , Follinett, Follinyl + , Gentrol + , Gravistat, Gravistat 250, Mithuri + , Monovar, Neogentrol, Neogentrol 250/50, Neogynon, Neogynona, Neo-Primovlar, Neovlar, Noral, Nordiol, Norginor, Normanor, Novogyn 21, Novogynon, Ologyn, Ovadon, Ovidon, Ovlar, Ovoplex, Ovral + , Ovral 0.25 mg, *Ovran*, Pil KB, Planovar + , Primovlar + , Promovlar 50 + , Profan, Stediril + , Stediril-d.

| EE 30 | + | LNG 250 | Combination 5, *Eugynon 30*, Nordiol 30, *Ovran 30*, Primovlar 30 |
| EE 30 | + | LNG 150 | Ciclo, Combination 3, Contraceptive LD, Egogyn, Follimin, Gynatrol, Levlen, Lo-Femenal +, Lo-Gentrol +, Lo-Ovral +, Lo/Ovral +, Lo-Rondal +, Mala D, Microgest, Microgyn 30, *Microgynon 30*, Microvlar, Minibora, Minidril, Minigynon 30, Minivlar, Min-Ovral +, Neo-Gentrol 150/30, Neomonovar, Neovletta, Nordet, Nordette, Norgestrel Pill, Norvetal, Ologyn-micro, Ovoplex 30/150, Ovoplexin, Ovral L +, Ovranet, *Ovranette*, Rigevidon, Stediril-30, Stediril-d 150/30, Stediril-M, Suginor |

Triphasic formula

EE 30	+	LNG 50	⎫ Fironetta, *Logynon, Logynon ED*, Triagy-
EE 40	+	LNG 75	⎬ non, Triciclor, Trigynon, Trikvilar, Tri-
EE 30	+	LNG 125	⎭ Levlen, *Trinordiol*, Triogyn, Trionetta, Tri-ovlar, Triphasil, Triquilar, Triquilar ED, Tri-Regol, Trisiston.

Group E (norethisterone, NET)

| MEE 50 | + | NET 1000 | Anogenil, Combiginor, Conceplan, Conlumin, Duofem, Floril, Genora 1 + 50, Gulaf, Maya, Nelova 1/50, Nor-50, Norethin 1/50 M, NorFor, Noriday, Noriday 1 + 50, Norimin, Norinyl, *Norinyl-1*, Norinyl 1 + 50, Norit, Novulon 1/50, Orthonett, Orthonett 1/50, Ortho-Novin, *Ortho-Novin 1/50*, Ortho-Novum, Ortho-Novum 1/50, Ortho-Novum 1 + 50, Perle, Plan mite, Regovar, Regovar 50, Ultra-Novulane |
| EE 35 | + | NET 1000 | Brevicon-1, Brevicon 1 + 35, Brevinor-1, Genora 1 + 35, Gynex 1/35 E, Kanchan, Membrettes, N.E.E. 1/35, Nelova 1 + 35 E, Neocon, *Neocon 1/35*, Neo-Norinyl, Norcept-E 1/35, Norethin 1/35 E, |

			Norimin, Norinyl 1 + 35, Norquest, Norquest-Fe, Ortho 1 + 35, Ortho 1/35, Ortho-Novum 1 + 35, Ortho-Novum 1/35, Ovysmen, Ovysmen 1/35
EE 35	+	NET 500	Brevicon, *Brevinor*, Conceplan Mite, Genora 0.5/35, Gynex 0.5/35 E, Mikro Plan, Modacon, Modicon, Nelova 0.5/35 E, Neo-Ovopausine, Nilocan, Norminest, Norminest-Fe, Orthonett-Novum, Ovacon, *Ovysmen*, Ovysmen 0.5/35, Perle LD

Biphasic formula

EE 35	+	NET 500	*Binovum*, Jenest, Nelova 10/11, Ortho 10/11, Ortho-Novum 10/11 (similar to *Binovum*, but giving 3 extra days at the lower dose)
EE 35	+	NET 1000	

Triphasic formulae

EE 35	+	NET 500	Ortho 777, Ortho-Novum 7/7/7, Triella, *Trinovum, Trinovum ED*
EE 35	+	NET 750	
EE 35	+	NET 1000	
EE 35	+	NET 500	Synfase, Synfasic, *Synphase*, Synphasec, Synphasic, Tri-Norinyl
EE 35	+	NET 1000	
EE 35	+	NET 500	

Group D (norethisterone acetate, NEA)

EE 30	+	NEA 1500	*Loestrin 30*, Loestrin 1.5/30, Loestrin Fe 1.5/30, Logest 1.5/30, Minestril-30, Zorane 1.5/30
EE 20	+	NEA 1000	Loestrin, *Loestrin 20*, Loestrin 1/20, Loestrin Fe 1/20, Lostrin 1/20, Minestril-20, Minestrin 1/20, Nogest, Zorane 1/20

Group E (ethynodiol diacetate, EDDA)

EE 30	+	EDDA 2000	Conova, *Conova 30*, Demulen 30

Continuous progestagen – only pills (POPs)

Group D	LNG 37.5	*Neogest* + , Ovrette + , Postinor
	LNG 30	Follistrel, Microlut, Microluton, *Microval*, Mikro-30, *Norgeston*.
Group E	NET 350	Conceplan-Micro, Dianor, Micronett, *Micronor*, Micro-Novum, Micronovum, *Noriday*, Noriday 1, Noridei, Nor-QD
Group E	EDDA 500	Continuin, *Femulen*

Phasic pills

For comparison with monophasic brands, the *average* daily doses given in the British phasic brands are shown below:

Tri–Minulet, Triadene	EE 32.4 + DSG 78.6
Logynon, Trinordiol	EE 32.4 + LNG 92
Binovum	EE 35 + NET 833
Trinovum	EE 35 + NET 750

Index

Page numbers in italics refer to figures and tables.